Infection Prevention
in Surgical Settings

Infection Prevention

in Surgical Settings

Barbara J. Gruendemann,
RN, MS, FAAN, CNOR

Principal and Project Director
G4 Productions
Dallas, Texas

Sandra Stonehocker Mangum,
RN, MN, CNOR

Professor, College of Nursing
Brigham Young University
Provo, Utah

SAUNDERS

An Imprint of Elsevier

SAUNDERS
An Imprint of Elsevier
The Curtis Center
Independence Square West
Philadelphia, PA 19106

Library of Congress Cataloging-in-Publication Data

Gruendemann, Barbara J.
Infection prevention in surgical settings/Barbara J. Gruendemann, Sandra
Stonehocker Mangum.
p.   cm.

Includes bibliographical references and index.

ISBN 0-7216-9035-1 (alk. paper)

1. Surgical wound infections—Prevention.   2. Surgery, Aseptic and
    antiseptic.   3. Nosocomial infections—Prevention.   4. Hospitals—Sanitation.
    I. Mangum, Sandra Stonehocker.   II. Title

RD91.G78 2001   617'.01—dc21   00-052958

Vice President and Publishing Director, Nursing: Sally Schrefer
Senior Editor: Michael S. Ledbetter
Senior Developmental Editor: Laurie K. Muench
Project Manager: Deborah L. Vogel
Production Editor: Kelley Barbarick
Design Manager: Bill Drone

INFECTION PREVENTION IN SURGICAL SETTINGS   ISBN 0–7216–9035–1

Permissions may be sought directly from Elsevier's Health Sciences Rights
Department in Philadelphia, USA: phone: (+1)215-238-7869, fax: (+1)215-238-2239,
email: healthpermissions@elsevier.com. You may also complete your request on-line via
the Elsevier Science homepage (http://www.elsevier.com), by selecting 'Customer
Support' and then 'Obtaining Permissions'.

Printed in the United States of America

Last digit is the print number: 9   8   7   6   5   4   TG/FF

Reviewers

Cecil A. King, RN, BSN, CNOR
Assistant Nurse Manager, Surgical Services
University of Washington Medical Center
Seattle, Washington

Susan McBride, RN, MS
Director of Clinical Outcomes
Texas Health Resources
Dallas, Texas

Jeanne Pfeiffer, RN, BSN, MPH, CIC
Infection Control Program Director
Hennepin County Medical Center
Minneapolis, Minnesota

Deborah Y. Phillips, RN, MPH, CIC
Infection Control Coordinator
Parkland Health & Hospital System
Dallas, Texas

Mark L. Phippen, RN, MN, CNOR
Clinical Educator
Valleylab
Boulder, Colorado

Donna M. DeFazio Quinn, BSN, MBA, RN, CPAN, CAPA
Director, Orthopedic Surgery
Concord Hospital
Concord, New Hampshire

Susan Sebazco, RN, BS, CIC
Infection Control/Employee Health Director
Arlington Memorial Hospital
Arlington, Texas

Victoria Steelman, RN, BSN, MA, PhD, CNOR
Advanced Practice Nurse, Surgical Services
University of Iowa Hospitals and Clinics
Iowa City, Iowa

Preface

This book represents a marriage between infection prevention and control and perioperative nursing. It is a book about the myriad infection prevention practices that are carried out each day in surgical settings. As a reference guide, it is designed to assist the practitioner in making infection prevention and control decisions that affect surgical patient care.

This book is also intended to motivate infection control and perioperative practitioners to increasingly collaborate and communicate about infection control issues that arise each and every day in surgical settings, particularly in the operating room (OR). There are very few practices and issues in a surgical setting that do not have infection control implications. Truly, an OR represents the best and the most frequent use of infection prevention practices.

The following quote emphasizes the marriage between these two disciplines: "A critical bridge of cooperation must exist between OR and infection control professionals. Infection prevention of an intense nature is practiced by perioperative nurses in an OR. Infection control professionals are valuable consultants and watchdogs for OR personnel and vice versa. The synergy that exists between these two groups must be nourished and strengthened. I challenge you, as professionals, to study and learn together!"[1]

New Focus

This book is different from other infection control and perioperative practice texts in that it spells out, *in one place,* principles of and reasons for infection control practices. These practices are supported by references that apply to surgical settings. Each related topic is introduced, discussed from a practice perspective, and referenced from the literature and textbooks written by leaders and experts in both fields. All topics are presented in a user-friendly format (see Format).

Prevention and Control

The book's title represents the trend toward using the term *infection prevention* rather than *infection control,* even though both terms are used throughout the literature and, therefore, in this text. Since the Centers for Disease Control and Prevention (CDC) changed its name

---

[1]Gruendemann BJ: Editorial, *Asepsis: The Infection Prevention Forum* 16(1):1, 1994.

to include the word *prevention,* the goal has been geared to prevention as well as control. Certainly, prevention practices should take precedence in surgical settings, but controls are still needed to reinforce certain practices and deal with the infections that do occur.

Format

This book is divided into the following general sections for ease of reading and categorizing infection prevention and control practices:

Preoperative Preparation of Patients
Surgical Environments and Traffic
Preparation of Personnel
Surgical Practices
Special Considerations

Chapters contain the following:

1. **Introductory statements** that set the scene for the ensuing discussion and state why the topic is important in surgical settings.
2. **Headings** relating to usage, practices, procedures, and other necessary specifics of the topic.
3. **Content** that is bulleted, where appropriate, and paragraphs or issues that are referenced from available literature, textbooks, or the Internet, enabling the reader to do further study or to refine techniques according to practice setting and need. This is the meat of the book. In the content, **several similar references on a particular topic are often cited and discussed together.** It is our hope that readers will receive adequate information on practices and procedures to justify (or refute) their clinical use *and thus will be able to make informed decisions.* **References** and **suggested reading** are listed at the end of each chapter.

Statements, paragraphs, and introductions that are not referenced as such are generally the comments of the authors. Also, the notation "NOTE:" usually indicates that an author explanation is needed or that a section contains information that may seem confusing or conflicting to the reader. The overall goal of this method of writing is ease in reading and understanding.

Two **appendixes** are included. Of all the relevant guidelines available today, the two that are most widely used as references, and as bases for recommended practices, are *Guideline for Isolation Precautions in Hospitals* (Standard Precautions), and *Guideline for Prevention of Surgical Site Infection.* Both are reprinted CDC guidelines. Appendix A contains relevant highlights from the guideline for Standard Precautions (SP); Appendix B contains relevant highlights from the Surgical Site Infection (SSI) guideline.

The objective of this format is to give the reader a **quick reference** to "what the experts say," without having to consult four or five other sources. Adding to this is another objective—to **save time** for clinicians who are often woefully short of minutes and hours in today's practice settings, and who would rather use one source for infection prevention practices and rationales than have to do a time-consuming library or Internet search. Questions such as, Can I sterilize wood? Should food be allowed in the OR? or Do tacky mats serve a useful purpose? can be answered quickly by referring to the respective topics in this book.

Target Audience

This book is intended for use by perioperative and infection control professionals who practice, manage, or provide consultation in surgical settings. Surgical settings include traditional ORs; ambulatory surgery centers; cardiac catheterization, endoscopy, and gastrointestinal (G-I) laboratories; interventional radiology units; physician offices; and other clinical areas where surgical asepsis is used in setting up sterile fields for operative and other interventional procedures.

This book can also be a helpful reference for physicians and surgeons, anesthesia providers, assistants, students, and even sales representatives. Governmental officials could also find useful information in this text relating to infection control issues. Because infection control and perioperative concepts apply to many clinical settings, a wide audience of readers will find the content helpful and informative.

Issues and Observations

Several issues and observations related to the subject of this book arose as the chapter topics were studied and the literature exhaustively searched:

1. *Infection control and perioperative practices are not always black and white.* There are many gray areas. Some topics, such as principles of asepsis, have been quite consistent over the years and have not changed radically. Others, such as high-level chemical disinfection practices (e.g., acceptable soak times for immersion of instruments), have undergone changes as new disinfectants have been introduced into the marketplace, and as standards are being re-examined for relevancy in the practice setting. Also, the discussion continues regarding high-level disinfection versus sterilization for certain devices (e.g., endoscopes). The use of laminar airflow systems in ORs is another gray area with strong proponents on each of the sides

"yes, necessary" and "no, not needed." These gray areas are discussed in this text.

2. *Recommendations of professional organizations and other standard-setting bodies are occasionally inconsistent.* This inconsistency can confuse the practitioner at times, but it can also encourage greater examination of the principles involved and the reasons for following a particular procedure. From this examination, then, comes decision making by clinicians who are informed. For example, in our discussion of bacterial filters on anesthesia equipment (see the chapter "Disinfection"), differing recommendations from professional organizations and other influential bodies are included. Also included is a note alerting practitioners that there is not total agreement on this issue. Practitioners can choose the direction they wish to take based on their examination of the recommendations.

3. *Many practices do, however, have almost unanimous agreement from the experts.* The need for protection from bloodborne pathogens, for example, receives consistent attention in journal articles and on websites, resulting in a similarity of advice given on the use of personal protective equipment (PPE). Another example is the importance of pre-cleaning instruments before disinfection or sterilization, which is a practice that is globally supported by the experts.

4. *We want quick answers.* Living in a time of bullet-speed changes in technology, infection control and perioperative professionals often want instant answers to emerging millennium-age questions. One comment commonly heard is, "How does this practice affect SSI rates?" We focus on infection rates because rates are measurable and comparable. We want to make direct (sometimes causal) associations between a practice and an infection rate without examining the evidence, the total picture, or the research studies, if done. Associations and causal relationships often cannot be made without a study design and a thorough analysis of the data. SSIs are multifactorial and often cannot even be studied, either because of the large numbers of subjects needed, or because there might not be a logical and direct relationship between the practice and the infection rate. Assuming that a change in a practice or procedure will automatically show up in infection rates is, in and of itself, false thinking. Certainly, we do and should monitor infection rates very closely, but they can only provide one piece of the puzzle. Pittet and Ducel say it succinctly: "Critical factors to prevent infection spread by OR personnel are personal integrity and work ethics. The entire surgical team—from cleaning personnel

to staff surgeons—should adhere to standardized, *though not always scientifically proven,* guidelines for infection prevention in the operating room."[2] It is our hope that this book will assist the reader in sorting out which recommendations and practices are science-based and can be associated with infection rates, which are "best" practices that seem to work, and which practices just make good sense.

Beyea and Nicoll speak of the value of using scientific principles and rationales when there may be no research. There are many unclear and untested practices in healthcare, but all of us have the responsibility to know the scientific principles that guide our practice. Until sound research evidence is available, we must rely on scientific principles and existing knowledge, adhering to practices that are tried and true. This is not to ignore change; but change in practices should occur based on new information, facts, or evidence generated from research.[3]

Today, many clinical practices are being questioned. Some, such as home laundering of scrubs and using surgical masks, are being labeled as "sacred cows." We want scientific research that would support or not support such practices, but conducting research that definitively decides these issues would be labor intensive and prohibitively expensive. So, in situations like this, we must rely on scientific principles and existing knowledge to guide practice.[4]

It is our hope that this book will help in identifying not only the relevant scientific principles, rationales, and research, but also the tried and true practices that may or may not be "sacred cows."

5. *"Follow manufacturers' written instructions"* is an admonition seen more and more in published studies and guidelines. Authors of textbooks and journal articles, and developers of professional and governmental guidelines, seem to be giving more general rather than specific information and advice. When clinicians look for specific guidelines and practice procedures, they are less apt to see them in the scientific literature today, compared with 10 years ago. Two reasons for the shift of the responsibility for specific usage information to manufacturers could be avoidance of liability and that manufacturers are best

---

[2]Pittet D, Ducel G: Infectious risk factors relating to operating rooms, *Infect Control Hosp Epidemiol* 15(7):456-462, 1994.

[3]Beyea SC, Nicoll LH: Using scientific principles when there is no research, *AORN J* 69(5):1037-1038, 1999.

[4]Beyea SC, Nicoll LH: Using scientific principles when there is no research, *AORN J* 69(5):1037-1038, 1999.

equipped to deal with the intricacies of the hundreds of new devices and the variations in products and designs. It is nearly impossible for a busy clinician to know the specifications and operating instructions for each new device that appears so frequently in ORs. An overall "should" for this book could be: *Always follow manufacturers' written instructions, first.*

6. *The speed with which new research, information, and guidelines appear is mind-boggling.* During the 10 months we have spent writing this book, at least four important new guidelines, and several new book editions, have been published. This has made for frequent and challenging revisions of a text like this one. All attempts have been made to include the latest editions and revisions. For example, one new draft guideline, the Food and Drug Administration (FDA) Reprocessing and Reuse of Single-Use Devices (SUDs), appeared on the Internet during this initial period. The final guidance document was released on August 2, 2000, during the editing stage of this text. Because of the importance of this document, the chapter on Reuse and Reprocessing of Single-Use Devices (SUDs) was rewritten to reflect this new FDA guidance document. The rapid appearance of new information in healthcare only highlights the need (for both readers and authors) to continuously stay updated on the newest trends, findings, and guidelines—sometimes an almost impossible task!

7. *The tendency to consider the relevancy of studies published **only** in the last five years is debunked.* The newest literature did receive the most attention in this book, but there were other studies and textbooks, written even in the late 1980s and early 1990s, that are very applicable today; these are included where appropriate. For example, the Occupational Safety and Health Administration (OSHA) Bloodborne Pathogen Final Rule was published in 1991 and is still used in every surgical setting today. The CDC guidelines for care of patients with tuberculosis were published in 1994 and are still relevant, although a new guideline is now being drafted. Principles of scrubbing, gowning, and gloving, some published in the 1980s and early 1990s, are still being used in most surgical settings. Two of the mainstays of infection control, the Association for Professionals in Infection Control and Epidemiology (APIC) guidelines on hand antisepsis, and disinfection, both used today as highly regarded references, were published in 1995 and 1996, respectively. Beck and Collette's treatise on strike-through, the first of its kind, was published in 1952. As a classic, this reference is cited throughout this book.

Summary

This book is a reference guide to infection prevention and control thinking and practices that take place in surgical settings. We originally thought that this information could be contained in a small pocket handbook. However, we soon discovered that this was impossible because of the large amount of infection control and perioperative information available. As a result, we chose the present format and content.

Our goal is to provide information and references that will enable readers to make informed decisions about infection prevention and control practices. We hope we have met this goal in a time-efficient and helpful manner for the readers.

Our wish is that this book will be a useful and handy bible of infection control and perioperative practices, one that is used often and well.

Barbara J. Gruendemann

Sandra S. Mangum

Abbreviations Used in This Book

AAMI	Association for the Advancement of Medical Instrumentation
ACS	American College of Surgeons
AIDS	Acquired immunodeficiency syndrome
AORN	Association of periOperative Registered Nurses
APIC	Association for Professionals in Infection Control and Epidemiology
CDC	Centers for Disease Control and Prevention
EPA	U.S. Environmental Protection Agency
FDA	U.S. Food and Drug Administration
HBV	Hepatitis B virus
HCV	Hepatitis C virus
HCW	Healthcare worker
HEPA	High-efficiency particulate air
JCAHO	Joint Commission on Accreditation of Healthcare Organizations
NIOSH	National Institute for Occupational Safety and Health
OR	Operating room
OSHA	Occupational Safety and Health Administration
PACU	Post-anesthesia care unit
PPE	Personal protective equipment
SP	Standard Precautions
SSI	Surgical site infection
UP	Universal Precautions

Contents

APPENDIXES

1

Preoperative Preparation of Patients

A. Preoperative Patient Preparation

Use of certain key principles of patient preparation is essential to infection prevention. These principles should be considered as essential to assure the patient the best possible infection-free outcome of the surgical intervention. It is important to understand that all patients should receive the same consideration and attention to infection prevention strategies, including strict aseptic technique. However, assessment and recognition of those who are at increased risk may heighten the healthcare team's awareness of the importance of strategies that decrease risk of surgical site infection (SSI) so that care can be planned and given accordingly.

The importance of risk assessment; the use of appropriate antimicrobial prophylaxis (AMP), before and during surgery; and pre-

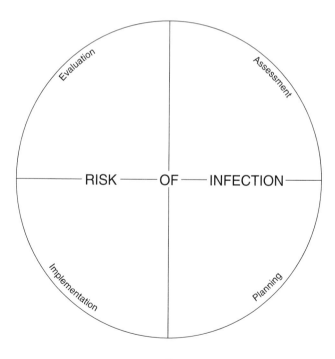

operative preparation of the skin by showering, bathing, and hair clipping or shaving cannot be underestimated.

CAUSES OF INFECTION

For most SSIs, the source of pathogens is the endogenous flora of the patient's skin, mucous membranes, or hollow viscera. When an incision is made, the exposed tissues are at risk for contamination with endogenous flora. These organisms are usually gram-positive cocci (e.g., staphylococci), but may include fecal flora (e.g., anaerobic bacteria and gram-negative aerobes) when incisions are made near the perineum or groin. Exogenous sources of pathogens usually come from the surgical environment (e.g., circulating air, surgical personnel, or instruments). Exogenous flora is primarily aerobic, especially gram-positive organisms (e.g., staphylococci and streptococci) (19, p. 421; 16, p. 254).

Early study of infection control found that the risk of SSI is directly proportional to the dose of the bacterial contaminant and the virulence of the organism. This risk is inversely proportional to both the ability of the patient or host to control microbial contamination and the condition of the wound at the completion of the procedure (23, pp. 157-158).

A formula explains how microbial contamination of the surgical site is a precursor of SSI:

$$\frac{\text{Dose of bacterial contamination} \times \text{virulence}}{\text{Resistance of the host patient}} = \frac{\text{Risk of surgical site}}{\text{infection (16, p. 253)}}$$

Awareness of the interplay of these factors leads clinicians to a better understanding of the importance of putting in place infection control measures with every patient and every surgical procedure.

WOUND CLASSIFICATION

The following is a standardized classification system for surgical wounds. This classification system describes levels of wound contamination from the lowest to the highest levels and is thought to be one of the main predictors of the possibility of postoperative SSI.

Clean wounds are uninfected operative wounds in which no inflammation is encountered and the respiratory, alimentary, genital, or urinary tract is not entered (23, p. 154). Examples: hernia repair; breast biopsy.

Clean-contaminated wounds are operative wounds in which the respiratory, alimentary, genital, or urinary tract is entered under controlled conditions and without unusual contamination (23, p. 154). Examples: cystoscopy; gastrectomy.

Contaminated wounds include open, fresh, accidental wounds; operations with major breaks in sterile technique or gross spillage from the gastrointestinal tract; and incisions in which acute, nonpurulent inflammation is encountered (23, p. 154). Examples: appendectomy for ruptured appendix; ruptured diverticulum of bowel.

Dirty or infected wounds include old traumatic wounds with retained devitalized tissue and those that involve existing clinical infection or perforated viscera (23, p. 154). Examples: incision and drainage of infected hip; debridement of infected pressure ulcer.

ASSESSMENT OF RISK

Recent clinical and epidemiological studies have demonstrated the complexity and variety of additional risk factors that affect the incidence of SSI (23, pp 157-158; 16, p. 254). Knowledge of these risk factors before certain operations may allow surgeons and staff to take targeted prevention measures. For example, if the surgeon knows that a patient has a remote site infection, then the surgeon may reduce SSI risk by postponing the procedure until after the remote infection has resolved (16, p. 254).

The Centers for Disease Control and Prevention (CDC) published a risk assessment guideline with the following categories of recommendations:

Category IA: Analysis of multiple research studies that give enough evidence supported by well-designed experimental, clinical, or epidemiological studies to strongly recommend implementation.

Category IB: Analysis of some experimental, clinical, or epidemiological studies and strong theoretical rationale to strongly recommend implementation.

Category II: Analysis of clinical or epidemiological studies or theoretic rationale to suggest implementation.

Unresolved issue: Review of practices for which there is insufficient evidence or no consensus regarding efficacy. No recommendation made (16, p. 266). See Appendix B.

This guideline provides a basis for evaluating risk factors and implementation strategies.

Diabetes

The contribution of diabetes to SSI risk is controversial. However, recent preliminary findings from a study of patients who underwent coronary artery bypass grafts showed a significant relationship between increasing levels of glycated hemoglobin and SSI rates. Also, increased glucose levels (>200 mg/dl) in the immediate postoperative period (<48 hours) were associated with increased risk.

CDC recommendation: Category IB. Adequately control blood glucose levels in all diabetic patients and particularly avoid hyperglycemia perioperatively (16, pp. 254, 266).

Nicotine Use

Studies have shown that nicotine use delays primary wound healing and may increase the risk of SSI. Nicotine use is an independent risk factor for sternal and/or mediastinal SSI following cardiac surgery. Other studies have corroborated that cigarette smoking is an important risk factor.

CDC recommendation: Category IB. Encourage tobacco cessation. At minimum patients should be instructed to abstain from smoking cigarettes, cigars, and pipes and from any other forms of tobacco consumption for at least 30 days before elective surgery (16, pp. 254, 266).

Steroid Use

Patients receiving steroids or other immunosuppressive drugs preoperatively may be predisposed to developing SSIs. Data supporting this recommendation are contradictory.

CDC recommendation: unresolved issue. No recommendation to taper or discontinue steroid use prior to surgery (16, pp. 254-255, 267).

Malnutrition

Total parenteral nutrition (TPN) and total enteral alimentation (TEA) have enthusiastic acceptance by surgeons and critical care specialists. However, the benefits of preoperative nutritional repletion of malnourished patients in reducing SSI risk are unproven. Administering TPN or TEA may be indicated in a number of circumstances (e.g., major oncological operations, severe malnutrition, or major traumatic injuries), but doing so does not necessarily decrease the risk of SSI.

CDC recommendation: unresolved issue. No recommendation to enhance nutritional support for surgical patients solely as a means to prevent SSI (16, pp. 256, 267).

Prolonged Preoperative Hospital Stay

Prolonged hospital stay is commonly suggested as a patient characteristic associated with increased SSI risk. However, a lengthy preoperative stay is more likely due to the severity of the illness and comorbid conditions requiring inpatient work-up and/or therapy before surgery.

CDC recommendation: Category II. Keep preoperative stay as short as possible while allowing for adequate preoperative preparation of the patient (16, pp. 256, 267).

Preoperative Nares Colonization with *Staphylococcus aureus*

Staphylococcus aureus is commonly found in the nares of 20% to 30% of healthy humans. Preliminary analysis of multiple studies shows an association between nasal carriage of *S. aureus* and subsequent SSI development.

Colonization in the nares has been found to have a definite impact on postoperative SSI, especially in cardiothoracic operations. It has been determined that the application of mupirocin to the nares preoperatively has reduced the incidence of SSI in cardiothoracic patients (4, pp. 775-779; 15, p. 783).

The most important reservoirs of methicillin-resistant *Staphylococcus aureus* (MRSA) are infected or colonized patients. Use of Standard Precautions should control the spread of MRSA in most instances. If the MRSA infection is judged by the hospital's infection control program to be of special clinical or epidemiological significance, then Contact Precautions should be considered. Colonized or infected patients should be identified as quickly as possible, appropriate barrier precautions instituted, and handwashing by medical personnel before and after all patient contacts strictly adhered to (5).

CDC recommendation: unresolved issue. No recommendation to preoperatively apply mupirocin to the nares to prevent SSI (16, pp. 256, 267).

Perioperative Transfusion

Perioperative transfusion of leukocyte-containing allogenic blood components, including whole blood, is an apparent risk factor for the development of postoperative bacterial infections, including SSIs. However, when a detailed review of multiple studies was conducted, any effect of perioperative transfusion on SSI risk was found to be either small or nonexistent.

CDC recommendation: Category IB. Do not withhold necessary blood products from surgical patients as a means to prevent SSI (16, pp. 256, 267).

The CDC and other authors list the following additional risk factors that should be considered.

Obesity

Obesity (>20% above ideal body weight) and morbid obesity (>100% above ideal body weight) are strong and independent risk factors for SSI. The increased risk is thought to be due to diminished blood flow, increased wound area, and the added technical difficulty of handling adipose tissue (16, p. 254; 14, p. 846).

Age

Extremes of age are considered to predispose patients to increased risk of SSI. The very young have an immature immune system, and the very old may have altered immune system function (16, p. 254; 14, p. 846).

ASA Score

This scoring system, developed by the American Society of Anesthesiologists (ASA), assesses the overall physical status of patients. The scoring range is from 1 (healthy patient) to 5 (patient not expected to survive 24 hours). The ASA score has been shown to be highly predictive of the development of SSI (14, p. 846). The ASA score has also been shown to be in interrelationship with other factors, such as the disease severity score and the wound classification system; however, it appears that the ASA score is the most definitive predictor of the risk of development of SSIs (7, p. 75).

No single risk factor will consistently lead to infection, but when multiple risk factors are present, the likelihood of developing a SSI increases (14, p. 846).

USE OF ANTIMICROBIAL PROPHYLAXIS

Surgical antimicrobial prophylaxis (AMP) is defined as a brief course of an antimicrobial agent initiated just before an operation begins (13, p. 1135; 16, p. 258). This therapy is not meant to sterilize tissues but to act as a critically timed adjunct used to reduce the microbial burden of intraoperative contamination to a level that cannot overwhelm host defenses. AMP is most often delivered by intravenous infusion. Four main guidelines are suggested to maximize the benefits of AMP.

1. AMP should be used for all operations and all classes of operations in which its use has been shown to reduce SSI rates by evidence from clinical trials or for those operations after which incisional or organ/space SSI would represent a catastrophe.
2. The antimicrobial used should be safe, inexpensive, bactericidal, and cover the most probable intraoperative contaminants for the operation.
3. The initial dose of the AMP by infusion should be timed so that a bactericidal concentration of the drug is established in serum and tissues by the time the skin is incised (30 and 60 minutes prior to incision are timing examples given for two specific antibiotics).

4. A therapeutic level of antimicrobial should be maintained in the tissues throughout the procedure and until a few hours after the incision is closed (16, pp. 259-260; 22, p. 56; 11, p. 356).

Indications For and Against AMP

AMP is indicated in the following surgical procedures:
- Entry into a hollow viscus under controlled conditions. Additional antimicrobials may be necessary for certain procedures such as colectomy or abdominal-perineal resection to prepare the colon by emptying the bowel of its contents and to reduce the level of live microorganisms. This is done by enema and cathartic administration and the use of oral antimicrobials in divided doses the day before surgery (16, p. 259).
- Implantation of any intravascular prosthetic material or prosthetic joint (16, p. 259).
- Operation in which an incisional or organ/space SSI would pose catastrophic risk (16, p. 259).
- High-risk cesarean section, when an antimicrobial agent should be given immediately after the umbilical cord is clamped (16, p. 259).
- Surgery of proximal femoral and other closed long bone fractures. A single dose of an antimicrobial prophylactic is an effective intervention if the agent used provides tissue levels exceeding the minimum inhibitory concentration over a 12-hour period or when the agent chosen is given on a 12-hour dosage schedule if the short half-life does not allow adequate concentrations in the blood from incision to wound closure (10, p. 8).

AMP is not indicated in the following procedures:
- Routine laparoscopic cholecystectomy. The vast majority of patients will have no infectious problems of any sort, regardless of whether antibiotics are given, even in the presence of acute inflammation found intraoperatively. However, thorough skin preparation should be performed (11, p. 88).
- Contaminated or dirty procedures when these patients are already receiving antimicrobial therapy for established infection (16, p. 259).

Controversy remains regarding the types of procedures in which prophylactic antibiotics are indicated. Their use in contaminated and dirty-infected surgeries is considered therapeutic. The consensus is that prophylactic antibiotics are indicated in all clean-contaminated procedures and high-risk clean procedures (22, p. 52).

Choice of Antimicrobial Agent

Cephalosporins are the most thoroughly studied and used antimicrobial agents as the first choice for clean operations. These drugs are effective against many gram-positive and gram-negative microorganisms. They are safe, have acceptable pharmacokinetics, and are reasonable in cost (20, p. 233; 16, p. 259).

- Other antimicrobials may be used as indicated by special needs and circumstances (20, p. 233).
- Vancomycin should not be used routinely for antimicrobial prophylaxis (16, p. 267).

Use of Intraoperative Antimicrobial Agents

Antimicrobial agents have been used during surgery for prophylaxis.

- One or a combination of antimicrobials, mixed in 1000 ml of 0.9% sodium chloride solution, is used to soak and prepare grafts and implants prior to implantation as well as for irrigation of wounds in orthopedic surgery and neurosurgery. Commonly used antimicrobials are bacitracin, polymyxin B, and gentamicin (18, p. 119).
- The arguments in favor of local irrigation in vascular surgery are: (1) high concentrations of antibiotics for a prolonged period at higher levels than those obtained by intravenous route and (2) high antibiotic levels in inert zones as well as in wound hematomas. Local irrigation, however, may not be any more effective than intravenous prophylaxis. The value of a combination of both techniques (local plus intravenous) has not been established (17, pp. 539-540).
- Antibiotic irrigation in obstetric procedures has been shown to result in therapeutic levels of antibiotic. Controversy surrounds the efficacy of antibiotic irrigation as compared with systemic antibiotic administration and, therefore, antibiotic irrigation for prophylaxis has not become popular (22, p. 53).
- Antimicrobials used in ophthalmological surgery are given by injection into the sclera, while others are administered topically (18, p. 118).

USE OF ANTIMICROBIAL AGENTS FOR REDUCTION OF SKIN MICROORGANISMS

The patient's own normal flora, particularly *S. aureus,* can be a primary endogenous source of wound contamination during surgery. Carriers of *S. aureus* in the nares are at increased risk for SSI. This pathogenesis takes place most likely when colonization of the deeper layers of the skin in carriers, not reached effectively by preoperative disinfection, causes contamination of the incision (14, p. 846). In certain patients, it seems reasonable to attempt reducing the microbial count before surgery.

Skin Preparation with Showers or Baths

Showers or baths using antimicrobial agents have been suggested as a means of reducing SSI risk, especially in patients who are *S. aureus* carriers or for those at significant risk because of the type of surgery anticipated (e.g., joint replacement or coronary artery bypass graft).

- The surgical site should be free of soil and debris. Cleansing can be accomplished before the surgical prep by the patient's showering and/or shampooing before arriving at the practice setting (1, p. 329).
- Several studies observed lower SSI rates when the patient showered preoperatively with chlorhexidine gluconate-containing agents. Other studies failed to show a reduction in the wound infection rate using whole-body disinfection (14, p. 850).
- Good evidence exists that skin flora may be reduced effectively and that wound contamination is lessened when chlorhexidine detergent is used for a preoperative bath. Again, results of studies have varied (21, p. 703).
- A preoperative antiseptic shower or bath decreases skin microbial colony counts. In a study of >700 patients who received two preoperative antiseptic showers, chlorhexidine reduced bacterial colony counts 9-fold, while povidone-iodine and triclocarban-medicated soap reduced colony counts by 1.3- and 1.9-fold, respectively. Other studies corroborate these findings. It is important to consider that repeated showers are needed because chlorhexidine gluconate-containing products require several applications to attain maximum antimicrobial benefit. Even though preoperative showers reduce the skin's microbial colony count, they have not definitively been shown to reduce SSI rates (16, p. 257).

CDC recommendation: Category IB. Patients should shower or bathe with an antiseptic agent on at least the night before the operative day (16, pp. 257, 267). The incision site should be washed and cleaned to remove gross contamination before performing antiseptic skin preparation (16, p. 267).

OTHER CONSIDERATIONS
Preoperative Hair Removal

Removal of hair at the surgical site is a time-honored tradition that has come under scrutiny in the past few years. Though it may be aesthetically more acceptable and satisfy the surgeon's desire for a smooth, clean skin surface, shaving the evening before surgery is associated with increased rates of SSI. The lowest infection rates are found in those patients whose hair is left intact (12, p. 258). If hair must be removed, following these guidelines may help to minimize SSI risk:

- Hair removal should be performed by personnel skilled in hair removal techniques. Use of inappropriate hair removal techniques may traumatize the skin and provide an opportunity for colonization of microorganisms at the surgical site. Hair should be removed as close to the time of surgery as possible, and the hair removal procedure should be performed away from the room where the surgery will take place (1, p. 330; 16, pp. 257, 267).
- Hair should be removed in a manner that preserves skin integrity. Hair removal with a razor can disrupt skin integrity. Use of an electric shaver or a depilatory cream is preferred, although depilatory creams can cause skin irritation (16, pp. 257, 267).
- Wet shaving is preferred over dry shaving (1, p. 330).
- Preoperative shaving of the surgical site the night before surgery is associated with a significantly higher SSI risk than either the use of depilatory agents or no hair removal. The increased risk has been attributed to microscopic cuts in the skin that later serve as foci for bacterial multiplication. When compared with shaving within 24 hours of surgery, shaving immediately before the operation was associated with decreased SSI rates. Clipping the hair immediately before an operation also has been associated with a lower risk of SSI than shaving or clipping the night before an operation. Other studies showed that preoperative hair removal by any means was associated with increased SSI rates (16, pp. 257, 267).

CDC recommendation: No preoperative removal of hair unless the hair at or around the incision site will interfere with the operation. If hair is removed, it should be done immediately before the operation, preferably with electric clippers (16, pp. 257, 267).

Patient Attire

It has long been standard policy that patients remove all clothing prior to surgery. Adherence to this policy eliminates unclean clothing—a source of the patient's endogenous microorganisms, especially *S. aureus.* However, many surgical centers allow patients to wear some of their own clothing, especially if the clothing does not interfere with the procedure and the procedure is of short duration (e.g., cataract surgery). The following recommendations should be considered during the decision-making process:

- AORN recommends that patients wear a gown and hair covering in both semirestricted and restricted areas of the surgical suite. Patients are not required to wear a mask (2, p. 365; 12, p. 286).
- Patients should don a clean gown prior to surgery (9, p. 357).
- AORN states that the matter of attire for outpatients is a facility decision. The AORN recommendation that patients wear clean gowns, be covered with clean linens, and have their hair covered does not specifically state that patients must remove all clothing. Most persons feel more comfortable if allowed to wear their underwear. However, in some situations the patient's underwear may not be clean and it would be preferable for the patient to remove all clothing and to be clothed only in clean, hospital-approved attire. For the sake of consistency, AORN states that their recommendation should be considered as a minimum. If it is judged by the caregiver that more clothing needs to be removed, that can be accommodated on a patient-by-patient basis (3).

Patient Jewelry

Jewelry should be removed because it carries microorganisms into the restricted area. Other reasons for removal of jewelry are issues of safety and security. Jewelry also presents a potential risk of burn from direct current if electrocautery is used (8, pp. 120-121; 9, p. 317).

The Emergency Care Research Institute states that removal of jewelry is not necessary to avoid patient burns during electrosurgery. The conductivity of jewelry poses no significant increase in the likelihood of alternative site burns or any other electrosurgical skin injuries (6, p. 441).

The following information applies to body jewelry:

- Jewelry that pierces the skin should be removed and the pierced area cleansed thoroughly prior to surgical skin preparation.
- Most body jewelry can be removed by hand, using the same threading principle with which it was inserted. Other body jewelry must be removed by using ring spreaders and closers that are available in different sizes from a body jewelry store. Ring spreaders and closers can be kept in the holding or preoperative preparation area. They must be disinfected following use.
- Healthcare facilities should have written policies regarding body jewelry.

- If a patient refuses to remove body jewelry, a written release should be signed prior to surgery.
- A question regarding body jewelry might be included in the preoperative interview so that patients would be informed and able to remove jewelry before arrival at the surgical facility. Physicians' office staff could also inform patients to leave jewelry at home (8, pp. 120-121).

References

1. AORN: Recommended practices for skin preparation of patients. In *Standards, recommended practices and guidelines,* Denver, 2000, Author, pp 329-333.
2. AORN: Recommended practices for traffic patterns in the perioperative practice setting. In *Standards, recommended practices and guidelines.* Denver, 2000, Author, pp 365-367.
3. AORN Online Clinical Practice FAQ Database, 1999: www.aorn.org/_results/clinical.asp (accessed 2000).
4. Boyce JM: Preventing Staphylococcus infection by eradicating nasal carriage of *Staphylococcus aureus:* proceeding with caution, *Infect Control Hosp Epidemiol,* 17(12):775-779, 1996.
5. Centers for Disease Control and Prevention: *Methicillin-resistant Staphylococcus aureus,* 1999, www.cdc.gov/ncidod/hip/aresist/mrsa.htm (accessed 2000).
6. Emergency Care Research Institute: Allowing patients to wear jewelry during surgical and electrosurgical procedures, *Health Devices* 26(11):441-442, 1997.
7. Eschenbach DA: Preventing and managing incisional surgical site infections, *Contemporary OB/GYN,* pp 69-85, March 1998.
8. Fogg DL: Clinical issues, *AORN J* 70(1):120-121, 1999.
9. Fortunato N: *Berry & Kohn's operating room technique,* ed 9, St Louis, 2000, Mosby.
10. Gillespie WJ, Walenkamp G: Antibiotic prophylaxis for surgery for proximal femoral and other closed long bone fractures, *The Cochrane Library 1999,* Issue 4:1-16, Oxford Update Software (CD-ROM), 1999.
11. Illig KA et al: Are prophylactic antibiotics required for elective laparoscopic cholecystectomy? *J Am Coll Surg* 184:353-356, 1997.
12. Gruendemann BJ, Fernsebner B: Infection prevention and control. In *Comprehensive perioperative nursing,* vol 1, *Principles,* Boston, 1995, Jones & Bartlett.
13. Kaiser AB: Antimicrobial prophylaxis in surgery, *N Engl J Med* 315(18):1129-1138.
14. Kluytmans AWJ: Surgical infections including burns. In Wenzel RP, editor: *Prevention and control of nosocomial infections,* ed 3, Baltimore, 1997, Williams & Wilkins, pp 841-865.
15. Kluytmans AWJ et al: Reduction of surgical-site infection in cardiothoracic surgery by eliminating nasal carriage of *Staphylococcus aureus, Infect Control Hosp Epidemiol* 17(12):780-785, 1996.
16. Mangram AJ, Hospital Infection Control Practices Advisory Committee (HICPAC), Centers for Disease Control and Prevention: Guideline for prevention of surgical site infection 1999, *Infect Control Hosp Epidemiol* 20(4):247-278, 1999. (Reprinted, in part, in Appendix B.)
17. Martin C, Viviand X, Potie F: Local antibiotic prophylaxis in surgery, *Infect Control Hosp Epidemiol,* 17(8):539-544, 1996.

18. Martinelli AM: Administering drugs and solutions. In Phippen ML, Wells MP, editors: *Patient care during operative and invasive procedures,* Philadelphia, 2000, WB Saunders, pp 113-135.
19. Nichols RL: The operating room. In Bennett JV, Brachman PS, editors: *Hospital infections,* Philadelphia, 1998, Lippincott-Raven, pp 421-430.
20. Platt R: Guidelines for perioperative antibiotic prophylaxis. In Abrutyn E, Goldmann DA, Scheckler WE, editors: *Saunders infection control reference service,* Philadelphia, 1998, WB Saunders, pp 229-280.
21. Rotter M: Hand washing, hand disinfection and skin disinfection. In Wenzel RP, editor: *Prevention and control of nosocomial infections,* ed 3, Philadelphia, 1997, Lippincott-Raven, pp 691-709.
22. Sheridan RL, Tompkins RG, Burke JF: Prophylactic antibiotics and their role in the prevention of surgical wound infection. In *Advances in surgery,* Chicago, 1994, Year Book Medical, pp 43-65.
23. Wong ES: Surgical site infections. In Mayhall CG, editor: *Hospital epidemiology and infection control,* Baltimore, 1996, Williams & Wilkins, pp 154-175.

Suggested Reading

1. Classen D et al: The timing of prophylactic administration of antibiotics and the risk of surgical-wound infection, *N Engl J Med* 326(5):281-286, 1992.
2. Simmons M: Update, preoperative skin preparation, *Prof Nurse* 13(7):446-447, 1998.

Surgical Environments and Traffic

A. Floors, Walls, and Ceilings

Floors, walls, and ceilings are made of various materials and installed with many specifications. It behooves infection control and surgical personnel to be knowledgeable about these materials and specifications and to properly care for and closely monitor operating room (OR) floors, walls, and ceilings for any changes that may signal possible risks for infection. This chapter includes a discussion of materials and specifications for floors, walls, and ceilings in ORs.

FLOORS
Materials
- Flooring is available in many materials suitable for the OR, including asphalt tile, vinyl, and terrazzo. The most common flooring used today is seamless vinyl. The surface of all floors must not be porous but instead be suitably hard, particularly for cleaning by the flooding, wet-vacuuming technique. Cushioned flooring is available (5, p. 155).
- Floors in an OR should be hard, seamless, and easy to clean and should not be affected by germicidal cleaning solutions (e.g.,

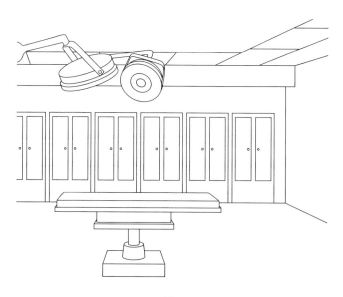

staining, degrading). Plastic terrazzo floor covering should not be used because the surface becomes pockmarked during installation and, therefore, hinders adequate cleaning (2).

- Floor materials should be easily cleanable and appropriately wear-resistant for the location. In new construction or after major renovation work, the floors and wall bases of all ORs and any delivery rooms used for cesarean sections should be monolithic and joint free (1, pp. 7-86—7-87).
- Self-coving floors are often used in ORs, post-anesthesia care units, and clean and soiled utility rooms. When self-coving is used, the flooring continues up the wall for 3 to 4 inches. This prevents the accumulation of debris and microorganisms in the crevices where the floor and wall would join if the floor were not self-coving. Sheet vinyl with heat-welded seams is a preferred material for a self-coving floor. Neither waxing nor buffing is recommended for sheet vinyl floors (4, pp. 1017-1018).

Floor Drains

Floor drains should not be installed in operating and delivery rooms. If a floor drain is installed in cystoscopy, it should contain a nonsplash, horizontal-flow flushing bowl beneath the drain plate (1, p. 7-102).

Conductive Floors

- Floors in areas and rooms in which flammable anesthetic agents are stored or administered shall comply with NFPA (National Fire Protection Agency) 99. Conductive flooring may be omitted in anesthetizing areas where a written resolution is signed by the hospital board stating that no flammable anesthetic agents will be used and appropriate notices are permanently and conspicuously affixed to the wall in each such area and room (1, p. 7-86).
- Conductive floors and conductivity are no longer prime considerations because explosive anesthetic gases are no longer used (5, p. 155).

  note: If conductive flooring is of concern, the reader is referred to reference 3, p. 135, for more information.

WALLS

- The floor and the bases of walls in an OR should be one continuous surface and free of seams. Walls should have a satin or matte finish because reflection and glare can be disturbing to the OR team (2).
- In ORs, delivery rooms for cesarean sections, isolation rooms, and sterile processing rooms, wall finishes shall be free of fissures, open joints, or crevices that may retain or permit passage of dirt particles (1, p. 7-87).

- Wall paneling made of hard vinyl materials is easy to clean and maintain. A plastic filler can seal seams. Laminated polyester or smooth, painted plaster provides a seamless wall, but epoxy paint on walls has a tendency to flake or chip. Wall tiles can present problems such as cracking and breaking, collecting dust and microorganisms in areas between the tiles, and having porous grout lines that harbor microorganisms (5, p. 155).

CEILINGS

- Finishes of all wall and ceiling surface materials should be hard, nonporous, fire resistant, waterproof, stainproof, seamless, nonreflective, and easy to clean. The ceiling should be a minimum of 10 feet high, depending on ceiling-mounted equipment, and may have soundproof, acoustic tiles (5, p. 155).
- Ceiling-mounted equipment is common in ORs. Suspended track mounts, however, can release dust and microorganisms when moved. Movable track-ceiling devices should not be mounted directly over the OR bed but instead be recessed into the ceiling to minimize dust accumulation fallout (5, p. 155).

References

1. American Institute of Architects Academy of Architecture for Health, U.S. Department of Health and Human Services: *Guidelines for design and construction of hospital and health care facilities, 1996-1997,* Washington, DC, 1996, American Institute of Architects Press. Online: www.e-architect.com/resources/hdfg1.asp
2. AORN Online Clinical Practice FAQ Database, 1999: www.aorn.org/_results/clinical.asp (accessed 2000).
3. Atkinson LJ, Fortunato NH: *Berry & Kohn's operating room technique*, ed 8, St Louis, 1996, Mosby.
4. Fogg DL: Clinical issues, *AORN J,* 69(5):1014, 1017-1018, 1999.
5. Fortunato N: *Berry & Kohn's operating room technique*, ed 9, St Louis, 2000, Mosby.

B. Temperature and Humidity

The operating room (OR) is a controlled environment and all practices, including those related to environmental control, are focused on the same desired outcome: absence of postoperative infection. This chapter contains discussions on two important aspects of environmental control: temperature and humidity. A closely related topic—ventilation—is discussed in the chapter "Airborne Contamination, Ventilation Systems, and Laminar Airflow."

TEMPERATURE

- The temperature of the OR should be maintained between 68° F and 75° F (20° C and 24° C). Keeping the OR temperature in this range may help to inhibit bacterial growth. This range is one that most patients can tolerate, and one that is also comfortable for personnel. Certain patients (e.g., infants, children, and burn patients) require a warmer environment for the purpose of preventing hypothermia. Each OR should have its own controls for adjusting the temperature (4, p. 284).
- Room temperatures of 68° F to 76° F (20° C to 24.4° C) inhibit bacterial growth. Except in extenuating circumstances, such as an emergency situation or when the room temperature is raised to accommodate a patient at risk for alteration in body temperature, procedure rooms that cannot be maintained at these ranges should not be used. Room temperatures and humidity levels that vary from the recommended norm may lead to alterations in the patient's body temperature, and also to discomfort and stress to the surgical team. Supplies and equipment necessary for regulating temperature and humidity are available (6, p. 147).

HUMIDITY

- A relative humidity of 50% to 60% inhibits bacterial growth and decreases the potential for static electricity (6, p. 147).
- The Association of periOperative Registered Nurses (AORN) does not prescribe any specific humidity level for ORs but does subscribe to recommendations from the American Institute of Architects Academy of Architecture for Health (AIAAAH) and the U.S. Department of Health and Human Services. AIAAAH recommends a humidity range of 30% to 60% for the OR. Providing a range of acceptability is more reasonable than requiring an absolute of 50% because there are always variations, depending on temperature fluctuation (1; 3, p. 500).

- The Joint Commission on Accreditation of Healthcare Organizations (JCAHO) indicates that facilities should use healthcare community design criteria. JCAHO specifies the AIAAAH publication, stating that maintenance of OR humidity between 30% and 60% indicates compliance with JCAHO standards (1; 3, p. 500; 5).
- Recommended relative humidity levels may be difficult to maintain in some geographic locations. In this case, special centralized units are needed to maintain the recommended level. Such units should be self-regulating to maintain a constant level within the recommended range. Room units of any kind in individual ORs are not recommended because they create unwanted dust and turbulence and/or dispense harbored mold and bacteria into the environment. A relative humidity that is too high can result in damp or moist supplies with added opportunities for mold growth. A relative humidity that is too low can result in excessive bacteria-carrying dust within the surgical environment (2).
- When explosive anesthetics were used, humidity control was necessary to help reduce the presence of static electricity. Today, humidity is controlled to provide a comfortable environment for personnel and a humidity level below that which is conducive to bacterial growth (60%) (4, p. 284).

References

1. American Institute of Architects Academy of Architecture for Health, U.S. Department of Health and Human Services: *Guidelines for design and construction of hospital and health care facilities, 1996-1997,* Washington, DC, 1996, American Institute of Architects Press. Online: www.e-architect.com/resources/hcfg1.asp
2. AORN Online Clinical Practice FAQ Database, 1999: www.aorn.org/_results/clinical.asp (accessed 2000).
3. Fogg DM: Clinical issues, *AORN J* 70(3):498, 500-501, 1999.
4. Gruendemann BJ, Fernsebner B: *Comprehensive perioperative nursing,* vol 1, *Principles,* Boston, 1995, Jones & Bartlett.
5. Joint Commission on Accreditation of Healthcare Organizations: Management of the environment of care. In *Comprehensive accreditation manual for hospitals: the official handbook, EC-9,* Oakbrook Terrace, Ill, 1998, Author.
6. Rhyne L, Ulmer BC, Revell L: Monitoring and controlling the environment. In Phippen ML, Wells MP, editors: *Patient care during operative and invasive procedures,* Philadelphia, 2000, WB Saunders, pp 147-166.

C. Airborne Contamination, Ventilation Systems, and Laminar Airflow

The beneficial effects of clean air with regard to prevention of contagious diseases were documented throughout the early ages, including in the works of such leaders as Lister, Hippocrates, and Florence Nightingale. Many of these leaders thought that exposure to fresh air minimized disease (7, pp. 841-842).

Since early times, the topic of airborne contamination has received variable emphasis, which is surprising considering that it is a potential risk factor in the genesis of SSIs. Even today, in some parts of the world a great deal of emphasis is placed on the airborne contamination factor; in other parts, very limited emphasis is placed.

This chapter includes a discussion of airborne contamination and a related topic—ventilation—in surgical settings. This chapter also includes another closely related topic—laminar airflow (LAF)—and the role it is thought to play in reducing airborne contamination. There is no clear-cut decisive mandate for either using or not using LAF systems in operating rooms (ORs); in fact, the studies on these

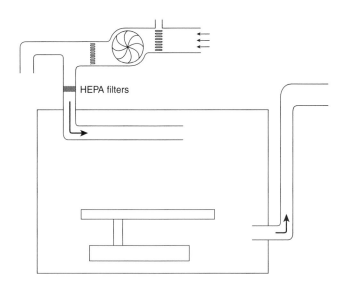

HEPA filters

systems are often conflicting. The reader is urged to consider all aspects of LAF and to temper decision-making by: (1) considering the current ventilation system in use, the types of procedures performed, and the types of patients cared for and (2) performing a risk analysis after thoroughly reviewing the literature.

AIRBORNE CONTAMINATION

Many factors affect the patient's risk for infection during surgical procedures; therefore every step taken to minimize postoperative infections and patient suffering is valuable. It is thought that airborne contamination from bacteria-carrying particles is one of the causes of postoperative infection in clean surgery. Therefore one of the major goals of surgical team members is to reduce or minimize the counts of bacteria-carrying particles in the air, which are generated almost exclusively by OR staff members (7, pp. 841-842).

Operating Room Airflow

- Much effort and many resources have been devoted to improving airflow in the OR. Even though it was well documented in the 1960s that multiple air changes were associated with decreased infection rates, most current infection control practices emphasize contact as the major mechanism for the spread of nosocomial infections. Despite this, some research demonstrates that if there is a widespread presence of organisms, such as staphylococci, in the OR, a biomaterial surface can become contaminated, leading to late-onset infections (5).
- Surgical personnel should consider methods of reducing the levels of airborne particulates that may serve as vectors to increase the transport of microbes in the OR environment. It is suggested, for example, that prosthetic grafts and other implantable devices not be left exposed (uncovered) for long periods before insertion. Also, aerosols need further study (5, p. 1182).
- Interest in airborne sources of infection in the hospital environment continues. These sources are primarily related to the spread of multidrug-resistant tuberculosis, aerosol spread of saprophytic fungi in the transplant population, and the potential spread of multidrug-resistant microorganisms in healthcare facilities (5, p. 1179).
- Infections are usually multifactorial. The importance of environmental factors in the origin of postoperative surgical infection is difficult to assess in prospective, well-designed studies. Patient-associated risk factors for infection certainly remain predominant in the infectious process. Thus the importance of patient-

associated, environment-associated, and procedure-associated factors may be difficult to assess apart from certain clean surgeries associated with low rates of surgical wound infection (10, p. 460).

- According to Pittet and Ducel (10, p. 460), who conducted studies on total joint replacements, a significant number of infections in these types of surgeries might be associated with airborne transmission. This potential mode of transmission does not seem to have as significant an importance in other types of surgery, according to these authors. Overall efforts aimed at preventing surgical wound infections, however, should concentrate on the importance of other, nonairborne, risk factors for infectious complications.

VENTILATION SYSTEMS

- According to the American Institute of Architects Academy of Architecture for Health (AIAAAH) (1, p. 58), design of an OR ventilation system should consider comfort as well as asepsis and should provide air movement that is from clean to less-clean areas. If any form of variable air volume or load shedding system is used for energy conservation, it must not compromise the corridor-to-room pressure balancing relationships or the minimum air changes required (e.g., 15 total air changes per hour), with a minimum of three of these being outdoor air changes.
- The Centers for Disease Control and Prevention (CDC) Surgical Site Infection (SSI) guideline specifies that OR ventilation should be maintained at positive pressure with respect to the corridors and adjacent areas because positive pressure prevents airflow from less clean areas into more clean areas. The guideline also reiterates the AIAAAH specifications of 15 air changes per hour, of which at least 3 (20%) should be fresh air. All air should be introduced at the ceiling and exhausted at the floor. All recirculated and fresh air should be filtered through appropriate filters, according to AIAAAH recommendations (1; 9, pp. 260, 267).
- All ventilation or air conditioning systems in hospitals, including those in ORs, should have two filter beds in series, with the efficiency of the first filter bed being ≥30% and that of the second filter bed being ≥90%. Detailed ventilation parameters for ORs can be found in reference 1 (9, p. 260).
- OR air may contain microbial-laden dust, lint, skin squames, or respiratory droplets. Since the microbial level in OR air is directly proportional to the number of people moving around in the room, efforts should be made to minimize personnel traffic during operations. OR doors should be kept closed except as needed for passage of equipment, personnel, or the patient (9, pp. 260, 267).

LAMINAR AIRFLOW SYSTEMS

- Controversy exists about the efficacy of LAF in decreasing wound infections. Researchers conclude that a clean wound infection rate of less than 1% to 2% should be achievable with standard OR air handling. It is not reasonable to consider adding on the capital cost, maintenance expense, and noise and communication problems of LAF rooms until the less expensive infection control measures are rigorously applied in daily practice, and infection rates are at or above the standard. These less expensive measures include good surgical technique; meticulous hemostasis; gentle handling of tissue; reduction of traffic, use of appropriate antibiotic prophylaxis, and avoidance of surgery when the patient has infected skin lesions, dermatitis, or a urinary tract infection (8, pp. 285-286).
- LAF is an option to be considered when addressing ventilation in the surgical suite. However, surgical infections could be reduced in rooms with modern standard ventilation systems and meticulous aseptic techniques (4, p. 95-1).
- The consequences of infection are greater with certain surgical procedures, such as total joint replacement or bone marrow transplantation, than with others, owing to the devastating effect an infection would have on these patients. In addition to scrupulous surgical technique, some facilities have installed LAF systems simply to provide a clean-air environment (8, p. 285).

Purpose and Use

NOTE: There is disagreement among several of the authors concerning LAF.
- LAF is defined as an airflow in which the entire body of air within a confined area moves with uniform velocity along parallel flow lines (i.e., laminar) with a minimum of eddies (7, p. 845).
- The purpose of OR ventilation is to dilute and remove airborne bacteria-carrying particles. LAF units recirculate excessive volumes of high-efficiency particulate air (HEPA), filter sterile air, and usually have up to 400 to 500 air changes per hour. If used correctly, LAF systems provide $<$10 CFU/m^3 during surgical procedures. This usually will result in an infection rate of $<$1%, even after infection-prone, clean surgery (7, p. 842).
- Ultraclean air systems have the potential to protect the patient, but users need to wear proper basic OR attire (see the chapter "Surgical Attire"), manage intraoperative activities correctly, and respect the aseptic zones (7, p. 850).
- LAF is designed to move particle-free (ultraclean) air over the aseptic operating field at a uniform velocity, sweeping away parti-

cles in its path. LAF can be directed vertically or horizontally, and recirculated air is usually passed through a HEPA filter (9, pp. 260-261).

- Performance of orthopedic implant operations in ORs supplied with ultraclean air should be considered (9, p. 267).
- The CDC SSI guideline states that most of the studies examining the efficiency of ultraclean air involve only orthopedic operations. Findings suggest that both ultraclean air and antimicrobial prophylaxis can reduce SSI following orthopedic implant operations, but antimicrobial prophylaxis is more beneficial than ultraclean air (9, p. 261).
- Results of studies on the value of an LAF system in reducing airborne contamination are inconclusive. Other types of filtered air-delivery systems that have a high rate of airflow are as effective in controlling airborne contamination (6, p. 154).
- It is clear that airborne bacteria-carrying particles play a role in causing wound infections. A reduction in the number of these particles is definitely beneficial; however, there is a threshold below which further reduction in colony-forming units (CFUs) fails to yield a corresponding reduction in wound infection rates (11, p. 366).
- LAF systems will reduce CFUs. The question remains, however, regarding whether this practice translates into a lower infection rate. Studies during the past 25 years have failed to show that LAF systems are necessary when prophylactic antibiotics are used in conventional ORs. The need for the expensive ultraclean LAF OR in an era of restricted financial resources is not warranted (11, p. 366).
- The ultraclean LAF system has yet to demonstrate its value. As a rule, consensus holds that airborne organisms are an important factor in causing wound infection only in the folowing scenarios:
  - When an air-handling system is grossly contaminated
  - When an otherwise effective air-handling system is abused
  - During highly specialized surgical procedures in which a large foreign body is implanted (2, p. 274)

The following sections on garb and body exhaust systems are included for the benefit of those who choose to use, or are investigating the use of, LAF systems.

Garb

The combination of disposable noncotton, nonwoven clothing with modern face masks and wide surgical hoods that reach out over the shoulder to prevent skin bacteria emission spread from the neck, worn in conventional ORs, has been found to be as efficient as body exhaust systems worn in ORs with vertical or horizontal LAF systems. Reusable, tightly woven clothing may offer comparable results but so far have not been adequately evaluated. In addition, the barrier efficiency of woven clothing may decrease when washed and, if so, the number of washings must be tracked (7, pp. 848-849).

Body Exhaust Systems in Laminar Airflow Operating Rooms

The late British orthopedic surgeon Sir John Charnley championed ultraclean air in the OR to prevent deep joint sepsis following total hip replacement. He developed a total body exhaust system that had an impervious gown, visored hood, and total body aspiration via a nonportable filtered blower. Various types of body gear have been developed since Charnley's time and are still being used today (3, p. 421).

- Laminar and exponential airflow systems offer significant reductions in air contamination, and further reduction is possible with body exhaust apparatus. The value of these body suits, however, continues to be questionable (3, p. 421).
- An ultraclean air system (LAF system) may be used for high-risk procedures such as total joint replacement, cardiac surgery, or organ transplantation. In addition to the LAF air system, sterile team members wear total body exhaust gowns resembling space suits and covering the whole body. Air is piped into the headpiece and removed through filtered tubes; the hood or helmet is equipped for hearing and speaking. Negative pressure is maintained under the gown by a vacuum hose and body cooling is provided for the wearer (6, pp. 226-227).
- LAF with a total body exhaust system reliably reduces bacterial contamination at the wound site. The LAF system is an adjunct to the control of airborne contamination, not a substitute for meticulous surgical technique (6, p. 227).

Body Exhaust Systems in Conventional Operating Rooms

There are few data regarding the performance of body exhaust suits in conventional ORs, without ultraclean air systems. To this end, Bohn, et al. (3, p. 421), assessed the effect of a portable HEPA-filtered body exhaust system on OR airborne microbial contamination. Equivalent levels of airborne contamination, with and without these portable body exhaust systems, were found in a conventional OR during total knee and hip replacement surgeries. The conclusion was that these air exhaust hoods did not further lower airborne microbial contamination compared with standard head covers and masks in a modern conventional OR.

References

1. American Institute of Architects Academy of Architecture for Health, US Department of Health and Human Services: *Guidelines for design and construction of hospital and health care facilities, 1996-1997,* Washington, DC, 1996, American Institute of Architects Press. Online: www.e-architect.com/resources/hcfg1.asp
2. Belkin NL: Laminar airflow and surgical wound infections, *AORN J* 68(2):273-275, 1998.
3. Bohn WW et al: The effect of a portable HEPA-filtered body exhaust system on airborne microbial contamination in a conventional operating room, *Infect Control Hosp Epidemiol* 17(7):419-422, 1996.
4. Earl A: Operating room. In Olmsted R, editor: *APIC infection control and applied epidemiology, principles and practice,* St Louis, 1996, Mosby, pp 95-1—95-7.
5. Edmiston C et al: Airborne particulates in the OR environment, *AORN J* 69(6):1169-1183, 1999.
6. Fortunato N: *Berry & Kohn's operating room technique,* ed 9, St Louis, 2000, Mosby.
7. Friberg B: Ultraclean laminar airflow ORs, *AORN J* 67(4):841-851, 1998.
8. Gruendemann BJ, Fernsebner B: *Comprehensive perioperative nursing,* vol 1, *Principles,* Boston, 1995, Jones & Bartlett.
9. Mangram AJ, Hospital Infection Control Practices Advisory Committee (HICPAC), Centers for Disease Control and Prevention: Guideline for prevention of surgical site infection, 1999, *Infect Control Hosp Epidemiol* 20(4):247-278, 1999. (Reprinted, in part, in Appendix B.)
10. Pittet D, Ducel G: Infectious risk factors related to operating rooms, *Infect Control Hosp Epidemiol* 15(7):456-462,1994.
11. Turpin IM: Laminar airflow systems, *AORN J* 68(3):366, 1998.

Suggested Reading

1. Charnley J: A clean air operating enclosure, *Br J Surg* 51:202-205, 1964.
2. Cole EC, Cook CE: Characterization of infectious aerosols in health care facilities: an aid to effective engineering controls and preventive strategies, *Am J Infect Control* 26(4):453-464, 1998.
3. Eftekhar NS: The surgeon and clean air in the operating room, *Clin Orthop* 96:188-194, 1973.
4. Grab L: Controlling airborne microorganisms in the healthcare environment, *Infection Control Today* 2(7):12, 16, 1998.
5. Hambraeus A: Aerobiology in the operating room—a review, *J Hosp Infect* 11(suppl A):68-76, 1988.
6. Howorth FH: Prevention of airborne infection during surgery, *Lancet* 1:386, 388, 1985.
7. Howorth FH: Prevention of airborne infection in operating rooms, *J Med Eng Technol* 11(5):263-266, 1987.
8. Howorth FH: Prevention of airborne infection in operating rooms, *NATN News* 13-15, Feb 1987.
9. Humphreys H, Stacey AR, Taylor EW: Survey of operating theatres in Great Britain and Ireland, *J Hosp Infect* 30:245-252, 1995.

10. Joint Commission on Accreditation of Healthcare Organizations: Management of the environment of care. In *Comprehensive accreditation manual for hospitals: the official handbook, EC-9,* Oakbrook Terrace, Ill, 1998, Author.

11. Laufman, H: Airflow effects in surgery, *Arch Surg* 114:826-830, 1979.

12. Lidwell OM: Clean air at operation and subsequent sepsis in the joint, *Clin Orthop* 211:91-102, 1985.

13. McQuarrie D, Glover JL, Olson MM: Laminar airflow systems, *AORN J* 51(4):1035-1048, 1990.

14. Ritter MA et al: The surgeon's garb, *Clin Orthop* 153:204-209, 1980.

15. Ritter MA, Marmion P: The exogenous sources and controls of microorganisms in the operating room, *Orthop Nurs* 7(4):23-28, 1988.

16. Walter CW, Kundsin RB: The airborne component of wound contamination and infection, *Arch Surg* 107:588-595, 1973.

D. Ultraviolet Irradiation and Lights

The use of ultraviolet (UV) irradiation in surgical settings is controversial. Most commonly UV irradiation has been used for treatment of the tubercle bacillus of tuberculosis (TB) or other airborne contaminants. In operating rooms (ORs) where airborne contamination is a major concern, UV irradiation as an engineering control has been used as a form of germicidal disinfection or air treatment. Currently UV lights are seldom used in the United States for germicidal effects, but occasionally interest in their use is rekindled.

DESCRIPTION AND USE

NOTE: In the following discussion the reader will find conflicting recommendations with regard to whether the use of UV irradiation leads to reductions in surgical site infection (SSI) rates. There is no one generally accepted recommendation for the overall use of UV irradiation.

- Not long after the recognition of bacteria, it was observed that exposure to sunlight killed many organisms. After the discovery of UV radiation in 1801, researchers learned that certain wavelengths of this type of energy were lethal to microorganisms, especially wavelengths between 250 and 265 nm. Although UV germicidal lamps produce some visible violet-blue light, the UV radiation emissions are not visible and technically should not be referred to as "lights" (3, p. 724).
- The ability of UV irradiation in ventilation ducts to kill airborne tubercle bacilli generated by patients has been demonstrated (5, p. 160).
- UV lights, generated by low-pressure mercury vapor bulbs, produce nonionizing radiant energy in sufficient wavelengths and intensity for low-level disinfection. The rays can kill selective vegetative bacteria, fungi, and lipoprotein viruses on contact in air or water. UV irradiation is not sporicidal and hepatitis B virus can survive exposure to it (2, p. 288).
- UV lights have been installed in a few ORs to decrease airborne microorganisms to low levels. However, UV rays can cause skin burns, similar to sunburn, and conjunctivitis. Protective skin coverings and goggles or a visor over the eyes must be worn. When used, UV lights are usually turned on only when the room is unoccupied. This practice is thought to reduce airborne and surface contamination (2, p. 288).
- The practical usefulness of UV irradiation is limited because the rays must make direct contact with the organisms. Moving across

the ray of UV light, pathogens may be exposed for too short a time for effective contact with the radiant energy (2, p. 288).

- Because of the results of numerous studies (references 3 and 5; suggested reading 1) and the experiences of TB clinicians during the past several decades, the use of ultraviolet germicidal irradiation (UVGI) has been recommended as a supplement to other infection control measures. UVGI can be used inside air ducts, for upper-room air irradiation, or as a supplement to portable or fixed high-efficiency particulate air HEPA filtration units (6, p. 28).
- There is a use for upper-room air UVGI irradiation in areas that are difficult to ventilate, such as waiting rooms, emergency rooms, corridors, and other central areas of a facility where patients with undiagnosed TB could contaminate the air. Potential hazards (e.g., keratoconjunctivitis) to patients and visitors must be considered (6, p. 28).
- UV light is an alternative to clean air control systems to reduce infection in prosthetic joint replacement. UV systems are inexpensive and easy to install, but their usefulness is limited. The primary limitations are the hazards to patients and personnel. Conjunctivitis, skin erythema, and corneal burns have been reported. These effects can be minimized or avoided by wearing hoods, gowns, and protective glasses with side shields. Patients may need to wear sunscreen preparations to protect exposed areas of the skin (1, pp. 441-442).
- Use of a UV device should always be supplemented with the usual methods of reducing airborne contamination (e.g., reducing personnel numbers and movements, limiting unnecessary conversation, excluding personnel with infections, and maintaining adequate positive air pressure in the OR) (1, pp. 441-442).
- Intraoperative UV irradiation has not been shown to decrease overall SSI risk. UV irradiation should not be used in the OR to prevent SSI (4, pp. 261, 267; 7, pp. 85-93).

References

1. Conner R: Clinical issues, *AORN J* 69(2):438, 441-442, 1999.
2. Fortunato N: *Berry & Kohn's operating room technique,* ed 9, St Louis, 2000, Mosby.
3. Macher JM: The use of germicidal lamps to control tuberculosis in healthcare facilities, *Infect Control Hosp Epidemiol* 14(12):723-729, 1993.
4. Mangram AJ, Hospital Infection Control Practices Advisory Committee (HICPAC), Centers for Disease Control and Prevention: Guideline for prevention of surgical site infection, 1999, *Infect Control Hosp Epidemiol* 20(4):247-278, 1999. (Reprinted, in part, in Appendix B.)
5. Nardell EA: Interrupting transmission from patients with unsuspected tuberculosis: a unique role for upper-air ultraviolet air disinfection, *Am J Infect Control* 23(2):156-164, 1995.

6. Pugliese G: Preventing nosocomial transmission of tuberculosis, *Infection Control Today* 3(6):22-34, 1999.
7. Taylor GJ, Bannister GC, Leeming JP: Wound disinfection with ultraviolet radiation, *J Hosp Infect* 30(2):85-93, 1995.

Suggested Reading

1. Nardell EA: Fans, filters, or rays? pros and cons of the current environmental tuberculosis control technologies, *Infect Control Hosp Epidemiol* 14(12):681-685, 1993 (editorial).
2. Rutala WA et al: Efficacy of portable filtration units in reducing aerosolized particles in the size range of *Mycobacterium tuberculosis, Infect Control Hosp Epidemiol* 16(5):391-398, 1995.
3. Sheretz RJ, Belani A, Kramer BS: Impact of air filtration on nosocomial *Aspergillus* infections, *Am J Med* 83:709-718, 1987.

E. Contaminated or Dirty Procedures

The concept of *contaminated* or *dirty* procedures has historically meant that patients with certain suspected or diagnosed conditions (e.g., those with draining infected wounds) were treated differently than other patients. Extraordinary precautions such as removing all room furniture before the procedure, having an extra or outside circulator, decontaminating instruments differently, scheduling procedures at the end of day, or only using certain rooms would be taken. Often, this so-called treatment would be used for patients with bloodborne diseases such as hepatitis B or acquired immunodeficiency syndrome (AIDS).

We now know that this "extra treatment" was very time consuming, often caused discrimination among patients, and furthermore was not considered an efficacious infection control process. Also, patients with unknown infections were not appropriately treated. In other words, this treatment was neither cost effective nor advantageous. *Dirty-case technique has no place in modern surgical settings.*

The advent of Universal Precautions (UP) (6) has helped to put this practice to rest, even though Standard Precautions (SP) do stipulate that patients with documented or suspected highly transmissible or epidemiologically significant pathogens receive care patterned after Transmission-Based Precautions, namely Airborne, Droplet, and Contact Precautions (2, p. 65).

UP, as advocated by the Centers for Disease Control and Prevention (CDC) and regulated by the Occupational Safety and Health Administration (OSHA) in the 1991 Bloodborne Pathogen Rule, are not particularly difficult to implement in perioperative settings. The concept of treating *all patients* as though they are potentially infectious has become the impetus for eliminating the practice of dirty-case management (3, p. 246).

DEFINITIONS AND DISCUSSION

The word *contaminated* does have a place in surgical terminology. In the operating room (OR), *contaminated* refers to items that are no longer sterile. Contaminated items are never introduced into a sterile field (3, p. 291). The word *contaminated* also appears in the title of two of the four classifications of surgical patient risk (see the section on wound classification in the chapter "Preoperative Patient Preparation").

- *Contaminated* is defined by AORN as the presence of potentially infectious pathogenic microorganisms on animate or inanimate objects (1, p. 259).

- In the regulatory arena, the word *contaminated* refers to a surface or an object that was in contact with an infectious agent, as in contaminated sharps. In the OSHA Bloodborne Pathogen Rule, *contaminated* is defined as the presence of blood or other potentially infectious materials on an item or surface. It is important that staff be familiar with the various meanings of *contaminated* and *dirty* and use the terms appropriately in surgical settings (3, p. 291).
- Practices such as scheduling dirty operative procedures for the end of the day are no longer necessary (7, p. 459).
- Practices aimed at scheduling dirty operations at the end of the day or in a specific room (septic room) should be discouraged. In a modern, well-managed OR, the chance of environmentally spread infection remains remote because of the vigorous processes of cleaning and sterilizing instruments, the efficient ventilation systems that provide clean air, and the adequacy of the techniques of cleaning the OR environment between patients and procedures (5, p. 468).
- There are no data to support the use of special cleaning procedures or the closing of an OR after a contaminated or dirty operation has been performed (4, p. 261). NOTE: See the chapters "Standard Precautions" and "Tuberculosis" for environmental decontamination protocols for ORs following procedures on patients who are known to have diseases caused by airborne or small droplet particles.
- In support of the CDC guidelines, AORN's recommended practices advocate that all surgical patients be considered potentially infected with bloodborne pathogens. All surgical procedures, therefore, are considered contaminated, and the same environmental cleaning protocols should be implemented for all surgical procedures (1, p. 255).

NOTE: For more information about SP, antibiotic-resistant organisms (including methicillin-resistant *Staphylococcus aureus* and vancomycin-resistant *enterococcus*), TB, and cleaning of rooms, see these chapters. For a discussion on UP, see the chapter "Bloodborne Pathogens and Safety Issues."

References

1. AORN: Recommended practices for environmental cleaning in the surgical practice setting. In *Standards, recommended practices and guidelines,* Denver, 2000, Author, pp 255-260.
2. Garner JS, Hospital Infection Control Practices Advisory Committee, Centers for Disease Control and Prevention: Guideline for isolation precautions in hospitals, *Infect Control Hosp Epidemiol* 17(1):53-80, 1996. (Reprinted, in part, in Appendix A.)

3. Gruendemann BJ, Fernsebner B: *Comprehensive perioperative nursing,* vol 1, *Principles,* Boston, 1995, Jones & Bartlett.
4. Mangram AJ, Hospital Infection Control Practices Advisory Committee (HICPAC), Centers for Disease Control and Prevention: Guideline for prevention of surgical site infection, 1999. *Infect Control Hosp Epidemiol* 24(4):247-278, 1999. (Reprinted, in part, in Appendix B.)
5. Nichols RL: The operating room. In Bennett JV, Brachman PS, editors: *Hospital infections,* ed 3, Boston, 1992, Little Brown, pp 461-473.
6. Occupational Safety and Health Administration: Occupational exposure to bloodborne pathogens: final rule, *Federal Register* 56(235):64175-64182, 1991.
7. Pittet D, Ducel G: Infectious risk factors related to operating rooms, *Infect Control Hosp Epidemiol* 15(7):456-462, 1994.

F. Tacky (Sticky) Mats

Tacky floor mats with sticky surfaces were historically placed at the entrance of operating rooms (ORs). The intent was for the mats to collect dust, dirt, and microorganisms from shoes and gurney wheels. The mats were thought to reduce the amount of dirt and debris being carried into a surgical setting and therefore contribute to cleanliness and, possibly, a decrease in surgical site infection (SSI) rates.

Tacky mats are not commonly used today. Their use is not normal practice and is not recommended. However, this chapter is included because tacky mats are still occasionally seen in surgical areas.

USAGE

- It is thought that few bacteria are brought into the OR on the feet of personnel; therefore using tacky mats to reduce floor contamination is unnecessary and the practice should be abandoned (4, p. 531).

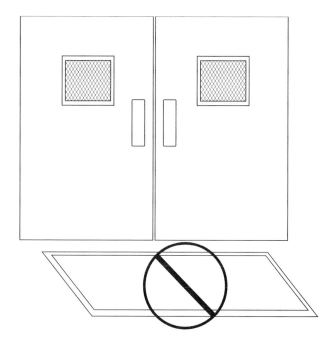

- The use of tacky, or antiseptic, mats at the entrance of the OR for infection control is contraindicated (3, p. 465).
- Tacky mats placed outside the entrance to OR suites have not been shown to reduce the number of organisms on shoes or stretcher wheels, nor do they reduce the risk of SSI. Therefore the Centers for Disease Control and Prevention (CDC) recommends that tacky mats not be used at the entrance to OR suites, or individual ORs, for infection control (1, pp. 261, 268).
- Tacky mats are ineffective and expensive. There is no evidence that their use reduces postoperative wound infection rates. Also, the use of mats soaked with disinfectant is ineffective in preventing contamination of floors in the OR. Such mats may also be hazardous because the floor becomes slippery after the disinfectant is tracked onto the surface adjacent to the mat (2, pp. 632-633).

References

1. Mangram AJ, Hospital Infection Control Practices Advisory Committee (HICPAC), Centers for Disease Control and Prevention: Guideline for prevention of surgical site infection, 1999, *Infect Control Hosp Epidemiol* 24(4):247-278, 1999. (Reprinted, in part, in Appendix B.)
2. Mayhall CG: Surgical infections including burns. In Wenzel RP, editor: *Prevention and control of nosocomial infections,* ed 2, Baltimore, 1993, Williams & Wilkins, pp 614-664.
3. Nichols RL: The operating room. In Bennett JV, Brachman PS, editors: *Hospital infections,* ed 3, Boston, 1992, Little Brown, pp 461-473.
4. Roy MC: The operating theater: a special environmental area. In Wenzel RP, editor: *Prevention and control of nosocomial infections,* ed 3, Baltimore, 1997, Williams & Wilkins, pp 515-538.

G. Construction and Renovation

In the past few years, much progress has been made in healthcare facility construction/renovation (C/R), but risks related to possible hazards and contaminants still remain. Balancing indoor air quality health risks with the challenges of managing construction costs is always a challenge.

This chapter includes a discussion of some of the C/R guidelines, risks, and interventions that relate to prevention of exposure to infectious agents. It is imperative that infection control and surgical personnel work together, especially when C/R involves operating rooms (ORs) and other surgical settings.

GUIDELINES AND INFECTION CONTROL INVOLVEMENT

Infection control professionals play a crucial role in minimizing risks to patients and staff in facilities where C/R projects are taking place. Infection control personnel can be valuable educators and advisors during C/R.

- Infection control personnel should collaborate with the facilities, engineering, nursing, and administration departments in developing construction-related policies, educational materials, and survey tools. Infection control personnel educate the hospital staff, architects, engineers, construction crew, and maintenance personnel about infection risks associated with construction, and they collaborate with specific departments to monitor compliance with infection control standards (7, p. 60).
- The Association for Professionals in Infection Control and Epidemiology (APIC) State-of-the-Art Report (SOAR) points to the need for infection control personnel to be actively involved in construction projects from the inception, planning, and design stages through the implementation stage. The SOAR includes a discussion of an infection control risk assessment, also recommended by the American Institute of Architects Academy of Architecture for Health (AIAAAH). Also discussed in the report are the following major design components, which need to be addressed at the beginning of any C/R project:
  - Design to support infection control practice
  - Design, number, and type of isolation rooms
  - Heating, ventilation, and air conditioning systems (HVAC)
  - Mechanical systems involving water supply and plumbing
  - Number, type, and placement of handwashing fixtures, clinical sinks, dispensers for handwashing soap, paper towels, and lotion

- Sharps disposal unit placement
- Accommodation for personal protective equipment
- Surfaces, such as ceiling tiles, walls, counters, floor coverings, and furnishings
- Utility rooms
- Storage of movable and modular equipment (2, pp. 156, 159-160)
- The AIAAAH suggests, among other things, that qualified risk assessment personnel be included in the planning and design process for any C/R project (1; 9, p. 1).
- The AIAAAH guidelines are a valuable resource during any C/R project. The guidelines cover many topics in detail, including HVAC requirements, filter efficiencies, electrical standards, and construction guidelines for general hospitals and outpatient facilities (1). In addition to the AIAAAH guidelines (as interpreted by federal or state jurisdictions, and as adopted in the Joint Commission on Accreditation of Healthcare Organizations [JCAHO] Environment of Care Standards), compliance with federal, state, county, and local codes, standards, and regulations must be ensured (3, p. 104-2).

RISKS

- The patient risk with greatest consequence in C/R is infection, followed by allergic reaction or irritation. The inclusion in the planning and design process of medical staff, infection control staff, safety personnel, planning departments, contractors, and subcontractors is critical in carrying out any C/R project (9, p. 1).
- *Aspergillus* spp. is one of over 20 construction-related organisms. The infection risk associated with *Aspergillus* spp. is critical, especially to immunocompromised patients (e.g., bone marrow transplant patients). The control of all construction-related airborne pollutants is critical in any C/R project. This issue is supremely important, particularly given the current trend of increased numbers of both older and seriously ill patients, along with emerging infectious diseases (6, p. 1).
- Major hazards result from designs that lack infection control personnel input during C/R. Insufficient planning can lead to the compromise of air quality and the potential for continued environmental contamination from fungi (*Aspergillus* spp.) or from water contaminated with *Legionella* spp. (3, p. 104-1).
- Risks associated with C/R include the following:
  - Construction dust and debris that can carry microorganisms into patient care areas

- Roof leaks caused by construction that can lead to water damage with subsequent mold formation
- Plugging of ventilation system filters, leading to decreased airflow
- Penetration of exterior of building, disrupting normal airflow
- Interruption of utilities, leading to insufficient airflow to critical facility areas, lack of exhaust air for removal of airborne pathogens, and lack of water for sanitation and disinfection (10, p. 111-6)

INTERVENTIONS

- An important intervention is to monitor patients for possible construction-related infections, especially *Aspergillus* spp. Any clusters of fungal infection potentially caused by air contamination should be investigated immediately (8, pp. 173-174).
- During C/R, healthcare and construction staff should be educated to consider dust, footprints, open doors, flies, and wet ceiling tiles as infection risks. Immunocompromised patients should be admitted or relocated to areas away from construction (8, p. 173).
- Suggested interventions to prevent risks of C/R are as follows:
  - Assuring clean-to-dirty airflow in and around construction areas
  - Erecting barriers to contain dust and debris
  - If possible, removing patients from C/R area
  - Assuring window seals that minimize infiltration of outside dust and debris
  - Recognizing that simple procedures (e.g., removing old water-damaged ceiling tile) might cause significant mold exposure
  - Advising on infection prevention implications of ventilation systems maintenance
  - Providing input regarding scheduling of C/R interruptions and provision of back-up strategies, such as potable water supply (10, p. 111-6)
- Construction areas must be separated from patient care areas, pharmaceuticals, and sterile supplies by barriers that dust and dirt cannot penetrate. Framed plasterboard, sealed with duct tape or spackling compound and incorporating a tight-fitting, closable door sealed with weather-stripping, should be used for all demolition and reconstruction projects expected to exceed 48 hours. Plastic sheeting and duct tape may be used for small projects that last no more than 48 hours (7, p. 60).
- Walk-off mats with adhesive floor strips should be placed just outside the construction site to trap dust. Signs should be posted at the work site stating, "Construction zone, authorized entry

only." Housekeeping should remove debris in covered containers and wet mop the area around the construction site at least once daily (7, p. 60).

· Airtight barriers used in temporary walls and plastic sheeting should be set up in construction zones. Airflow should be exhausted in order to maintain negative air pressure in zones of construction. Doors should be kept closed. Dust at doorways and construction sites should be removed routinely. Mats for wiping feet should be placed at construction exits. Pedestrian traffic flow should be redirected away from construction sites (8, pp. 173-174).

· Dust in ceilings and construction debris contains fungus spores. Construction activities causing disturbance of existing dust or creating new dust or other airborne contaminants must be conducted in tight enclosures cutting off any flow of particles into patient areas (5, p. 3).

· Renovation areas should be isolated from occupied areas during construction using airtight barriers, and exhaust airflow should be sufficient to maintain negative air pressure in the construction zone. The potential exists for disturbances from adjacent construction to dislodge dust collected above suspended or false ceilings. Contained areas should be checked frequently for penetrations, and monitoring for open windows must be ongoing (3, pp. 104-4—104-5).

· Infection control areas of concern during C/R include the following: availability of sinks; traffic control; negative-pressure isolation rooms; adequate waste management; water; heating and air conditioning; and protection of surfaces, specifically ceilings and carpets. For example, acoustic ceiling tiles and/or fireproofing and filter materials may become wet after water breaks or floods, becoming a reservoir for fungal spores. Also, *Aspergillus* spp. and other fungi may contaminate carpets and become a reservoir if carpet cleaning agents interfere with the antimicrobial compound incorporated into carpets, and if carpets become contaminated after an event such as a fire (3, pp. 104-3—104-4).

· Carpeting is not recommended in areas of frequent spillage or heavy soilage, or where odor control may be necessary (e.g., ORs, obstetrics, intensive care units, laboratories, chemotherapeutic units, or utility rooms) (3, p. 104-4). Carpeting, although not generally associated with infection, has a higher potential risk of contamination than hard-surface floors. Carpeting must be considered a potential harbor for fungal infection during demolition and after events such as fires (8, p. 173).

· Carpets have not generally been associated with nosocomial infection, even though studies have found that bacterial contamination per unit of carpet may be higher than that of hard-surface floors. Carpets do require regular vacuuming, shampooing, or extraction depending on use, material, and degree of soiling (3, p. 104-4).

DESIGN AND CONSTRUCTION ERRORS

- Carter and Barr (4, p. 590) have encountered the following design and construction errors in their infection control practice:
  - Air intakes placed too close to exhausts, or other mistakes in the placement of air intakes
  - Incorrect number of air exchanges
  - Air handling systems that function only sporadically
  - Air vents not reopened after construction completed
  - Large new inpatient facility built without negative-air–pressure rooms
  - Carpet placed where vinyl should be used
  - Wet-vacuum system in an OR that pulls water up one floor into a holding tank rather than down one floor
  - Aerators on faucets
  - Sinks located in inaccessible places
  - Patient and treatment rooms without sinks in which healthcare workers can wash their hands
  - Doors too narrow to allow beds and equipment to be moved in and out of rooms
- Infection control personnel should be involved in all phases of C/R projects to ensure that patients, visitors, and staff are protected from unnecessary exposure to infectious agents. Infection risks posed by each project must be identified, and ways to minimize risks and avoid errors must be planned (4, p. 587).

References

1. American Institute of Architects Academy of Architecture for Health (AIAAAH), U.S. Department of Health and Human Services: *Guidelines for design and construction of hospital and healthcare facilities, 1996-1997,* Washington, DC, 1996, American Institute of Architects Press. Online: www.e-architect.com/resources/hcfg1.asp
2. Bartley JM, APIC Guidelines Committees: APIC state-of-the art report: the role of infection control during construction in health care facilities, *Am J Infect Control* 28(2):156-169, 2000.
3. Bartley J: Construction. In Olmsted R, editor: *APIC infection control and applied epidemiology, principles and practice,* St Louis, 1996, Mosby, pp 104-1—104-6.
4. Carter CD, Barr BA: Infection control issues in construction and renovation, *Infect Control Hosp Epidemiol* 18(8):587-596, 1997.
5. Cheple M, editor: Did you know . . . *Indoor Air Quality Project, University of Minnesota* 1(4):3, 1999.

6. Cheple M, editor: Healthcare facility construction management: indoor air quality workshop highlights, *Indoor Air Quality Project, University of Minnesota,* 1(5):1, 1999.

7. Finkelstein LE, Mendelson MH: Challenges during hospital renovation, *Am J Nurs* 97(12):60-61, 1997.

8. Jennings J, Manian FA, editors: *APIC handbook of infection control and epidemiology,* ed 2, Washington, DC, 1999, Association for Professionals in Infection Control and Epidemiology.

9. Streifel A: Establishing risk assessment, *Indoor Air Quality Project, University of Minnesota* 1(4):1, 1999.

10. Streifel AJ: Maintenance and engineering: biomedical engineering. In Olmsted R, editor: *APIC infection control and applied epidemiology, principles and practice,* St Louis, 1996, Mosby, pp. 111-1—111-7.

Suggested Reading

1. Are patients at risk from the hospital environment? *Hosp Infect Control* 26(12):164-166, 1999.

2. CDC at work on new environmental guidelines, *Hosp Infect Control* 26(12):166-167, 1999.

3. Rutala WA, Weber DJ: Water as a reservoir of nosocomial pathogens, *Infect Control Hosp Epidemiol* 18(9):609-616, 1997.

4. Vesley D, Streifel AJ: Environmental services. In Mayhall CG, editor: *Hospital epidemiology and infection control,* ed 2, Philadelphia, 1999, Lippincott Williams & Wilkins, pp 1047-1053.

H. Traffic Patterns

Use of aseptic principles begins when personnel enter the doors of the surgical area. The entire area has been designed to facilitate movement of patients, personnel, equipment, and supplies in a manner that protects the safety and privacy of patients and the cleanliness and integrity of the environment. Traffic patterns have been established to limit access by outsiders and increase the control of contact as patients and personnel move closer to restricted areas that include the rooms where sterile procedures take place.

DISTINCT AREAS AND ATTIRE REQUIREMENTS

Surgical suites and traffic patterns are designed to facilitate movement of patients and personnel into, through, and out of defined areas within the surgical suite. Increasing environmental controls and the use of additional surgical attire as the progression is made from unrestricted to restricted areas decreases the potential for cross-contamination (2, p. 365; 1, pp. 22-25). Signs should be posted that clearly indicate the appropriate environmental controls and surgical attire required (2, p. 365; 1, pp. 22-25). All persons (staff, patients, and visitors) should follow the delineated patterns in appropriate attire (3, pp. 149-150).

Unrestricted Area

The unrestricted area includes a control point that serves to monitor the entrance of patients, personnel, and materials. Street clothes are

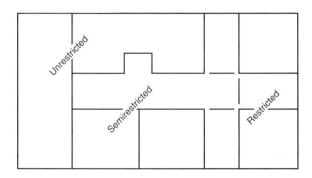

permitted in this area, and traffic is not limited (2, p. 365). A corridor on the periphery accommodates traffic from the outside, including patients. This area is isolated from the main hospital corridor and elevators and from other areas in the operating room (OR) suite (3, p. 150).

Transition Zone

The transition zone allows for movement of personnel from unrestricted areas to either the semirestricted or restricted areas inside the surgical suite. This zone (locker and dressing rooms) allows personnel to enter in street clothes and exit into a semirestricted or restricted area with proper attire. It also allows for security because people can be monitored before admission to the surgical suite (2, p. 365).

Semirestricted Area

The semirestricted area includes the peripheral support area of the surgical suite that may have storage space for clean and sterile supplies, work areas for storage and processing of clean instruments, and corridors leading to the restricted area of the surgical suite. Traffic in this area is limited to patients and authorized personnel. Persons who work in this area are required to wear surgical attire and cover all head and facial hair, including sideburns and necklines, by a surgical cap or hood. Nonscrubbed personnel should wear long-sleeved jackets that are buttoned or snapped closed during use (2, p. 365).

Because coughing or sneezing explodes droplets into the environment, persons with respiratory infections should not be permitted in the surgical suite (3, p. 224; 4, p. 157). NOTE: Persons with skin infections should not be permitted in the semirestricted area of the surgical suite.

Restricted Area

The restricted area includes operating and procedures rooms, the sterile core, and scrub sink areas. Persons in this area are required to wear full surgical attire and cover all head and facial hair including sideburns and necklines. Nonscrubbed personnel should wear long-sleeved jackets that are buttoned or snapped closed during use. Masks are required where open sterile supplies or scrubbed persons are located (2, p. 365; 3, p. 150). Sick personnel, or those with skin infections, should not work in restricted areas (4, p. 157).

ADDITIONAL ATTIRE CONSIDERATIONS

Patients entering the surgical suite should be clean, be wearing clean gowns, be covered with clean linens, and have their hair covered. This practice will minimize particulate shedding during surgical procedures. During transport, patients are not required to wear masks unless they are under respiratory precautions (e.g., with active tuberculosis [TB] or other airborne respiratory disease) (2, pp. 365-366; 3, p. 150).

Persons from other departments (e.g., maintenance technicians, computer support personnel) entering the semirestricted or restricted areas of the OR for a brief time for a specific purpose may don a disposable coverall suit, designed to totally cover outside apparel, or a cover gown that covers outside apparel. Shoe and hair covers should be donned as well (2, p. 365).

FLOW OF SUPPLIES

Separation of sterile supplies and equipment from soiled materials by space, time, and traffic patterns decreases the risk of infection (2, p. 366).

- Supplies in external shipping containers should be removed from the container in an unrestricted area or transition zone before transfer into the surgical suite. External shipping containers may collect dust, debris, and insects during shipment and could carry contamination into the surgical suite (2, p. 366).
- Supplies prepared for surgical procedures should be transported to the OR in a manner that maintains cleanliness and sterility and prevents physical damage. Protecting items from contamination facilitates their safe use and preserves the qualities of the clean and sterile (restricted) environment (2, p. 366). NOTE: Examples of this practice would be to cover unopened sterile items that must be transported from a semirestricted or restricted area to another restricted area in the hospital.
- The flow of clean and sterile supplies and equipment should be separated from contaminated supplies, equipment, and water by space, time, and traffic patterns. The flow of supplies should proceed from the sterile core through the operating room to the peripheral corridor following use. Soiled supplies, instruments, and equipment should not reenter the sterile core area. They should be contained in closed or covered carts or containers for transport to a designated decontamination area (2, p. 366).
- Decontamination and collection areas for soiled linen and trash should be separated from personnel and patient traffic areas (2, p. 366).
- Contaminated objects and waste disposal operations should be kept out of patient care areas (4, p. 157).

- Contamination can be contained by transporting trash, soiled linen, soiled instruments, and nonsterile equipment and supplies in an enclosed cart or an impervious system (4, p. 157).

ACTIVITY WITHIN SEMIRESTRICTED AND RESTRICTED AREAS

Because air is a potential source of microorganisms that can contaminate surgical wounds, and microbial shedding from surgical personnel is known to increase with activity, greater amounts of airborne contamination can be expected with increased movement of surgical team members.

- Careful assessment of and planning for patient care needs by surgical team members can reduce the need for excess movement or activity during procedures. Increased activity has been found to cause airborne contamination of the sterile field (2, p. 366).
- Doors to the ORs should be closed except during movement of patients, personnel, supplies and equipment (2, p. 366).
- Doors should be kept closed. Doors are only opened when transporting patients, supplies, or equipment (4, p. 157). NOTE: Open doors, or cupboards being opened and closed, causes disruption of the air currents. Instead of going from intake ducts in the ceiling to exhaust ducts near the floor, the air is pulled more laterally toward the open door or cupboard. This alteration in air flow can cause airborne contamination from personnel, supplies, and equipment in the OR.
- Talking and the number of people present should be minimized (2, p. 366).

References

1. American Institute of Architects Academy of Architecture for Health (AIAAAH), U.S. Department of Health and Human Services: *Guidelines for design and construction of hospital and healthcare facilities, 1996-1997,* Washington, DC, 1996, American Institute of Architects Press. Online: www.e-architect.com/resources/hcfg1.asp
2. AORN: Recommended practices for traffic patterns in the perioperative practice setting. In *Standards, recommended practices and guidelines,* Denver, 2000, Author, pp 365-367.
3. Fortunato N: *Berry and Kohn's operating room technique,* ed 9, St Louis, 2000, Mosby.
4. Rhyne L, Ulmer BC, Revell L: Monitoring and controlling the environment. In Phippen ML, Wells MP: *Care of the patient during operative and invasive procedures,* Philadelphia, 2000, WB Saunders, pp 147-166.

I. Visitors

Maintaining safety in surgical settings where patients are undergoing surgical procedures that put them at risk for developing surgical site infections requires careful monitoring of infection control practices. For this reason, hospital policy and procedures for visitors and observers in the surgical suite should provide guidelines that help maintain the integrity of the surgical environment. All areas should be carefully protected and monitored to ensure the highest level of quality patient care. Patient privacy must be maintained. For these reasons, special protocols for supervision of visitors should be followed.

Visitors may include those who are in the area to accompany patients (e.g., a family member, significant other, guard, or interpreter). Observers need access to the surgical suite as part of their educational experience (e.g., radiology, medical, and nursing students). Professionals (e.g., visiting surgeons, residents and interns, sales representatives) may request entrance to the operating room (OR) suite as part of their work. Other hospital employees (e.g., biomedical equipment technicians, maintenance or computer support personnel) may need entrance to repair equipment.

GENERAL GUIDELINES

Policies or guidelines regarding visitors in the surgical setting may vary, but they should be based on institution policy and on established infection control practices regarding surgical attire and restriction of traffic in the surgical suite. Infection control considerations include the following:

- Persons with an acute infection such as a cold or sore throat should not be permitted within the surgical suite (6, p. 239).
- All persons within semirestricted and restricted areas should wear clean, freshly laundered attire intended for use in the OR. In addition, hair and shoe covers should be worn within these areas (6, p. 239).
- Visitors whose presence in the OR will be brief may don a one-piece coverall, in addition to hair and shoe covers (6, p. 240). NOTE: Individual healthcare agencies may establish guidelines and policies based on sound infection control principles but still allow adjustment for individual circumstances. Parents accompanying a child to a preoperative preparation or holding area may be asked to wear cover gowns and hair and shoe covers instead of full OR garb.

GAINING ACCESS

Agency policy should require visitors to check in and obtain administrative permission from the facility administrator or designee, such as the surgical services manager, before entering the surgical area (5, pp. 657-658). NOTE: A name badge for identification may be issued. Depending on agency policy and the purpose of the person's visit, the patient may be asked to sign a written consent before the visitor is allowed in the OR suite (5, pp. 657-658).

FOLLOWING DESIGNATED TRAFFIC PATTERNS

Visitors should follow the delineated traffic patterns and wear the proper attire. Areas should be marked and signs posted that clearly indicate what attire and environmental restrictions are required (6, pp. 149-150).

> *Unrestricted areas* include a central control point established to monitor the entrance of patients, personnel, and materials. Street clothes are permitted and traffic may not be limited. A *transition zone* exists for staff and visitors to change into surgical attire and proceed to semirestricted and restricted areas of the OR suite (3, p. 365; 6, p. 150).

> *Semirestricted areas* are designated peripheral support areas and access corridors to the ORs. Traffic is limited to persons wearing surgical attire, shoe and hair covering, and a long-sleeved jacket that is buttoned or kept closed (3, p. 365; 7, p. 286).

> *Restricted areas* are the OR and procedure rooms, the sterile core, and the scrub sink areas. Persons in these areas are required to wear full surgical attire and cover all hair, including facial hair, sideburns, and necklines. Masks are required to be worn where open sterile supplies or scrubbed persons are located (3, p. 365; 6, p. 150).

Visiting Physicians and Residents

Physician visitors should be credentialed and/or given temporary privileges through the medical staff office (5, pp. 657-658).

Students

Medical, nursing, or radiology students should have received information regarding aseptic technique. In addition, they must have current immunizations, cardiopulmonary resuscitation (CPR) certification, negative tuberculosis (TB) test results, and carry malpractice insurance. Students must be adequately supervised while in the surgical setting. Agreements between educational programs and hospitals should specifically give details outlining expectations of both students and faculty (8, p. 428).

Sales Representatives

Sales representatives are allowed in surgical areas, but only under defined conditions and systems that are developed by each facility. Some facilities require that the patient be informed of the sales representative's presence and purpose of the visit and provide written permission that becomes part of the patient's medical record.

Table 2-1 compares official statements from the Association of periOperative Registered Nurses (AORN) and the American College of Surgeons (ACS).

TABLE 2-1	AORN and ACS Policy Statements on Sales Representatives in the Operating Room
Association of periOperative Registered Nurses (AORN)	**American College of Surgeons (ACS)**
Policy development Policy should be developed in collaboration with the facility's risk management and/or legal counsel to ensure compliance with applicable laws.	Healthcare organizations (e.g., hospitals and outpatient OR facilities) should establish written policies defining (1) requirements and procedures for MRs to be present in the OR and (2) restrictions to govern MR activities in the OR. Policies should comply with applicable state laws and regulations and should be consistent with an organization's existing policies.
Approval Each facility should develop a system that documents that the HCIR has completed instruction in the principles of asepsis, fire and safety protocols, infection control practices, bloodborne pathogens, and patients' rights. The RN should monitor the HCIR's activities whenever possible and facilitate the HCIR's service to the patient and the perioperative team during the procedure.	Each institution should delegate an authority for approving a MR's presence in the OR. A time-frame for securing this approval should also be established. The MR's orientation, training, and credentialing should include documented knowledge of patients' rights and confidentiality; appropriate conduct in the OR; aseptic principles and techniques; fire, electrical, and other safety protocols; infection control; and other applicable practices related to the operation.

HCIR, Health care industry representative; *MR,* manufacturer representative; *OR,* operating room; *RN,* registered nurse.

TABLE 2-1	AORN and ACS Policy Statements on Sales Representatives in the Operating Room—cont'd

Association of periOperative Registered Nurses (AORN)	American College of Surgeons (ACS)
Consent requirements	
Surgeon approval—The HCIR's presence and purpose should be prescheduled with the designated OR management authority and the surgeon in accordance with the facility policy. The RN should be notified prior to the procedure that a HCIR will be present and the purpose for being there.	*Surgeon approval*—If the surgeon did not initiate the request, the surgeon should be notified and approve the visit prior to the operation.
Patient approval—Each facility should develop a system that addresses informed patient consent regarding the presence and role of a HCIR in the OR during a surgical procedure in both routine and emergency situations; this system should include documentation in the medical record.	*Patient approval*—The patient should be notified of the presence and purpose of the representative in the OR and give written, informed consent.
Representatives' role, responsibilities, and restrictions	
Each facility should develop a system that clearly delineates limits on the HCIR's activities in the OR based on community standards. The HCIR should not scrub in. The HCIR with specialized training may perform calibration to adjust devices to the surgeon's specifications (e.g., pacemakers, lasers). The HCIR should wear identification while in the facility.	MR conduct in the OR should be defined in the written policy. MRs should wear identification during their visit to the OR and other patient care areas. They should not be permitted to participate directly in any procedures performed on the patient.
Documentation	
The presence of the HCIR should be documented in the medical record. (1, p. 1158; 2, pp. 266-273)	Documentation of a MR's presence during the procedure and the patient's consent regarding the MR's presence should be included in the permanent medical record. (4, pp. 31-32)

LIMITING THE NUMBER OF OBSERVERS

- Policies may be needed that limit the number of observers. Reducing the number of persons in the surgical suite is known to decrease the amount of bacterial shedding and the possibility of accidental contamination of sterile items (7, p. 288).
- Movement within the OR should be kept to a minimum while invasive procedures are in progress (3, p. 366).

References

1. AORN: Position statement on the role of the health care industry representative in the operating room, *AORN J* 71(6):1158, 2000.
2. AORN: Position statement: applying the health care industry statement to your setting, *AORN J* 72(2):226-273, 2000.
3. AORN: Recommended practices for traffic patterns in the perioperative practice setting. In *Standards, recommended practices and guidelines,* Denver, 2000, Author, pp 365-367.
4. Committee on the Operating Room Environment (CORE) of the American College of Surgeons: Statement on health care industry representatives in the operating room, *Bull Am Coll Surg* 85(5):31-32, 2000.
5. Fogg DM: Clinical issues, *AORN J* 69(3):652-658, 1999.
6. Fortunato N: *Berry and Kohn's operating room technique,* ed 9, St Louis, 2000, Mosby.
7. Gruendemann BJ, and Fernsebner B: *Comprehensive perioperative nursing,* vol 1, *Principles,* Boston, 1995, Jones & Bartlett.
8. Ziel S: Spectators in the OR, *AORN J* 65(2):427-430, 1997.

Suggested Reading

1. Applegeet C: Clinical issues, *AORN J* 61(1):254-255, 1995.
2. Giganti AW: Families in pediatric critical care: the best option, *Pediatric Nursing* 24(3):261-265, 1998.
3. Schulenburg P: Spectators in the operating room? *Nursing 98* 28(7):32hn13, 1998.

J. Alternative Surgical Settings

Infection control issues have been pushed to the forefront of healthcare practice concerns for the following reasons: re-emergence of infectious diseases such as hepatitis, acquired immunodeficiency syndrome (AIDS), and multidrug-resistant tuberculosis (TB); earlier discharge from acute care settings; reduction in lengths of stay; and patient care moving to ambulatory, subacute, rehabilitation, and home settings. All of these factors are *increasing the risk of infection at all points in the care continuum,* and many nosocomial infections are now being identified (17, pp. iv, 20).

Governmental and regulatory agencies are requiring that more stringent attention be paid to the rapid spread of infectious diseases. At the same time, the growth of managed care has increased the pressure to reduce costs in all settings, and program cuts have sometimes included infection control personnel and activities. Because of these challenges, it is essential for providers in *all settings* to review, revise, and improve their programs for infection surveillance, control, and prevention (and adapt the programs to out-of-hospital settings, even when resources for infection prevention may be scarce). Furthermore, lines of communication must be established and promoted among all healthcare organizations along the entire continuum of care so that infection prevention and control programs remain viable wherever patients are located (17, p. 20).

Because of the previously mentioned issues, and because surgery is now often performed in settings other than acute care hospital operating rooms (ORs)—settings such as ambulatory surgery centers, endoscopy and gastrointestinal (G-I) laboratories, cardiac catheterization laboratories, dialysis centers, interventional radiology units, and physician offices—we deem this chapter necessary. Discussion will focus on (1) general guidelines for effective program planning that can apply to all out-of-hospital settings, regardless of locale, size, specialization, or governance, and (2) comments from textbooks and the literature regarding specific setting recommendations.

It is important to realize that infection risks in surgical settings outside of the hospital are usually related more to patient populations and procedures than to designated settings; therefore we begin with a section on general guidelines. However, certain settings, such as cardiac catheterization laboratories, have unique structural and procedural characteristics that have implications for infection risks; therefore we have included a section on recommendations for infection prevention practices applicable to multiple settings.

GENERAL GUIDELINES

Hospitals comprise different units (e.g., neonatal and the intensive care unit [ICU]), each with a specific set of patient populations and surveillance procedures. However, infection control surveillance is more difficult in nonacute settings, which often combine a number of services and serve medically complex patients (17, p. 4).

The delivery of health care in the outpatient setting is very different from that in the acute care facility. The patient mix and interactions are more varied, patient clinical statuses can range from healthy to acutely ill, and visits can range from brief to all day. Infection control professionals have usually considered the risk for infection in the outpatient setting to be low. However, as more invasive procedures are performed in the ambulatory care setting, patients and healthcare workers (HCWs) alike are at risk for developing or transmitting infection (11, p. 421).

On the other hand, immunocompromised persons, the frail elderly, and newborns, regardless of the setting, are at high risk for infections. Others at high risk include cancer, transplant, radiation therapy, and trauma patients, and those with surgical wounds, pressure ulcers, invasive devices, and malnutrition (17, pp. 9, 15).

Nonacute care organizations should be careful of implementing acute care hospital infection control policies and procedures without special adaptation for use in other settings (17, p. 16). Because of the rapid and recent growth of ambulatory surgical care, time has not allowed for adequate validation of many procedures and guidelines that would apply to out-of-hospital settings. At this stage, we use the science that is available and continue to study its application to outpatients. The literature on infection prevention in alternative surgical settings continues to grow.

The Joint Commission on Accreditation of Healthcare Organizations (JCAHO) states that an effective infection control program, regardless of setting, must take into account the following:

- Patient population(s)
- Patients at high risk for infection
- Common patient diagnoses
- Types of care provided
- Risks of infection transmission
- Types of medical devices, equipment, and supplies used
- Types of medical waste generated
- Risks of employee and staff occupational exposures (17, p. 15)

High-risk, high-volume, problem-prone populations and procedures/treatments are usually the focus of infection control efforts because they have the greatest number of actual exposure and infection incidents, and they represent an organization's greatest investment of resources, both physical and financial (17, p. 15).

A healthcare organization with a successful infection control program will identify the following:
- At-risk patient populations (e.g., immunocompromised patients, or patients with multiple co-morbidities)
- At-risk procedures (e.g., those involving invasive devices)
- Causes, risks, and patterns of infections that can and do arise in a particular setting

Regardless of the setting, policies and procedures should address the following:
- Bloodborne pathogen exposure control
- Standard Precautions (SP), including handwashing
- TB exposure control
- An employee health program, including staff work restrictions, screening, and follow-up after occupational exposures
- Medical waste and specimen handling and disposal
- Surveillance and reporting activities for patients and staff (17, pp. 15-16)

Targeted surveillance is the monitoring of specific infections, populations, or types of care or procedures. This is the most commonly used type of surveillance, providing monitoring of the high-risk, high-volume, problem-prone populations and procedures identified in the design process. Surveillance should be appropriate, simple, and pragmatic; data are collected and then used in devising policies and procedures. *Prevention* is a proactive strategy aimed at avoiding the occurrence or decreasing the possibility of infection. *Control* is a reactive strategy that uses prevention measures to stop or reduce the transmission of infections that have been identified during surveillance (17, p. 16; 3).

A qualified, designated individual must oversee and manage all infection prevention and control efforts; this person may have other responsibilities, too, especially if the facility is small. Regulations, standards, and professional guidelines and recommendations must be up to date and made relevant to the setting. Education must be ongoing and appropriate, ensuring that employees are knowledgeable about trends and practices. An infection control coordinator will provide this education and information. Access to infection control and epidemiologic expertise and resources is a necessity for any alternative surgical setting, regardless of size, type of organization, or distance from a hospital or other resource center (17, p. 22).

INFECTION PREVENTION PRACTICES APPLICABLE TO MULTIPLE SETTINGS

In both ambulatory surgical and inpatient settings, the same major infection prevention concerns must be addressed and goals must be met: to protect the patients, HCWs, visitors, and others in the healthcare environment and to deliver services in a timely, efficient, and cost-effective manner (20, p. 422).

Aseptic practices such as opening and setting up rooms and sterile fields, scrubbing, gowning, gloving, prepping the patient's skin, wearing proper attire (depending on the procedure and its risks), and using SP should be faithfully followed and role modeled throughout the facility (13, p. 487). Patient care during invasive procedures, whether they occur in an ambulatory surgery facility or physician's office; in an endoscopy and G-I, cardiac catheterization, or interventional radiology laboratory, should be based on the principles of aseptic technique delineated in related association guidelines, current articles, national accreditation standards, and state regulations (17; 6; 3). NOTE: Adaptations can be made depending on the individual facility's needs, the degree of invasiveness of the procedure, and the special needs of the patient. However, rationale for these adaptations must be made based on sound infection prevention practices and the use of aseptic principles and technique. Guidelines for specific surgical settings include discussion of how standard procedures are adapted or apply to a variety of alternative surgical settings.

Ambulatory Surgery Centers

The risk of nosocomial infection has been thought to be minimal in ambulatory surgical settings because of the short stay in the facility, the short duration of anesthesia, the "minor" nature of the surgical procedures, and the general good health of the patient (10, p. 336). However, surgical site infections (SSIs) remain an important cause of morbidity, mortality, and excess hospital costs during the postoperative period when patients must be admitted to an acute care facility for treatment of SSIs (18, p. 515). As the shift toward more ambulatory surgery continues and more procedures are performed on an out-patient basis, verification will be needed that high-quality services are being provided in same-day surgery centers (20, p. 270).

Although SSIs can develop from post-operative wound contamination, most infections result from introduction of bacteria into the wound during surgery. For this reason, the ambulatory surgical environment should adhere to and maintain standards similar to those promoted for inpatient ORs. The designated infection control practitioner and the surgical staff must ensure that the OR is safe and that principles of asepsis are maintained (20, p. 270).

- Ventilation requirements are similar to those needed in hospital surgical settings (5, Table 2).
- Traffic patterns should be planned that allow for even flow of traffic from the unrestricted area to semirestricted and restricted areas where special attire is required and surgical procedures are

performed (5, p. A-28; 7, pp. 62-63). The OR must be separate and segregated from the general office area (e.g., waiting rooms, examination rooms, physician offices, and staff lounge) (3, p. 9).

The following guidelines are based on accreditation standards for the ambulatory surgical setting:

- Use of a steam autoclave is preferred where all instruments must be sterilized. Alternative methods can be chemical autoclave or gas (ethylene oxide [EtO]). Gas sterilizers must be vented, if appropriate for the specific sterilizer. High-level disinfection is used only for nonautoclavable equipment such as certain endoscopes (3, p. 10).
- A sterile field is routinely used and aseptic technique is maintained during and between procedures (3, p. 11).
- Proper scrub facilities are provided. If there is a sink in the OR proper, there must be a written policy to prevent its use for surgical scrubbing, during surgery, or to clean dirty instruments after surgery. The sink must be removed when remodeling is done (3, p. 11). If there is one sink used both to clean dirty instruments and to scrub for surgery, there must be a written policy to clean and disinfect the sink prior to scrubbing (3, p. 11).
- Appropriate attire, consisting of scrub suit, cap or hair cover, gloves, operative gown, mask, and eye protection, is worn (3, p. 11).
- Maintenance and cleaning of the operating room should be done routinely, using appropriate germicides and a written protocol (3, p. 11).
- Patient screening should be done to identify patient risk factors such as hypertension, heart disease, obesity, and alcohol and drug use. A careful assessment can minimize unanticipated complications (7, p. 79). The Accreditation Association of Ambulatory Health Care (AAAHC) notes that an appropriate and current history, including a list of current medications and dosages; a physical examination; and pertinent preoperative diagnostic studies should be incorporated into the patient's medical record before surgery (1, p. 32). Information gained during admission can reveal infection-related problems such as an elevated temperature. A chest x-ray could reveal asymptomatic TB or pneumonia. NOTE: Additional risk factors specific to infection prevention issues are discussed in the chapter "Preoperative Patient Preparation." Also, refer to the chapters "Bloodborne Pathogens and Safety Issues" and "Tuberculosis" for special precautions for patients with communicable diseases. These guidelines should be similar to those in acute care settings.

- Postoperative teaching should include the proper care of the incisional area, identification of possible signs of infection, procedures for home wound care, and appropriate communication lines should complications occur (13, p. 487).
- Employee health issues must be addressed in the ambulatory surgical setting. It cannot be assumed that a HCW in an ambulatory facility is at a lower risk of acquiring occupational injury or disease than a HCW at an inpatient facility. Same-day surgery units should have a well-designed plan to safeguard employee health and safety (20, p. 271). Refer to the chapters "Employee Health" and "Bloodborne Pathogens and Safety Issues."
- Accreditation criteria for ambulatory surgical settings include quality of care and quality improvement, which are necessary for maintaining a continuing emphasis on infection prevention (9, pp. 814-821). Required are a designated infection control person and infection control processes. Often, in nonacute care organizations, staffing numbers are insufficient to support a full-time infection control practitioner. Staff members may perform double duty as the head of an infection control program and as surgical staff, making it difficult to maintain surveillance, prevention, and control activities (17, pp. 3-4). Perhaps the most difficult infection control issue for ambulatory surgery is that of collecting data on surgical wound infections. Such confounding factors as surgeons' nonvoluntary reporting of SSIs, patients' inability to ascertain the nature of a wound infection, and the problem of many patients returning to their primary care physician rather than their surgeon make consistent and accurate reporting difficult. It is critical that innovative and collaborative ways of detecting and reporting SSIs be implemented in ambulatory care facilities (20, pp. 272, 276, 279).

Physicians' Office-Based Surgery

Infection-associated complications from surgical procedures performed in physicians' offices can be minimized by a combination of appropriate sterile and surgical techniques. As practiced in office settings, infection prevention standards may vary from strict aseptic technique to a very low level of care where practically no sterile technique is practiced (22, p. 1364). Accreditation standards and recommended practices for environmental cleaning, sterilization, use of sterile technique, Universal Precautions (UP) and SP, attire, and waste management used in ambulatory surgical settings can and should be followed for office-based surgery (7, pp. 9-10, 26-29, 50-60; 3, pp. 9-14; 4, pp. 20-22).

The following infection control recommendations apply to office-based surgery:

- Building codes for licensed office-based ORs require that the ceiling be smooth and washable. Acoustic ceiling tile is not acceptable. Tile flooring must be sealed. Surfaces must be cleaned and disinfected on a predetermined schedule and whenever necessitated by exposure to contamination. There should be a minimum of one adequately sized OR that is used exclusively for surgery. A general treatment room is not adequate (4, p. 20).

- Any opening to the outer air must be adequately controlled to prevent the entrance of insects. Adequate lighting, ventilation, and temperature must be provided and controlled (4, pp. 20-21).

- All premises must be kept neat and clean, and a cleaning schedule must be maintained that is adequate to prevent cross-contamination (4, p. 21).

- Adequate space, equipment, and personnel must be provided for aseptic treatment and prevention of cross-contamination among patients (4, p. 20).

- Hand care should include scrubbing of hands and wearing of gloves. These practices protect both the patient from possible infection and the surgeon and personnel from exposures to blood and body fluids (22, p. 1370; 3 pp. 9-14).

- Masks should be worn to protect the patient, surgeon, and surgical staff. Patients should not be exposed to spray from the mouths of surgical personnel; personnel should not be unnecessarily exposed to patients' saliva droplets, which could contain viruses such as hepatitis B virus (HBV) and human immunodeficiency virus (HIV). Also, dermabrasion, electrosurgery, and laser procedures can produce aerosols and droplets that can be inhaled without the protection of a mask. During dermabrasion, a cover gown is essential to protect personnel from the spray of skin squames (22, p. 1370).

- Surgical drapes should be used to isolate the surgical area following standard skin preparation. The drape should provide barrier and moisture protection, though it may not cover the patient completely (23, p. 42).

- Lasers may be used in a sterile surgical field. A sterile sleeve drape can cover the wand so that it can be handled by the surgeon without contaminating the sterile field (23, p. 45).

- Photographs may be taken during the surgical procedure. This can be done without breaking sterile technique by having an assistant use a long focal length to take close-up photos while standing away from the sterile field (23, p. 45).

The American College of Surgeons recommends the following additional infection-control-related guidelines for office-based surgeries, including both major and minor procedures:

- Using an operative suite that includes separate areas for surgical instrumentation preparation and sterilization, and another for preparation and cleaning of used instruments and reusable materials (4, p. 26)
- Having acceptable standards of cleanliness and sterility, and adequate sterilization of OR materials (4, p. 19)
- Training all surgical personnel in basic aseptic techniques; isolation precautions; and the wearing of suitable surgical attire such as scrub suits, caps, masks, gowns, shoe coverings, and protective eye wear (4, pp. 21-22)
- Employing procedures to minimize the sources and cross-transmission of infections, including adequate surveillance techniques (4, p. 7)
- Using disposable items that are processed according to standard Occupational Safety and Health Administration (OSHA) regulations (4, p. 26)
- Having a system for the proper identification, management, handling, transport, treatment, and disposition of hazardous materials and wastes, whether solid, liquid, or gas (4, p. 7)
- Advising patients of continuity of care provided after surgery (e.g., discharge instructions) (4, p. 26)
- Adopting a quality assurance program that includes records of complications, such as infections and resultant outcomes (4, pp. 2, 26)

Endoscopy and Gastrointestinal Laboratories

Infections related to endoscopic procedures are caused by both endogenous and exogenous microbes. Infections caused by *endogenous* microbes develop when the microflora colonizing the mucosal surfaces of the G-I or respiratory tract gain access to the bloodstream or other normally sterile body sites as a consequence of the procedure. Endoscopy-related *exogenous* infections are caused by introduction of microbes transferred from patient to patient or from staff to patient by the endoscope or bronchoscope. The microorganisms may be gram-negative bacilli, mycobacteria, fungi, parasites, or viruses. Examples of endogenous infections include cholangitis after the manipulation of an obstructed biliary tract and pneumonia resulting from aspiration of oral secretions in a sedated patient (2, p. 138).

- Ventilation requirements in endoscopy and G-I labs vary from those in others areas of the hospital or ambulatory surgical center. In the endoscopy and G-I departments, air movement from adjacent areas should be into the rooms with a minimum of 2 air exchanges of outside air per hour and a minimum of 6 total air exchanges per hour. There should be no recirculation of air by room units (5, Table 2). In a bronchoscopy room, air movement should be into the room from outside areas with a minimum of 2 air exchanges of outside air per hour and a minimum of 12 total air exchanges per hour. Air should not be recirculated by room units (5, Table 2). Air ventilation should conform to the latest Centers for Disease Control and Prevention (CDC) guidelines for preventing the transmission of TB in healthcare facilities (2, p. 150). Space used for cleaning and disinfection or sterilization should have adequate ventilation to exhaust toxic vapors and airborne pathogens. If large volumes of glutaraldehyde in basins are used, covers with tight-fitting lids should be used. Consideration should be given to the installation of an exhaust hood, or ductless fume hood, with absorbents for the vapor and air systems that provide 7 to 15 air exchanges per hour (2, p. 150).
- Space considerations should include patient volume, traffic flow, and the types of endoscopic procedures (e.g., bronchoscopy, G-I endoscopy) performed (2, p. 150). Space for the performance of procedures should be separate from the space used for cleaning and disinfection or sterilization of equipment. There should be designated sinks for handwashing and separate sinks for cleaning endoscopes. There must be adequate space for the storage of chemicals and sterilants, some of which have special handling requirements as hazardous materials. The areas should be designed so that the workflow can facilitate sound infection control practices (e.g., avoiding the comingling of contaminated with clean equipment) (2, pp. 150-151).
- Storage cabinets or closets used for drying and storing clean endoscopes and accessories should be constructed of materials that can be easily cleaned. Endoscopes must not be stored in foam-lined cases because foam lining is impossible to clean should it become contaminated. Endoscopes should be stored in a manner that will protect the endoscope and minimize the potential for residual moisture accumulation (2, p. 151).
- Cleaning and high-level disinfection (HLD) or sterilization of endoscopes and endoscopic accessories is a major infection prevention focus for the staff in any department or office where endoscopy is performed (24, p. 279). (See the chapter "Disinfection.")

- Instruments that penetrate mucosal barriers, such as biopsy forceps, are considered critical items and must be sterilized before use (2, p. 146).
- Cleaning and disinfection of the water bottle and connecting tubing may be difficult because these are often colonized with *Pseudomonas* spp. Both should be sterilized or receive HLD at least once daily. Sterile water is used to fill the bottle for endoscopic irrigation (2, p. 152). One study showed no difference in infection rates when comparing the use of tap water with the use of sterile water for irrigation. Similar bacterial isolates were found in both tap and sterile water, and no measurable effect on clinical outcomes was found (27, p. 409).
- Procedure stretchers, x-ray tables, and other noncritical equipment should be wiped down between uses with an Environmental Protection Agency (EPA)-approved disinfectant (25, pp. 1-8).
- The clean up of splashes and spills of radiological contrast material, blood, or blood-contaminated body fluids should be done with EPA-approved disinfectants (24, p. 282).
- Endoscopic attachments (e.g., teaching heads, video attachments) should also be decontaminated (24, p. 282).

The effectiveness of all cleaning methods should be validated. Routine or frequent culturing of endoscopes is not recommended. However, the following infection control measures are advocated:

- Maintaining a log for all endoscopic retrograde cholangiopancreatographies (ERCPs) (e.g., instrument used, date, patient name) (24, p. 283)
- Taking periodic, unscheduled cultures of endoscopes and related equipment (24, p. 283)
- Designating an individual to be responsible for seeing that national and manufacturers' guidelines for cleaning and disinfection are complied with (21, p. 535)

OSHA's Bloodborne Pathogen Standard is followed to protect personnel from potentially infectious materials while cleaning and disinfecting equipment during and following procedures. The Standard states that all surgical facilities should do the following:

- Develop an exposure control plan (24, p. 281).
- Train all employees on occupational risks and methods to reduce risk of exposure to bloodborne pathogens and hazardous chemicals. Label all chemicals. Employee training must include an explanation of the Hazard Communication Standard and identification of the hazards and their health effects. Employees must also know the location of the written hazard communication program and material safety data sheets (MSDSs). Employees should be instructed on safe work prac-

tices, how to detect and measure contaminants, the use of appropriate personnel protective gear, and be given an explanation of the labeling system. Employees should be aware of the hazards associated with the materials used and how to manage any spills that may occur (24, p. 281; 2, p. 151).

- Maintain records of employees' training and medical evaluations (24, p. 281).
- Protect employees by implementing safe handling of sharp objects, specimens, contaminated laundry, and waste (24, p. 281).

In addition, all surgical facility personnel should do the following:

- Perform thorough handwashing before, during, and after endoscopic procedures, even if gloves are worn (2, p. 151).
- Use personal protective clothing and equipment. This includes the use of impervious gowns, gloves, masks, and eye protection. During cleaning of the endoscopes, wear gloves that are resistant to chemicals. Document cleaning procedures (24, p. 281; 16, p. 132; 2, p. 151).
- Understand the risk of infection from *Mycobacterium tuberculosis,* HBV, HIV, herpes simplex, and enteric pathogens. Understand that the patient's infectious status may be unknown at the time of the procedure (2, p. 151). Hepatitis B vaccine must be made available to employees at no cost (24, p. 281).

Cardiac Catheterization Laboratories

The availability of literature describing the frequency, prevention, and outcome of infections associated with cardiac catheterization is limited. This makes it difficult to direct infection control recommendations at specific techniques used in the cardiac catheterization laboratory. However, infection control guidelines related to the insertion, use, and maintenance of any central vascular device apply. These devices give direct access of microorganisms to the bloodstream. It is critical that all precautions and guidelines for the prevention of SSIs be followed (26, p. 85-1). These guidelines are similar to those suggested for procedures in other ambulatory surgical areas. Specific guidelines for the cardiac catheterization laboratory are as follows:

- Air movement should be out of the cardiac catheterization room to adjacent areas. There should be a minimum of 3 outside air exchanges per hour and a minimum of 15 total air exchanges per hour (5, Table 2).
- Sterile equipment and solutions should be opened immediately before use in the room where they will be used (19, p. 268; 26, p. 85-4).

- Solutions used to flush the cardiac catheter should be prepared for individual procedures only. They should be dated, timed, and initialed when opened. Solutions should be discarded and not saved for another patient (26, p. 85-4).
- If syringes are filled from bowls of flush solution, care should be taken during filling to immerse only the tip of the syringe. The operator's gloves do not dip into the flush solution while filling a syringe (26, p. 85-4).
- Meticulous sterile technique should be used at all times, including during the application or change of dressings (26, p. 85-5).
- Sheaths that are left in place are to be maintained the same as any temporary vascular access catheter. They should be removed as early as possible. The site is cleansed every 72 hours using povidone-iodine, 70% isopropyl alcohol, or a 2% aqueous solution of chlorhexidine gluconate. Patients are taught to report any signs of infection (26, p. 85-6).

Dialysis Centers

Hemodialysis (HD), or the removing of toxins, electrolytes, and fluid by circulating the patient's blood through a hemodialyzer, requires either temporary or permanent access to the bloodstream by external or internal anteriovenous shunts, fistulas, or catheters. Because of the immunocompromised status of most patients and the inherent high risk of bloodstream infections associated with the use of these devices to access the bloodstream, the use of sterile technique is crucial (12, p. 89-1).

Specific guidelines for dialysis centers are as follows:
- Patients' personal hygiene is stressed because skin colonization of *Staphylococcus aureus* has been associated with access site infections. Persistence of *S. aureus* has been shown to be significantly higher in patients with poor hygiene. The access site should be kept clean and dry at all times (12, p. 89-2).
- Handwashing is essential when performing any procedure related to HD or continuous ambulatory peritoneal dialysis (CAPD) (16, p. 237).
- Clean procedure can be used for access to central venous catheters and dressing changes. This includes nonsterile gloves and clean technique (16, p. 237). NOTE: The port should be prepped with an antimicrobial solution, such as povidone-iodine or chlorhexidine gluconate. A gown and mask may be recommended, if risk of spray or splash exists.
- Sterile gloves, surgical masks, and sterile aseptic technique are used during initiation of CAPD treatments (16, p. 237).

- Skin is prepared using sterile technique and antimicrobial preparations (e.g., povidone-iodine or chlorhexidine gluconate) (12, p. 89-3).
- A sterile dressing is applied following dialysis. Patients are instructed to keep the site dry and change the dressing if it becomes wet or soiled. There is controversy regarding the use of occlusive dressings. Some experts have found an increase in the infection rate if the access site is kept moist (12, p. 89-3).
- Patient teaching prior to discharge should include instructions on caring for the access site and recognizing signs and symptoms of infection. Patients should report symptoms immediately. Remote site infections should be treated immediately so that seeding to the access site does not occur (12, p. 89-2).
- Hemodialyzers should be adequately labeled and used for one patient only. Although considered controversial, the reuse of the hemodialyzer for the same patient is accepted practice (12, p. 89-8). If the patient's dialyzer is to be reused, it is essential that the water used to prepare the germicide is of adequate quality and that the dialyzer is reprocessed appropriately (8, pp. 403-404). Pyrogenic reactions and bacteremia have occurred (12, p. 89-8).
- Reprocessing methods for dialyzers and sanitization of the water distribution and dialysis fluid proportioning system should be carefully standardized to provide effective concentrations of germicide. The water quality should be monitored monthly and the sample assayed by an appropriate culturing method. Dialysis personnel should be familiar with Association for the Advancement of Medical Instrumentation (AAMI) standards for water and dialysate and the correct methods for processing these specimens for microbiologic and endotoxin assay. Monitors used to assess water quality should be sufficiently sensitive to detect colony counts and endotoxin concentrations likely to result in infection or pyrogenic reaction (8, pp. 402-403).
- Policies and procedures for maintenance, cleaning, disinfection, membrane and catheter reuse should be developed in accordance with CDC recommendations as published in the AAMI standards (16, p. 237).
- Routine cultures are done quarterly, as recommended by AAMI standards, to check the integrity of the reverse osmosis (RO) membrane (16, p. 237).
- Cleaning of machine surfaces, monitors, blood pumps, and other related dialysis equipment should be thorough and accomplished with an appropriate disinfectant as recommended in the Association for Professionals in Infection Control and

Epidemiology (APIC) guidelines for disinfection and sterilization (16, p. 237).

- Syringes and needles are sterile and used only once. Reprocessing of small-bore needles is difficult and has been associated with outbreaks of infection (16, p. 237).
- Employee health issues should include staff education on performing dialysis procedures and the risks to patients and staff when established procedures are not followed (12, p. 89-8). Hepatitis B vaccine must be available to employees and should be made available to patients. Post-immunization and annual serological testing is performed and boosters administered as appropriate (16, p. 239). Staff members are instructed to follow UP when exposure to blood or other potentially infectious materials is likely. Personal protective equipment (PPE) should be made readily available to personnel and visitors. Use of PPE is monitored and enforced (12, p. 89-12).

Interventional Radiology Departments

The radiology or diagnostic imaging department is becoming an ambulatory surgical center as increasing numbers of minimally invasive procedures are being performed in this area.

Despite recommendations by the CDC and OSHA, use of UP remains highly variable in many healthcare settings. Interventional radiology is no exception (15, p. 4). Radiology is not traditionally thought of as an area of significant risk for exposure or transmission of pathogens. However, both patients and healthcare workers are concerned about the transmission of bloodborne pathogens during medical procedures in this setting (14, p. 209).

The potential for exposure to blood or other infectious materials by staff exists in virtually any invasive radiological procedure, from arteriography to image-guided biopsy. It is important that all radiology personnel are aware of the risks of transmission and exposure to bloodborne pathogens and observe pertinent safety and infection control recommendations (14, p. 209).

- Every effort should be made to reduce the risk of bloodborne pathogen transmission by attention to procedure safety and adherence to UP and SP and to be protected from possible exposure to bloodborne pathogens by wearing PPE whenever there is potential for exposure to blood or other body fluids. One of the most frequent violations of UP is the failure to remove gloves before touching telephones, doorknobs, film cassettes or films, and equipment control panels (14, p. 211).

- Sharps safety is important; therefore needles should not be recapped, and a safe or neutral zone should be established for the passing of sharps, allowing staff to avoid risky hand-to-hand exchanges (14, p. 211).
- Protective eyewear should be worn (15, p. 4).
- Infection prevention guidelines during radiological procedures include handwashing, patient skin preparation, hand scrubbing, use of sterile gloves, draping of the surgical area, and meticulous aseptic technique. These topics are covered throughout this book.

References

1. Accreditation Association for Ambulatory Health Care: *Accreditation handbook for ambulatory health care,* Skokie, Ill, 1998, Author.
2. Alvarado CJ, and Reichelderfer M: APIC guideline for infection prevention and control in flexible endoscopy, *Am J Infect Control* 28(2):138-155, 2000.
3. American Association for Accreditation of Ambulatory Surgery Facilities: *Standards and checklist for accreditation of ambulatory surgery facilities,* Mundelein, Ill, 1997, Author.
4. American College of Surgeons: *Guidelines for optimal office-based surgery,* ed 2, Chicago, 1996, Author.
5. American Institute of Architects Academy of Architecture for Health (AIAAAH), U.S. Department of Health and Human Services: *Guidelines for design and construction of hospital and health care facilities, 1996-1997,* Washington, DC, 1996, American Institute of Architects Press. Online: www.e-architect.com/resources/hcfg1.asp
6. Association for the Advancement of Medical Instrumentation (AAMI): *Steam sterilization and sterility assurance using table-top sterilizers in office-based, ambulatory care, medical, surgical and dental facilities,* Arlington, Va, 1998, Author.
7. Association of Operating Room Nurses: *Ambulatory surgery principles and practices,* Denver, 1999, Author.
8. Beck-Segue CM et al: Outbreak of gram-negative bacteremia and pyrogenic reactions in a hemodialysis center, *Am J Nephrol* 10:397-404, 1990.
9. Brown, S: Accreditation of ambulatory surgery centers, *AORN J* 70(5):814-821, 1999.
10. Flanders E, Hinnant JR: Ambulatory surgery postoperative wound surveillance, *Am J Infect Control* 18(5):336-339, 1990.
11. Friedman C et al: Requirements for infrastructure and essential activities of infection control and epidemiology in out-of-hospital settings: a consensus panel report, *Am J Infect Control* 19(1):418-430, 1999.
12. Garcia-Houchins S: Dialysis. In Olmsted RN, editor: *APIC infection control and applied epidemiology: principles and practice,* St Louis, 1996, Mosby pp 89-1—89-15.
13. Gruendemann BJ, Fernsebner B: *Comprehensive perioperative nursing,* vol 1, *Principles,* Boston, 1995, Jones & Bartlett.
14. Hansen ME: Bloodborne pathogens and procedure safety in interventional radiology, *Semin Ultrasound CT MRI* 19(2):209-214, 1998.
15. Hansen ME et al: Use of universal precautions in interventional radiology: results of a national survey, *Am J Infect Control* 22(1):1-5, 1994.

16. Jennings J, Manian FA editors: *APIC handbook of infection control and epidemiology,* ed 2, Washington, DC, 1999, Association for Professionals in Infection Control and Epidemiology.

17. Joint Commission on Accreditation of Healthcare Organizations (JCAHO): *Infection control: meeting Joint Commission standards,* Oakbrook Terrace, Ill, 1998, Author.

18. Manian FA, Meyer L: Comprehensive surveillance of surgical wound infections in outpatient and inpatient surgery, *Infect Control Hosp Epidemiol* 11(10):515-520, 1990.

19. Mangram AJ, Hospital Infection Control Practices Advisory Committee (HIPAC), Centers for Disease Control and Prevention: Guideline for prevention of surgical site infection, 1999, *Infect Control Hosp Epidemiol* 20(4):247-278, 1999. (Reprinted, in part, in Appendix B.)

20. Meier PA: Infection control issues in same-day surgery. In Wenzel RP, editor: *Prevention and control of nosocomial infections,* ed 3, Baltimore, 1996, Williams & Wilkins, pp 261-282.

21. Reeves DS, Brown NM: Mycobacterial contamination of fiberoptic bronchoscopes, *J Hosp Infect* 30:531-536, 1995.

22. Sebben JE: Sterile technique and the prevention of wound infection in office surgery, part 1, *J Dermatol Surg Oncol* 14(12):1364-1371, 1988.

23. Sebben JE: Sterile technique and the prevention of wound infection in office surgery, part 2, *J Dermatol Surg Oncol* 15(1):38-48, 1989.

24. Schaffner M: Infection control issues in the gastrointestinal endoscopy unit, *Gastroenterol Nurs* pp 279-284, Spring 1990.

25. Society of Gastroenterology Nurses and Associates (SGNA): Recommended guidelines for infection control in gastrointestinal endoscopy settings, *SGNA Monograph Series,* Nos. 1-8, 1990.

26. Vander Hyde K: Cardiac catheterization. In Olmsted RN, editor: *APIC infection control and applied epidemiology: principles and practices,* St Louis, 1996, Mosby, pp 85-1—85-8.

27. Wilcox CM, Waites K, Bookings ES: Use of sterile compared with tap water in gastrointestinal endoscopic procedures, *Am J Infect Control* 24:407-410, 1996.

Suggested Reading

1. Gorse G, Messner RL: Infection control practices in gastrointestinal endoscopy in the United States: a national survey, *Infect Control Hosp Epidemiol* 12(5):289-296, 1991.

2. Herwaldt LA, Smith SD, Carter CD: Infection control in the outpatient setting, *Infect Control Hosp Epidemiol* 19(1):41-74.

3. Humar A et al: Elimination of an outbreak of gram-negative bacteremia in a hemodialysis unit, *Am J Infect Control* 24(5):359-363, 1996.

4. Lee TB: Surveillance in acute care and nonacute care settings: current issues and concepts, *Am J Infect Control* 25(2):121-124, 1997.

5. Manian FA: Surveillance of surgical site infections in alternative settings: exploring the current options, *Am J Infect Control* 25(2):102-105, 1997.

Preparation of Personnel

A. Employee Health

Surgical personnel are at risk for occupational exposure to many bloodborne diseases such as hepatitis B and C (HBV and HCV) and human immunodeficiency virus (HIV). Exposure to tuberculosis (TB) is a possibility as well, as is exposure to other communicable diseases such as pertussis, varicella, rubella, and influenza. Ill personnel put their co-workers and patients at risk by coming to work with communicable diseases.

Following the basics of infection prevention and immunizations guidelines, using safe practices that protect the patient and the healthcare worker (HCW) by avoiding exposure and preventing risk to patients and self, is critical and cannot be overlooked or considered less important than other aspects of patient care. Following prevention guidelines is first and foremost an individual responsibility.

This chapter covers the responsibilities of employers and employees, immunizations and vaccine recommendations, immunization of immunocompromised HCWs, post-exposure and work exclusions recommendations, and special considerations for the pregnant HCW. In addition, TB as a special infection risk will be discussed, as well as exposure to bloodborne pathogens, procedure for immediate expo-

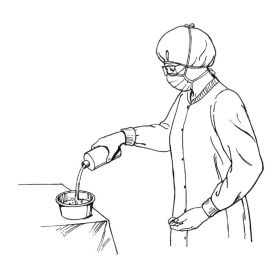

sure, post-exposure follow-up for needlestick and other percutaneous incidents, and post-exposure prophylaxis.

RESPONSIBILITIES
Employer
Responsibilities of the employer should include providing training programs that educate personnel about the principles of infection control and stressing individual responsibility for infection control, collaborating with the infection control department in monitoring and investigating potentially harmful infectious exposures and outbreaks among personnel, educating personnel about appropriate preventive measures for work-related illnesses and exposures, and containing costs by preventing infectious diseases that result in absenteeism and disability (3, pp. 292-293).

Employers must stay current with ever-changing regulations that set policy and protect employees (e.g., employers must follow the Occupational Safety and Health Administration's [OSHA's] recent compliance directives that emphasize the use of safer devices to prevent needlestick injuries) (22, pp. 18-19) and must provide hepatitis B vaccination at no cost to all HCWs (22, p. 37).

Specific policies should prevent HCWs from infecting patients and other HCWs and should cover management of (1) job-related illness and exclusion of ill personnel from work and (2) post-exposure prophylaxis when contact does occur. Policies should encourage personnel to report illnesses and exposures without fear of loss of wages, benefits, or job status (18, p. 258).

Healthcare Workers
HCWs who give direct patient care should be familiar with agency policies intended to protect them. Responsibilities should include protecting themselves and others from infection by frequent handwashing, keeping current on immunizations, and knowing how transmission can be prevented. HCWs should also be familiar with the latest information and agency policies regarding reporting of exposures and necessary follow-up care (11, pp. 19-20).

IMMUNIZATIONS
Because of contact with patients or infective material from patients, HCWs are at risk for exposure to and possible transmission of vaccine-preventable diseases. Maintenance of immunity is an essential part of infection prevention and control programs. Consistent immunization programs could substantially reduce both the number of susceptible HCWs and the accompanying risks for transmission of vaccine-preventable diseases in hospitals, physicians' offices, nursing homes, schools, ambulatory care centers, and laboratories.

All employees should be screened by way of history and/or sero-logic testing to document their immune status to diphtheria/tetanus, HBV (required by OSHA), rubeola, mumps, rubella, and varicella. Varicella immunization should be considered if the worker is non-immune (6, pp. 4-5; 11, p. 28).

Vaccine Recommendations

The following vaccines are strongly recommended and should be offered to all HCWs (3, p. 294):

Hepatitis B

Dose: 2 × 1 ml IM (deltoid) 4 weeks apart; third dose 5 months after second. Not contraindicated during pregnancy (3, p. 294).

Employers are required to make hepatitis B vaccine available to HCWs at no cost (22, p. 37). All personnel should be strongly encouraged to receive the hepatitis B vaccine because HBV presents the greatest risk of occupational disease (13, pp. 247-248). The risk for acquiring HBV from occupational exposures is dependent on the frequency of percutaneous and permucosal exposures to blood or body fluids containing blood (3, p. 303). It should be noted this immunization does not protect against HCV.

Influenza

Dose: 0.5 ml IM (deltoid), annual single dose (16, p. 94). Not contraindicated during pregnancy.

There is no evidence of maternal or fetal risk when this vaccine has been given to pregnant women with underlying conditions that render them at high risk for serious influenza complications (3, p. 294). Admitting patients infected with influenza to hospitals has led to nosocomial transmission of the disease, including transmission from staff to other patients. Influenza vaccine is strongly recommended for HCWs and others in close contact with persons in high-risk groups (8, pp. 9-10).

Rubella (German measles)

Dose: 0.5 ml SC. Contraindicated during pregnancy and within 3 months of planned pregnancy (3, p. 294). NOTE: HCWs should have documented evidence of having received live vaccine on or after their first birthday, or laboratory evidence of immunity.

Nosocomial rubella outbreaks involving both HCWs and patients have been reported. Although vaccination has decreased the overall risk for rubella transmission in all age groups in the United States by approximately 95%, the potential for transmission in hospitals and similar settings persists (6, p. 10).

Rubeola (measles)

Dose: 0.5 ml SC; booster: 0.5 ml SC no less than 1 month after primary dose (16, pp. 98-99). Contraindicated during pregnancy (3, p. 294).

All medical personnel beginning employment should have documentation of receipt of two doses of measles vaccine after their first birthday, or other evidence (e.g., physician-diagnosed measles or serologic evidence of immunity). If no documentation exists, the vaccine should be given (16, pp. 98-99). The risk for measles infection in medical personnel is estimated to be thirteen times that of the general population (6, p. 10).

Mumps

Dose: 0.05 ml SC. Contraindicated during pregnancy (3, p. 295).

Mumps transmission in medical settings has been reported nationwide (6, p. 11). NOTE: If measles or rubella immunity is in question, it is best to give measles/mumps/rubella (MMR) vaccine.

Varicella (chickenpox)

Dose: First dose 0.5 ml SC; second dose 4 to 8 weeks after first dose, if age 13 years or older. Contraindicated during pregnancy (3, p. 294).

Vaccination of susceptible HCWs is recommended. If seronegative and exposed, they can be furloughed (16, pp. 102-105). Sources of nosocomial transmission of varicella zoster virus have included patients, hospital staff, and visitors (6, pp. 11-12).

Other immunobiologic agents that should be available to HCWs in special circumstances are as follows:

Hepatitis A

Dose: 1 ml IM (deltoid); booster of 1 ml 6 to 12 months after primary dose (16, p. 92). Vaccine safety during pregnancy has not been evaluated (3, p. 295).

Tetanus and diphtheria

Dose: 0.5 ml IM; second dose 4 to 8 weeks after first dose; third dose should be given 6 to 12 months after second dose, then every 10 years (16, pp. 100-101). Contraindicated during first trimester of pregnancy (3, p. 295).

Immunocompromised Healthcare Workers

The degree of risk for developing infection in immunocompromised HCWs should be assessed by a physician who should consider the risk for exposure to a vaccine-preventable disease together with the risks and benefits of vaccination (6, p. 20).

POST-EXPOSURE RECOMMENDATIONS

- Infection control sources should be consulted and policies developed to assess exposures, evaluate risk of transmission, and implement steps to prevent further outbreaks (15, pp. 854-858).
- Post-exposure work restrictions ranging from restriction of contact with high-risk patients to complete exclusion from duty are appropriate for HCWs who are not immune to certain vaccine-preventable diseases (6, p. 32).

WORK EXCLUSION RECOMMENDATIONS

The following list provides work exclusion recommendations for ill HCWs. Illnesses not listed require that judgment and common sense be used so that patient and co-worker health is not compromised. Taking precautions and following work exclusion recommendations will protect patients as well as other HCWs (3, p. 329; 13, p. 851).

Acute infection: HCWs with acute infections such as the flu, a sore throat, or the common cold should not be permitted within patient care areas (13, p. 239).

Skin conditions: Persons with cuts, burns, rashes, or skin lesions should not be assigned as a scrub person or handle sterile supplies (circulating nurse) because serum may seep from the open wound. Open skin lesions may be portals of entry for contact with bloodborne pathogens (13, p. 239). Agents used for handwashing or scrubbing that are chemical or physical irritants can exacerbate skin conditions. Persons with chronic skin conditions should seek medical care and take measures to prevent future outbreaks (12, p. 248).

Conjunctivitis: Patient contact, as well as contact with patient environment, should be restricted until eye discharge ceases (16, p. 252).

Diarrheal disease: Acute illness: patient contact should be restricted, as well as contact with patient environment and food handling until symptoms resolve. Convalescent stage salmonella: HCWs should be restricted from care of high-risk patients. Local and state health authorities should be consulted regarding the need for negative stool cultures (3, p. 299).

Diphtheria: HCWs should be excluded from duty until antimicrobial therapy is completed and two cultures taken 24 hours apart are negative (3, p. 299).

Enteroviral infections: HCWs should be restricted from care of infants, neonates, and immunocompromised patients and their environments until symptoms resolve (3, p. 299).

Hepatitis A: HCWs should be restricted from patient contact, as well as contact with patient environment and food handling, until 7 days following the onset of jaundice (16, p. 252).

Hepatitis B: Depending on state regulations, there are no restrictions for persons who do not perform exposure-prone procedures (e.g., those during which reasonable anticipated skin, eye, mucous membrane, or parenteral contact with blood can occur). Infected persons should be restricted from performing exposure-prone procedures until hepatitis B antigen is negative (16, p. 253; 3, p. 299).

Hepatitis C: No recommendation for restricting professional activities of HCWs infected with HCV (16, p. 253). Those who are HCV positive should follow strict aseptic technique and Standard Precautions (SP), including appropriate use of handwashing and protective barriers and care in the use and disposal of needles and other sharp instruments (7, p. 17). NOTE: It may be considered prudent to restrict those infected with HCV from exposure-prone activities until more official guidelines are available.

Herpes simplex: Genital herpes: no restriction. Hand lesions: HCWs should be restricted from patient contact and contact with patient environment until lesions heal. Orofacial lesions: the need to restrict from care of high-risk patients should be evaluated (16, p. 253).

HIV: HCWs should not perform exposure-prone invasive procedures until counsel from an expert review panel has been sought. State regulations should be consulted and followed. No limit on duration (16, p. 254).

Rubeola: HCWs with active disease should be excluded from duty until 7 days after the rash appears. Exposed HCWs should be excluded from work from day 5 after the first exposure through day 21 after last exposure, or 4 days after the rash appears (16, p. 254).

Meningococcal infections: HCWs should be excluded from duty until 24 hours after start of effective therapy (16, p. 254).

Mumps: HCWs with active disease should be excluded from duty until 9 days after onset of parotitis (16, p. 254). HCWs who have been exposed should be excluded from duty from day 12 after first exposure through day 26 after last exposure, or until 9 days after onset of parotitis (3, p. 300).

Pertussis (whooping cough): HCWs with active disease should be excluded from duty from beginning of catarrhal stage through third week after onset of paroxysms, or until 5 days after start of effective antimicrobial therapy. Symptomatic personnel should be excluded from duty until 5 days after start of effective antimicrobial therapy. No restriction for asymptomatic exposed HCWs. Prophylaxis is recommended (16, p. 255).

Rubella: HCWs with active disease should be excluded from duty until 5 days after rash appears. Susceptible personnel who have been exposed should be excluded from duty from day 7 after first exposure through day 21 after last exposure (16, p. 255).

Tuberculosis: HCWs with active pulmonary disease should be excluded from duty until proven noninfectious. Purified protein derivative (PPD) converter: no restriction (16, p. 256). (See section on TB in this chapter.)

Varicella (chickenpox): HCWs should be excluded from duty until all lesions are dry and crusted. Susceptible HCWs who have been exposed should be excluded from duty from day 10 after first exposure through day 21 (day 28 if varicella zoster immune globulin [VZIG] given) after last exposure (16, p. 256).

Shingles: Healthy HCWs with localized lesions should be restricted from care of high risk patients (e.g., neonates, the elderly, and those who are immunocompromised) until all lesions are dry and crusted. Susceptible HCWs who have been exposed should be restricted from patient contact from day 10 after first exposure through day 21 after last exposure (day 28 if VZIG is given) or, if varicella occurs, until all lesions are dry and crusted (16, p. 257).

Viral respiratory infections—acute, febrile: HCWs should be screened for possible exclusion from the care of patients and contact with their environment if patients are at high risk for complications of influenza during community outbreak of respiratory syncytial virus and influenza (16, p. 257).

Staphylococcus aureus: NOTE: Factors related to *S. aureus* or methicillin-resistant *S. aureus* (MRSA) carriage and transmission are similar. The following recommendations relate to both.

• HCWs with active, draining lesions should be restricted from contact with patients and their environment or food handling until lesions have resolved. Carrier state: no restriction unless personnel are epidemiologically linked to transmission of the organism (16, p. 256). MRSA-carrier personnel who are epidemiologically linked to transmission should be removed from direct patient care until treatment of the carrier is successful (10). HCWs are known to have a higher *S. aureus* carriage rate (50% to 90%) than the general population.

S. aureus from the anterior nares can be transferred to skin and other body areas. Given a portal of entry (e.g., trauma to the skin or a surgical incision), *S. aureus* can cause infection. Eradication of nasal *S. aureus* carriage by the application of mupirocin often leads to elimination of the organism from other colonized body sites (10). However, nosocomial outbreaks have rarely been traced to a "shedder." *S. aureus* strains that cause infection are transmitted from patient to patient from the hands of HCWs (19, pp. 78-3—78-4). The main mode of transmission of MRSA is via the hands, especially the hands of HCWs. Contamination can occur from colonized or infected patients; infected body sites of the personnel themselves; or by devices, items, or environmental surfaces contaminated with body fluids containing MRSA. Following SP should control the spread of MRSA in most instances (10).

· Culturing of personnel who are *S. aureus* carriers should not be undertaken unless an epidemiologic investigation and organism typing indicate that cross-transmission is occurring and that staff may be an important reservoir (19, p. 78-6).

· The nasal application of mupirocin to eradicate nasal carriage of *S. aureus* has been used to reduce the chances that the organism will spread from one individual to another. Resistance development to the drug was not observed among *S. aureus* isolates when a single 5-day course of mupirocin was used (4, pp. 777-778).

THE PREGNANT HEALTHCARE WORKER

Pregnant women and women of childbearing age should be educated regarding the risk of transmission of particular infectious diseases (e.g., cytomegalovirus, hepatitis, herpes simplex, HIV, parvovirus, rubella, and varicella). If these diseases are acquired during pregnancy, there may be adverse effects on the fetus. Pregnant workers should be provided with information on SP and Transmission-Based Precautions appropriate for each infection. Women should not be routinely excluded on the basis of pregnancy, or the intent to become pregnant, from the care of patients with particular infections that have the potential to harm the fetus (3, p. 338).

TUBERCULOSIS AS A SPECIAL INFECTION RISK

TB is a recognized risk in healthcare facilities. The magnitude of this risk varies by the type of healthcare facility, the prevalence of TB in the community, the patient population served, the HCW's occupational group, the area of the hospital in which the HCW works, and the effectiveness of TB infection control interventions. Several outbreaks among persons in healthcare facilities have involved transmission of multidrug-resistant strains of *Mycobacterium tuberculosis* to both patients and HCWs (5, pp. 4-6).

- Persons who have become infected with *M. tuberculosis* have approximately a 10% chance of developing the active disease during their lifetime. This risk is greatest during the first 2 years after infection. The probability that a person who is exposed will become infected depends primarily on the concentration of infectious droplet nuclei in the air and the duration of the exposure (5, pp. 4-6).

- TB screening and risk assessment should be done on a regular basis as part of the employee health program. These measures should be based on a careful assessment of the risk for transmission in that particular setting because this risk will vary between settings (5, p. 8). Education should be provided for all HCWs on health maintenance, SP, and Transmission-Based Precautions that are relevant to their occupational group. Training should be conducted before initial assignment. The need for additional training should be reevaluated periodically (5, p. 36).

Reporting Exposures and Follow-up Care for Tuberculosis

Employees should be familiar with procedures for reporting and receiving post-exposure prophylaxis and follow-up (11, pp. 28-29). A PPD test should be performed immediately following exposure, with a follow-up at 12 weeks. The information from the tests will indicate whether infection occurred after the last known exposure (3, p. 318). Those with newly positive PPD test results or who have had PPD conversion (e.g., conversion to positive within 2 years, after a documented baseline negative PPD) should be evaluated promptly for active TB. This evaluation should include a clinical examination and a chest x-ray. If symptoms are compatible for active disease, the HCW should be excluded from the workplace until a diagnosis of active TB is ruled out, or, if a diagnosis of active disease is established, the treatment has rendered the HCW noninfectious (5, p. 40). If the chest x-ray is negative, a repeat chest x-ray is not needed unless TB symptoms develop. All HCWs with histories of positive PPD test results should be instructed about the symptoms of active TB and the need for prompt evaluation if symptoms occur (5, p. 40).

- HCWs with pulmonary or laryngeal TB pose a risk to patients and other HCWs until they are noninfectious (3, p. 336).

- The same work restrictions apply to all HCWs regardless of their immune status. Before returning to the workplace, the HCW should have documentation showing that adequate therapy is being received, the cough has resolved, and there have been three consecutive negative sputum smears collected on different days. A HCW with active laryngeal or pulmonary disease who discontinues treatment before he or she is cured should be evaluated promptly for infectivity (5, p. 41).

· A HCW with latent (nonactive) TB should not be restricted from usual work activities (5, p. 41).

· A HCW who has TB at sites other than the lung or larynx usually does not need to be excluded from the workplace if a diagnosis of concurrent pulmonary TB has been ruled out (5, p. 41).

Use of Bacille Calmette-Guérin Vaccine

TB vaccination with bacille Calmette-Guérin (BCG) vaccine has not been recommended for general use because the population risk for infection with TB is low and the protective efficacy of BCG vaccine is uncertain. The immune response to BCG vaccine also interferes with tuberculin skin testing. Instead, TB prevention and control efforts are focused on interrupting transmission from patients who have infectious disease, skin testing those at high risk for TB, and administering preventive therapy when appropriate (6, p. 14; 14, pp. 159-161). NOTE: In a few geographical areas of the United States, BCG vaccination may be an inexpensive and cost-effective intervention. However, the primary focus of TB prevention remains early detection, preventive therapy for infected persons, and appropriate infection control measures.

· The Centers for Disease Control and Prevention (CDC) recommends BCG vaccination for HCWs specifically at risk of exposure to patients with highly resistant strains of TB. BCG vaccination of HCWs has benefits superior to a program that depends on regular TB skin testing and isoniazid (INH) chemoprophylaxis (17, p. 192).

· BCG should not be used as a primary control strategy because the protective efficacy in HCWs is uncertain (3, p. 319). BCG vaccination should be considered on an individual basis in healthcare settings where the following conditions are met:

  · A high percentage of TB patients are infected with *M. tuberculosis* strains that are resistant to both isoniazid and rifampin. Transmission of such drug-resistant *M. tuberculosis* strains to HCWs is likely.

  · Comprehensive TB infection control precautions have been implemented and have not been successful (6, p. 26).

· Vaccination with BCG should not be required for employment or for assignment in specific work areas (6, p. 26). NOTE:

Special consideration should be given to immunocompromised HCWs, especially those infected with HIV, because TB infection in this population is associated with a high mortality rate. Discussion of prevention of TB transmission from patients to HCWs in surgical settings can be found in the chapter "Tuberculosis."

KNOWING AND REVEALING HUMAN IMMUNODEFICIENCY VIRUS AND HEPATITIS B VIRUS STATUS

- The Association of periOperative Registered Nurses (AORN) supports voluntary testing with informed consent and appropriate counseling for patients undergoing surgical intervention, regardless of the setting, and for all HCWs. If employees are HIV or HBV seropositive, they should modify participation in exposure-prone procedures (those during which reasonably anticipated skin, eye, mucous membrane, or parenteral contact with blood can be anticipated), except in extreme emergencies (1, pp. 135, 136).
- Personnel who participate in invasive procedures are encouraged to know their HIV and HBV status and voluntarily disclose a report of positive status to the appropriate facility authority (2, p. 336).
- Facilities should support employees' endeavors to remain employed when their health status does not impair performance or pose risks to patients (1, p. 136).
- Testing of the source's blood is required, and written consent is also required in some states. The employer must ask for consent from the source individual or anyone legally authorized to give consent on his or her behalf (22, p. 43).

EXPOSURES TO BLOOD AND OTHER INFECTIOUS SUBSTANCES

It has been estimated that 600,000 to 800,000 needlestick and percutaneous injuries occur annually. About half of these injuries go unreported. Some of these injuries expose workers to bloodborne pathogens that can cause infection (20, p. 2; 21, p. 2). Information on preventing needlesticks, percutaneous injuries, and mucocutaneous exposures is covered in the chapter "Bloodborne Pathogens and Safety Issues."

Procedure for Immediate Exposure

Immediately following an exposure to blood:
- Needlesticks and cuts should be washed with soap and water.
- Splashes to the nose, mouth, or skin should be flushed with water.

- Eyes should be irrigated with clean water, saline, or sterile solution.
- Exposures should be reported promptly because post-exposure treatment may be recommended and, if so, should be started as soon as possible (9, p. 2).

The following are not recommended after exposure to blood:

- The use of antiseptics and the squeezing of wounds, which have not been scientifically proven to reduce the risk of transmission of bloodborne pathogens.
- The use of a caustic agent such as bleach.

Post-Exposure Follow-up for Needlesticks and Other Percutaneous Incidents

Any exposure incident should be reported immediately after exposure and management should be conducted by a licensed healthcare professional as soon as possible (22, p. 42). Employers are required to document at a minimum the route of exposure and the circumstances under which the exposure incident occurred. Further documentation surrounding the incident allows identification and correction of hazards. It is helpful to document the following information:

- Engineering controls in use at the time
- Work practices followed at the time
- A description of the device
- A listing of protective equipment or clothing that was used at the time of the exposure incident
- Location of incident
- Procedure being performed
- The employee's training (22, p. 43)

POST-EXPOSURE PROPHYLAXIS

Most exposures do not result in infection. The risk of infection varies with the pathogen involved, the type of exposure, the amount of blood involved in the exposure, and the amount of virus in the patient's blood at the time of exposure (9, p. 1). The degree of risk also depends on the immune status of the worker, the severity of the exposure, and the availability and use of appropriate post-exposure prophylaxis (PEP).

Human Immunodeficiency Virus

PEP for exposure to HIV is recommended under certain circumstances. However, the drugs used for HIV post-exposure have many adverse side effects. Currently no vaccine exists to prevent HIV infection and no treatment exists to cure it (21, p. 6).

- HIV PEP recommendations are determined by analysis of the type of exposure and the virulence of the exposure source (16, pp. 247-251).
- Post-exposure treatment should begin as soon as possible after exposure, preferably within 2 hours. Starting treatment 1 to 2 weeks after exposure may be considered if the exposure was significant (9, p. 6).
- The Public Health Service recommends a 4-week course of two drugs, zidovudine and lamivudine, for most HIV exposures, or zidovudine and lamivudine plus a protease inhibitor, indinavir or nelfinavir, for exposures that may pose a greater risk for transmitting HIV (such as those involving a larger volume of blood or a concern about drug-resistant HIV). Differences in side effects associated with the use of these two drugs may influence which is selected in a specific situation. Side effects include nausea, vomiting, diarrhea, tiredness, and headache. Determining which drugs and how many drugs to use or when to change a treatment regimen is largely a matter of judgment (9, pp. 5-6).

Hepatitis B Virus

HBV rate of transmission to susceptible HCWs ranges from 6% to 30% after a single needlestick exposure to an HBV-infected patient. HCWs who have antibodies to HBV, either from vaccination or prior infection, are not at risk. If a susceptible worker is exposed to HBV, PEP with hepatitis B immune globulin and initiation of hepatitis B vaccine is more than 90% effective in preventing HBV infection. Administration of preexposure vaccination or PEP to workers can dramatically reduce this risk (21, p. 6). Recommendations vary depending on the immune status of the HCW and the infectious status of the source patient (16, p. 245).

Hepatitis C Virus

Currently, there is no recommended post-exposure treatment that will prevent HCV infection. Baseline antibody and liver enzyme tests should be done as soon as possible and again at 4 to 6 months after the exposure. Another test, hepatitis C virus ribonucleic acid (HCV RNA), may be recommended 4 to 6 weeks following exposure (9, pp. 5, 7).

References

1. AORN: AORN revised position statement on the patient and health care worker with bloodborne diseases including human immunodeficiency virus (HIV). In *Standards, recommended practices & guidelines,* Denver, 2000, Author, pp 135-137.

2. AORN: Recommended practices for Standard and Transmission-Based Precautions in the perioperative setting. In *Standards, recommended practices & guidelines,* Denver, 2000, Author, pp 335-340.

3. Bolyard EA: Hospital Infection Control Practices Advisory Committee (HICPAC), Centers for Disease Control and Prevention: Guideline for infection control in health care personnel, *Infect Control Hosp Epidemiol* 26(3):289-354, 1998.

4. Boyce JM: Preventing staphylococcal infections by eradicating nasal carriage of *Staphylococcus aureus:* proceeding with caution, *Infect Control Hosp Epidemiol* 17(12):775-779, 1996.

5. Centers for Disease Control and Prevention: Guidelines for preventing the transmission of *Mycobacterium tuberculosis* in health-care facilities, *MMWR* 43(RR-13):1-55, 1994.

6. Centers for Disease Control and Prevention: Immunization of health-care workers: recommendations of the Advisory Committee on Immunization Practices (ACIP) and the Hospital Infection Control Practices Advisory Committee (HICPAC), *MMWR* 46(RR-18):1-42, 1997.

7. Centers for Disease Control and Prevention: Recommendation for prevention and control of hepatitis C virus (HCV) and HCV-related chronic disease, *MMWR* 47(RR-19):1-39, 1998.

8. Centers for Disease Control and Prevention: Prevention and control of influenza: recommendations of the Advisory Committee on Immunization Practices (ACIP), *MMWR* 48(RR-04):1-28, 1999.

9. Centers for Disease Control and Prevention: *Exposure to blood: what health care workers need to know,* 1999, www.cdc.gov/ncidod/hip (accessed 2000).

10. Centers for Disease Control and Prevention: *Methicillin-resistant Staphylococcus aureus,* www.cdc.gov/ncidod/hip, 1999.

11. Donowitz LG: *Infection control for the health care worker,* Baltimore, 1994, Williams & Wilkins.

12. Fortunato N: *Berry and Kohn's operating room technique,* ed 9, St Louis, 2000, Mosby.

13. Gruendemann BJ, Fernsebner B: *Comprehensive perioperative nursing,* vol 1, *Principles,* Boston, 1995, Jones & Bartlett.

14. Henderson DK: Bacillus of Calmette and Guérin vaccination for tuberculosis prevention in healthcare workers: how good is good enough? *Infect Control Hosp Epidemiol* 19(3):159-161, 1998.

15. Herwaldt LA et al: Exposure workups, *Infect Control Hosp Epidemiol* 18(12):850-873, 1997.

16. Jennings J, Manian FA, editors: *APIC handbook of infection control and epidemiology,* ed 2, Washington, DC, 1999, Association for Professionals in Infection Control and Epidemiology.

17. Jenney WJ, Spelman DW: In support of bacillus of Calmette and Guérin for healthcare workers, *Infect Control Hosp Epidemiol* 19(3):191-193, 1998.

18. Mangram AJ, Hospital Infection Control Practices Advisory Committee (HICPAC), Centers for Disease Control and Prevention: Guideline for prevention of surgical site infection, 1999, *Infect Control Hosp Epidemiol* 20(4):247-278, 1999. (Reprinted, in part, in Appendix B.)

19. Mylotte JM: *Staphylococcus* species. In Olmsted RN, editor: *APIC infection control and applied epidemiology: principles and practice,* Washington, DC, 1996, Association for Professionals in Infection Control and Epidemiology, pp. 78-1—78-12.

20. National Institute for Occupational Safety and Health (NIOSH): *Preventing needlesticks in health care settings,* www.cdc.gov/niosh, 1999.

21. National Institute for Occupational Safety and Health (NIOSH): *Alert: preventing needlestick injuries in health care settings,* www.cdc.gov/niosh, 1999.

22. Occupational Safety and Health Administration (OSHA): *OSHA instruction: enforcement procedures for the occupational exposure to bloodborne pathogens,* U.S. Department of Labor, CPL 2-2, 44D, www.osha.gov, 1999.

Suggested Reading

1. Blumberg HM: Tuberculosis and infection control: what now? *Infect Control Hosp Epidemiol* 18(8):538-541, 1997.

2. Centers for Disease Control and Prevention: *Hepatitis C: what clinicians and other health professionals need to know* (web-based training program), 2000, www.cdc.gov/ncidod/diseases/hepatitis/c/index.htm (accessed 2000).

3. Centers for Disease Control and Prevention: *Influenza vaccine information for health care workers,* 1999, www.cdc.gov/ncidod/hip (accessed 2000).

4. Centers for Disease Control and Prevention: *Influenza,* 1999, www.cdc.gov/ncidod/hip (accessed 2000).

5. Diekema DJ, Doebbeling BN: Employee health and infection control, *Infect Control Hosp Epidemiol* 16(5):292-301, 1995.

6. Falk P: Infection control and the employee health service. In Mayhall CG, editor: *Hospital epidemiology and infection control,* Baltimore, 1996, Williams & Wilkins, pp 1094-1099.

7. Finney J: When a needle stick occurs, *Surgical Services Management* 6(3):41-43, 2000.

8. Johnson & Johnson Medical: *Preventing TB transmission in the operating room,* Arlington, Tex, 1995, Author.

9. Otero RB: Prevention of disease transmission in a healthcare setting, *Infection Control Today* 2(7):30-38, 1998.

10. Treharne P: Evaluation and management of occupational exposure to bloodborne pathogens, *Infection Control Today* 2(11):20-24, 1998.

11. Tydell P: Disease prevention in the workplace: focus on employee immunization, *Infection Control Today* 2(10):54-58, 1998.

12. Weber DJ, Rutala WA: Pertussis: an under-appreciated risk for nosocomial outbreak, *Infect Control Hosp Epidemiol* 19(11):825-827, 1998.

13. Weber DJ, Rutala WA, Weigle K: Selection and use of vaccines for healthcare workers, *Infect Control Hosp Epidemiol* 28(10):682-687, 1997.

B. Surgical Attire

Special clothing is required in surgical settings to protect patients from microorganisms brought in from the outside. The purpose of this long-standing practice is to prevent the spread of infection from staff to patient. The use of surgical attire (e.g., scrub suit, shoe covers, hair covering) minimizes patient exposure to microorganisms from skin, mucous membranes, or the hair of surgical team members. However, definitive studies have not shown that the use of special attire actually decreases infection rates.

Masks, shoe covers, hair covering, eye protection, nonsterile gloves, and sterile surgical gowns and gloves also protect personnel from possible contamination. These can be considered personal protective equipment (PPE) if they are specifically made and worn to prevent spread of contamination from the patient.

Additional topics related to surgical attire and PPE are covered in the chapters "Gowning," "Gloving," and "Surgical Scrubbing."

BASIC ATTIRE
The Scrub Suit

The scrub suit consists of a dress or pants and shirt. Policies vary regarding wearing, covering, changing, and laundering scrub suits. This variation exists because there are few definitive studies concluding that scrub suit use and particular methods of laundering decrease

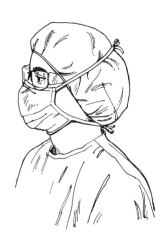

surgical site infection (SSI) risk (21, p. 262). Policies range from allowing home laundering of scrub suits to protecting scrub suits outside the surgical suite with a cover gown or lab coat. Some agencies require laundering of uniforms in a hospital-approved facility. Others allow staff to launder scrub suits at home. The following standards can provide guidelines until definitive studies provide more direction:

- All persons who enter the semirestricted and restricted areas of the surgical suite should wear attire intended for use within the surgical area. The attire should be approved, clean, and freshly laundered in a hospital-approved laundry facility (3, p. 199).
- The uniform should prevent shedding and promote environmental control (3, p. 199).
- Reusable, clean attire should be protected from contamination during transfer and storage (3, p. 199).
- Unless the style of scrub suit dictates otherwise, the shirt should be tucked in the pants to prevent the shedding of body scurf (flakes of dry skin) by surgical personnel (3, p. 200).
- When a scrub uniform becomes visibly wet or contaminated by blood, body fluid, sweat, or food, the attire should be changed as soon as possible to reduce the possibility of cross-contamination or spread of infection to the healthcare worker (HCW) (21, p. 262; 3, p. 199).
- The Occupational Safety and Health Administration (OSHA) states: "If a pull-over scrub becomes minimally contaminated, the employee should be trained to remove the pull-over scrub in such a way as to avoid contact with the outer surface. If the amount of blood exposure is such that the blood penetrates the scrub and contaminates the inner surface, it may be prudent to train employees to cut such a contaminated scrub to aid removal and prevent exposure to the face" (5, p. 403; 24).
- Used scrub suits should be placed in an appropriately designed container for washing or disposal and should not be hung in a locker for wearing at another time (3, p. 199).

Cover Gowns and Lab Coats

- Policy regarding the wearing of cover gowns and lab coats outside the surgical suite should be determined by the individual practice setting. Use of this apparel has not been shown to decrease the rate of surgical site infection (SSI) (3, pp. 199-200).
- The CDC has no recommendation regarding restricting use of scrub suits to the operating suite or wearing cover gowns over scrub suits outside of the surgical area (21, p. 268).

Warm-up Jackets

Warm-up jackets, either reusable or disposable, are used by non-scrubbed surgical staff to cover the arms and body for warmth in a cool environment and to prevent shedding. Long sleeved attire is advocated to prevent shedding from bare arms. Jacket sleeves should not be pushed up, but instead should cover the arms. Jackets should be buttoned or snapped closed during use. Rules for laundering or discarding warm-up jackets are the same as for the scrub suit (3, p. 200; 22, p. 65).

Shoes

Comfortable, supportive shoes should be worn for personal safety. Shoes should have enclosed toes and heels.

- Cloth shoes should not be worn because they do not protect from spilled liquids or from sharp items that may be dropped or kicked (8, p. 239; 3, pp. 202-203).
- Shoes worn in the operating room (OR) should provide protection from fluids and accidentally dropped items (11, p. 288).
- Clogs that have closed toes and heels are available for purchase and provide the same comfort advantages as those with open heels and toes. It is unlikely that clogs are less safe than any other footwear (7, p. 402).

HOME LAUNDERING

- Laundering of attire in a home laundry is not recommended.
- Attire becomes contaminated with microorganisms during wear. Taking soiled attire home may spread contamination to the home environment (3, p. 199; 8, p. 239).
- There are several problems with home-laundered surgical attire. In hospital-approved laundry facilities, conditions are monitored to meet specified standards. Linen may be washed in either hot or warm water, but there are defined concentrations of chemical additives that are used and monitored during the laundering process that are not possible at home. Clothing should be protected from possible contaminants. Unlike home laundry facilities, hospitals and hospital-approved facilities have processes in place to meet this requirement (2).
- If the scrub suit is contaminated with blood or other potentially infectious materials, the suit should be considered contaminated laundry that has to be handled according to Universal Precautions. Home laundering is not appropriate because laundry conditions cannot be controlled (6, pp. 21-22).

- Laundry is one link in the larger, potential chain of cross-contamination in the home. Pathogens of potential concern can survive the wash cycle of today's home laundry process (19, p. 3).
- Microorganisms that survive the wash cycle may be transferred from fabric to fabric in the wash, from the surfaces of the washer to other fabrics in the next load, and to human hands from wet laundry (18, p. S3).
- Microorganisms can survive today's laundry process (18, p. S1).
- There are certain groups within the overall population that are at increased risk of serious illness as a result of exposure to pathogenic microorganisms. There are also certain situations in the home in which the risk of exposure to pathogenic microbes is increased (e.g., when a household member is shedding an infectious agent) (18, p. S2).
- Various factors affect the inactivation of pathogens during the laundry process, including water temperature, the type of washing product used, and drying time. With the use of a sanitizing detergent in the wash, the risk of human exposure to laundry-borne pathogenic bacteria may be reduced significantly when compared with the use of a nonsanitizing detergent (18, p. S2).
- The risk for cross-contamination via household laundry was clearly demonstrated after an outbreak of *Staphylococcus aureus* skin infection among families sharing laundry facilities (26, p. S23).
- Hygiene failures in home and communal laundry practices can result in the cross-contamination of both viral and bacterial pathogens among different items of domestic laundry. Changes in household laundry practices (e.g., lower wash temperature, the use of a lower volume of water, and a reduction in the use of sodium hypochlorite additives) as a result of environmental and economic pressures may have had a negative impact on laundry hygiene ensurance (26, p. S23).
- Laundered fabrics may have a lower potential for contamination from the presence of microorganisms, but the possibility of cross-contamination via the hands to other surfaces and to food still exists (26, p. S23).
- The healthcare worker (HCW) may believe that normal laundering produces clean clothes, but this does not necessarily translate to *bacteriologically clean,* and the detergent used may have a wide range of efficacy in reducing the bacteria on contaminated clothing (9, p. S38).
- Good laundering practices may include the segregation of clothing items that may be at risk of contamination from other laundry items, as well as the use of a sanitizer (9, p. S38).

PERSONAL PROTECTIVE EQUIPMENT

Understanding the need to select and use PPE properly has grown over the past several decades as detailed research of the types of barriers that are most effective has become available (4, p. 18).

Hair Covering

- Surgical caps and hoods reduce contamination of the surgical field from microorganisms shed from the hair and scalp. SSI has been traced to organisms isolated from the hair or scalp even when caps were worn during the operation and in the OR suite (21, p. 262).
- Personnel should cover head and facial hair, including sideburns and necklines, when in semirestricted and restricted areas of the surgical area (21, p. 268).
- A surgeon's cap that does not cover the hair, beard, or sideburns entirely should not be worn. Instead, a bouffant cap or hood should be worn to fully cover hair on the head and face (11, p. 287; 21, p. 268).
- Hair covering should be applied first so that hair does not touch the scrub suit while it is being donned. Disposable covering is preferred, but a cloth cap is permissible if it is changed daily and laundered by an approved facility. Hair covering should be changed at least daily, and sooner if soiled (11, p. 287; 3, p. 200).

Masks

- Surgical masks have been categorized as PPE by OSHA (17, p. 25).
- OSHA's Bloodborne Pathogen Rule requires employers to provide masks and requires HCWs to wear a type of mask that prevents blood and other potentially infectious body fluids from penetrating the barrier (27, p. 28; 21, p. 268).
- Single disposable high filtration surgical masks should be worn in restricted surgical environments where open sterile supplies or scrubbed persons may be located (3, p. 200).
- A mask should be worn when entering the OR if an operation is about to begin, is already under way, or if sterile instruments and supplies are open. The mask should be worn throughout the surgical procedure (21, p. 268).
- Masks are designed to contain and filter droplets of microorganisms expressed from the mouth and nasal pharynx. *Double masking* acts as a barrier to exhaled air and droplets instead of a filter. This is an unacceptable practice because air vents to the side as it leaves the mask rather than being filtered by it (11, p. 288; 3, p. 200).

- Masks provide protection for the surgical staff by preventing blood and other potentially infective body fluids from penetrating and possibly contaminating mucous membranes of the nose and mouth under normal conditions of use. In addition, a face shield attached to some masks protects the eyes (17, p. 25).
- Masks should cover both the nose and mouth and be tied in such a manner that prevents venting at the sides. Strings should be tied tightly and the mask adjusted for fit to the facial contour so there is no venting (11, p. 288).
- Masks should be changed between procedures, or immediately if they become soiled (22, p. 66).
- When a mask is removed, it should be untied and handled by strings or elastic only. It should then be discarded, not hung around the neck or saved in a pocket (11, p. 288).
- Hands should be washed following removal and disposal of a mask (11, p. 288).
- Criteria for mask selection should be determined by performance requirements.
  - Some surgical procedures will require different types of performance than others. In procedures where there is a greater potential for exposure to blood and body fluids, masks should provide high fluid resistance performance. Specialized procedures involving electrocautery or laser surgery should require the mask to provide filtration of submicron particles as well as protection from spray. For other potential hazards, respiratory protection with particle filtration respirators may be necessary (27, p. 35).
  - It is important to specify minimum performance requirements before the selection process. Trade-offs may exist between different performance properties (e.g., increased fluid resistance and filtration efficiency) versus the ability to breathe (27, p. 35).
  - It is important to use a systematic approach in choosing masks to be used by surgical team members. Use of a checklist that details specific performance standards and methods of evaluation may be helpful (27, p. 34).

Shoe Covers

- The need to wear shoe covers to decrease the risk of SSI has not been proven. Shoe covers need not be worn if the intent is to decrease the risk of SSI or to limit bacterial counts on the OR floor (21, p. 262).
- Shoe covers protect surgical team members from exposure to blood and other body fluids during an operation (11, p. 288).

- Shoe covers are considered part of PPE and should be worn when it can be reasonably anticipated that splashes or spills may occur (3, p. 202).
- OSHA regulations require that disposable shoe covers or boots be worn in situations when gross contamination is likely to occur (21, p. 262).
- Shoe covers should be worn in semirestricted and restricted areas of the surgical suite, removed when leaving the area, and replaced when reentering or when they are wet, soiled, or torn (3, p. 202).
- Knee-high impervious boots should be used when a major blood spill or large amounts of irrigation drainage is anticipated (10, p. 288).

Gloves

No glove is appropriate for everyone in all situations. Nonlatex gloves are recommended for activities unlikely to involve contact with infectious materials. Typically, this would include food preparation, housekeeping, patient transport, and maintenance activities. Glove manufacturers cannot test all gloves for compatibility with all chemicals; therefore the recommended handling procedures from the material safety data sheet (MSDS) for the chemical in question should be consulted (20, p. 32).

The need for protection from potential contamination from contact with blood and body fluids has mandated the use of high-quality patient examination gloves. Furthermore, the increased incidence of allergy to natural rubber latex has led to the development and manufacture of latex gloves that are powder-free and have reduced protein content. Alternatives to latex gloves are those made of materials such as nitrile, vinyl, and chloroprene, as well as a combination of these materials.

- Test studies have shown that all medical gloves do not offer the same barrier protective qualities. It is important that the barrier integrity of the various materials be tested during actual use (1, pp. 27-32; 17, p. 26).
- Assorted gloves vary in performance characteristics under different circumstances. Where a glove made of a specific material may be inappropriate for use in one procedure, it may be the glove of choice in another (29, p. 42).
- Gloves should be evaluated for barrier efficacy, durability, and chemical permeability. With increased concern over safety, it is important to consult institutional safe gloving protocols reflecting infection control and safe gloving practice guidelines established by the Centers for Disease Control and Prevention

(CDC) and OSHA. Furthermore, latex avoidance and management guidelines should be taken into account to avoid the risk of continued patient and worker exposure (28, p. 28).

- Results of clinical research and manufacturers' information regarding glove uses, chemical composition, and the advantages and disadvantages of particular gloves should be studied before purchase (25, pp. 405-410; 14, pp. 20-26; 13, pp. 28-29; 10, pp. 30-31; 12, pp. 22-28).
- General purpose rubber utility gloves should be used for housekeeping chores involving potential blood contact and for instrument cleaning and decontaminating. These gloves can be decontaminated and reused unless they become cracked, punctured, or discolored, or if they show signs of peeling or other evidence of deterioration (16, p. 132).

Protective Eyewear

- Human immunodeficiency virus (HIV) has been contracted via eye splashes, yet compliance with protective eyewear recommendations is poor. Compliance failure may be due to insufficient time to don eye protection, interference with vision, discomfort of eyewear, or eye shields not being immediately available (17, p. 25).
- Staff may not be aware of splash potential until it is too late.
- Protective eyewear or a face shield should be worn whenever the possibility of splashing or spraying exists. This practice prevents risk of contamination of the mucous membranes of the mouth, nose, and eyes of healthcare personnel (3, p. 202; 22, p. 65).
- Eyes are particularly vulnerable to blood contact. The conjunctiva serves as a transmission route for HIV and hepatitis C virus HCV. This type of exposure is particularly high in surgical settings because often blood sprays and splashes occur at significant distances from the sterile field. Despite this, protection is usually worn only by scrub personnel. All personnel, regardless of proximity to the sterile field, should wear protective eyewear as routinely as surgical masks (15, p. 994).
- Face shields provide good eye protection, but only when used in conjunction with protective eyewear (23, p. 54). NOTE: The face shields described here are secured around the forehead and head and are open from below; therefore protective eyewear is needed to deter any spray that is projected upward.
- Protective eyewear or a face shield should be discarded or decontaminated as soon as possible after soiling (3, p. 203).

References

1. Aldape T: Examination gloves: quality pressures, *Infection Control Today* 3(7):27-32, 1999.
2. AORN Online Clinical Practice FAQ Database, 1999: www.aorn.org/_results/clinical.asp (accessed 2000).
3. AORN: Recommended practices for surgical attire. In *Standards, recommended practices & guidelines,* Denver, 2000, Author, pp 199-204.
4. Avalos-Bock S: Personal protective equipment: practices and problems, *Infection Control and Sterilization Technology* 5:18-23, 1999.
5. Belkin NL: Use of scrubs and related apparel in health care facilities, *Am J Infect Control* 25(5):401-404, 1997.
6. Editorial Consultants: Should scrub suits be laundered at home? *OR Manager* 12(8):21-22, 1993.
7. Fogg DM: Clinical issues, *AORN J* 71(2):398-403, 2000.
8. Fortunato N: *Berry and Kohn's operating room technique,* ed 9, St Louis, 2000, Mosby.
9. Gibson LL, Rose JB, Haas CN: Use of quantitative microbial risk assessment for evaluation of the benefits of laundry sanitation, *Am J Infect Control* 27(6):S34-S39, 1999.
10. Glove manufacturers' product matrix, *Infection Control Today* 4(4):30-31, 2000.
11. Gruendemann BJ, Fernsebner B: *Comprehensive perioperative nursing,* vol 1, *Principles,* Boston, 1995, Jones & Bartlett.
12. Hamann C, Long T, Rodgers P: Cost effective glove selection, *Infection Control Today* 4(4):22-28, 2000.
13. Higa L: Glove manufacturers' glove matrix, *Infection Control Today* 3(2):28-29, 1999.
14. Huggins KA: A hand in the glove: lessons learned about glove selection, *Infection Control Today* 3(2):20-26, 1999.
15. Jagger J, Bentley M, Tereskerz P: A study of patterns and prevention of blood exposures in OR personnel, *AORN J* 67(5):979-996, 1998.
16. Jennings J, Manian FA, editors: *APIC handbook of infection control and epidemiology,* ed 2, Washington, DC, 1999, Association for Professionals in Infection Control and Epidemiology.
17. Koch F: What's new in personal protective devices? *Infection Control Today* 3(7):22-28, 1999.
18. Larson E: Home hygiene: a reemerging issue for the new millennium, *Am J Infect Control* 27(6):S1-S3, 1999.
19. Larson E et al: *Perspectives on home hygiene: building a rational approach,* cpmcnet.columbia.edu/dept/nursing/hygiene.html, 1999.
20. Leakakos T: All gloves are not created equal, *Surgical Services Management* 5(7):29-32, 1999.
21. Mangram AJ, Hospital Infection Control Practices Advisory Committee (HICPAC), Centers for Disease Control and Prevention: Guideline for prevention of surgical site infection, 1999, *Infect Control Hosp Epidemiol* 20(4):247-278, 1999. (Reprinted, in part, in Appendix B.)
22. Mews PA: Establishing and maintaining a sterile field. In Phippen ML, Wells MP: *Patient care during operative and invasive procedures,* Philadelphia, 2000, WB Saunders, pp 62-67.

23. Michels M et al: Personal protective equipment for the eyes in a healthcare setting, *Infection Control Today* 2(3):54-56, 1998.
24. Occupational Safety and Health Administration: Occupational exposure to bloodborne pathogens: final rule, *Federal Register* 56(235):64175-64182, 1991.
25. Rego A, Roley L: In-use barrier integrity of gloves: latex and nitrile superior to vinyl, *Am J Infect Control* 27(5):405-410, 1999.
26. Scott E: Hygiene issues in the home, *Am J Infect Control* 27(6):S22-S25, 1999.
27. Stull JO: New developments in standards affecting the selection of surgical masks, *Surgical Services Management* 4(7):24-35, 1998.
28. Sullivan KM, Rodgers PA, Hamann CA: The right glove for the right job: just one is not enough, *Infection Control Today* 2(7):20-28, 1998.
29. Truscott W: Examination gloves selection criteria and infection control, *Infection Control Today* 2(5):40-56, 1998.

Suggested Reading

1. Carlson S: Single-use vs. multiple-use protective apparel, *Infection Control Today* 3(3):72-75, 1999.
2. Copp G et al: Cover gowns and the control of operating room contamination, *Nurs Res* 35(5):263-268, 1986.
3. Copp G et al: Footwear practices and operating room contamination, *Nurs Res* 36:366-369, 1987.
4. Donaldson K, Frederick D, Hodge M: Cover gown policy and postoperative infection rate, *Infection Control Today* 4(4):64, 70, 2000.
5. Douglas A, Simon TR, Goddard M: Barrier durability of latex and vinyl medical gloves in clinical settings, *Am Ind Hyg Assoc J* 58:672-676, 1997.
6. Garcia R: To attire or not to attire: the questions of what to wear in surgery, *Surgical Services Management* 6(3):30-35, 2000.
7. Humphreys H et al: Theatre over-shoes do not reduce operating theatre floor bacterial counts, *J Hosp Infect* 17:117-123, 1991.
8. Jurkovich P: Rationale for home laundering of scrub attire, *AORN J* 69(5):1024-1025, 1999.
9. Kiehl E, Wallace R, Warren C: Tracking perinatal infection: is it safe to launder your scrubs at home? *MCN Am J Matern Child Nurs* 22:195-197, July/August 1997.
10. Korniewicz DM et al: Integrity of vinyl and latex procedure gloves, *Nurs Res* 38(3):144-146, 1989.
11. Lutz C, Hagen L: OR garments and PPE, *Infection Control Today* 3(10):62-66, 1999.
12. National Institute for Occupational Safety and Health (NIOSH): *Report to Congress on workers' home contamination study conducted under the workers' family protection act,* September 1995, www.cdc.gov/niosh/contamin.html (accessed 2000).
13. Olson RJ et al: Examination gloves as barriers to hand contamination in clinical practice, *JAMA* 270(3):350-353, 1993.
14. Prust JM: Surgical masks: current issues and updates, *Surgical Services Management* 3(4):33-39, 1997.
15. Tydell P: Are you in compliance with personal protective equipment requirements? *Infection Control Today* 2(11):55-58, 1998.
16. Wong ES: Surgical site infection. In Mayhall CG, editor: *Hospital epidemiology and infection control,* Baltimore, 1996, Williams & Wilkins, pp 154-175.

C. Handwashing

Handwashing is the simplest of infection prevention practices, yet the most neglected. Effective handwashing, done at appropriate times, reduces cross-transmission of microorganisms from one person to another or from one place to another, even in surgical settings.

Since surgical scrubbing of hands and arms is frequently done in surgical settings, it is often assumed that routine handwashing is less important or not important at all. Nothing is further from the truth. It is just as important for personnel to wash hands between patient contacts in a surgical setting as it is in nonsurgical clinical areas.

The handwashing procedure has many variations that include a short wash (10 to 15 seconds) with plain soap, or a longer wash (30 seconds) with a topical antimicrobial agent. In a surgical setting, topical antimicrobial agents that remove both transient and resident microorganisms should be used for handwashing, as well as for surgical scrubbing.

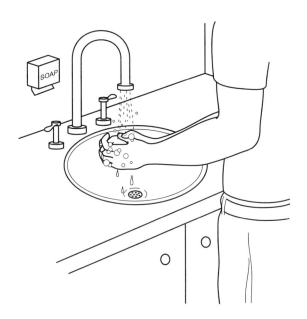

In this chapter we consider the principles of routine handwashing along with procedures, agents, and acceptable adjuncts to handwashing. Surgical scrubbing procedures and nail care are discussed in the chapter "Surgical Scrubbing."

TERMINOLOGY

- *Soaps* and *detergents* lower surface tension, thus helping to physically remove microbes and debris from the hands (6, p. 12).
- *Topical antiseptics* or *topical antimicrobials* (terms used interchangeably) are products applied to skin or other living tissue to disable, inactivate, or kill microorganisms and reduce total skin bacterial counts of both transient and resident flora (6, p. 12).
- *Disinfectants* are chemicals with higher potency than antiseptics and are used to eliminate many or all microorganisms, except bacterial spores, on surfaces of inanimate objects such as table tops and floors (6, p. 12).
- *Transient bacteria,* also called contaminating or noncolonizing flora, are loosely attached to the skin's surface; may be pathogenic; and can be removed quickly and easily with friction, soap or cleansers, and water (1, p. 8; 6, p. 4).
- *Resident bacteria,* also called colonizing flora, survive and multiply on the skin and can be cultured repeatedly. These microorganisms rarely cause infection except when introduced into the body through invasive means or trauma. They are not easily removed by handwashing but can be inactivated by topical antimicrobial agents (6, p. 4; 1, p. 8).

INDICATIONS

- Thorough handwashing is the most effective means of preventing nosocomial infection by removing both resident and transient microorganisms from the nails, hands, and arms. Superficial contact with a source not suspected of contamination, such as by taking a blood pressure, does not require handwashing. In contrast, prolonged and intense contact with any patient should be followed by handwashing (3, p. 7).
- Other authors concur that hands should be washed before and after each patient contact, when contamination has occurred, and when gloves are removed (4, p. 9; 17, p. 20).
- Lack of handwashing can increase the risk of contaminating a patient when gloves from multi-glove boxes are used for patient care. If gloves are used as a substitute for handwashing, there is a risk that both the areas at the opening to the multi-glove box and the gloves within the box will be contaminated with organisms transferred from the hands. The highest risk potential for

contamination occurs when individuals remove their gloves and reach into a glove box without first washing their hands (12, p. 36).

- The decision to wash hands depends on (1) the intensity of contact with patient or families, (2) the degree of contamination that is likely to occur with that contact, (3) the susceptibility of patients to infection, and (4) the procedure to be performed (9, p. 253; 1, p. 7).

Hands should be washed in the following situations:

- Between patient contacts, in the absence of a true emergency (3, p. 8).
- Before performing or assisting with invasive procedures (3, p. 8).
- Before taking care of particularly susceptible patients, such as those who are severely immunocompromised or newborns (3, pp. 8-9).
- Before and after touching wounds, whether surgical, traumatic, or associated with an invasive device (3, pp. 8-9).
- After touching inanimate sources that are likely to be contaminated with virulent or epidemiologically important microorganisms, such as devices for urine measuring or secretion collection (3, pp. 8-9).
- After taking care of an infected patient or one who is likely to be colonized with microorganisms of special clinical or epidemiological significance, such as multiple resistant bacteria (3, pp. 8-9).
- Between contacts with patients in high-risk units such as the intensive care unit or the operating room (3, pp. 8-9).
- Immediately after gloves are removed (9, p. 258; 7, p. 122).
- Before and after performing sterile procedures (7, p. 122).
- After contact with blood or body substances, mucous membranes, soiled linen, waste, or contaminated equipment (7, p. 122).
- Between patient contacts and when otherwise indicated to avoid transfer of microorganisms to other patients and environments (7, p. 122).
- Between tasks at different body sites on the same patient to prevent cross-contamination (7, p. 122).

PROCEDURE

The generally accepted correct handwashing method is as follows:

- Remove rings, bracelets, and watches.
- Wet hands with running water. Apply handwashing detergent and distribute thoroughly over hands (1, pp. 10-11).
- If necessary, remove debris from under fingernails because this area has higher microbial counts than other areas. Recontami-

nation of the hands can occur because of the moist, warm environment under the nails, especially if gloves are worn (9, p. 257).
- Use detergent during a 10- to 15-second vigorous rubbing together of all lathered surfaces (7, p. 122).
- Apply friction on all surfaces of the hands and fingers (7, p. 122).
- Wash all surfaces of the hands because parts of thumbs, backs of fingers and hands, and under nails are often missed (9, p. 257).
- Increase wash time if hands are visibly soiled (7, p. 122).
- Rinse thoroughly with a flowing stream of water (7, p. 122; 3, p. 10; 9, p. 257; 2, p. 12).

The faucet, if not foot or knee operated, should be turned off using a paper towel. The most common break in standard handwashing procedure is touching the faucet without paper protection while manually turning off the water. The increase of microorganisms after repeated handwashing with plain soap could be attributed to this break in technique (20, p. 261).

Detergents with water can remove only a certain level of microorganisms (transient bacteria) from the skin. They do not kill the resident bacteria released by the shedding of skin squames. Antiseptic agents may be necessary to kill or inhibit resident microorganisms and reduce the bacterial level still further. A characteristic of certain antiseptic agents that sets them apart from plain soap is the ability to bind to the stratum corneum, resulting in a persistent activity on the skin (9, p. 253).

DRYING

Many options are available for hand drying. Cloth towels, paper towels, and air dryers all have been shown to further reduce microorganisms following handwashing. However, cloth towels are rarely used because of the risk of contamination between healthcare workers (HCWs). There is no difference between paper towel drying and air drying in the numbers of bacteria remaining. Paper towels should be placed in a holder that dispenses one towel at a time. The dispenser should be placed near the sink but far enough away that towels are not contaminated by splash (9, p. 258).

FACILITIES

Handwashing facilities should be located throughout the hospital and inside or close to every patient room. They should be located in or adjacent to rooms where handwashing should be performed before and after diagnostic or invasive procedures such as cardiac catheterization or colonoscopy (3, pp. 8-9).

Sinks with faucets that can be turned off by means other than the hands and that are designed to minimize splashing can help personnel avoid recontamination of washed hands (3, p. 8).

CHOICE OF CLEANSING AGENT

The choice of plain soap, antiseptic or antimicrobial soaps, or hand rubs depends on the degree of hand contamination and the importance of effecting a reduction of minimal counts of resident flora and reducing the levels of transient flora (7, p. 122; 9, p. 254). This choice also may depend on the susceptibility of the patient. Handwashing with plain soap that reduces microorganisms to below the minimum infectious dose for one patient may not be adequate when caring for another more susceptible patient, in whom the same reduced level of microorganisms may be able to produce disease (16, p. 693). Topical antimicrobial agents should be used for handwashing in surgical settings (6, p. 10).

Plain Soap

NOTE: Plain soap is not recommended for use in surgical settings.
- The primary action of plain soap is the mechanical removal of viable transient microorganisms (9, p. 253). As a result of mechanical friction, microorganisms are emulsified, suspended, and rinsed off with water (8, p. 10).
- Research has shown that when plain soap and water are used for frequent daily handwashing they produce only minimal declines and at times even cause an increase in bacterial yield relative to baseline counts on clean hands (1, p. 15).
- If bar soap is used, it should be kept on racks that allow drainage of water. If liquid soap is used, the dispenser should be replaced or cleaned and filled with fresh product only when empty; liquids should not be added to a partially full dispenser (3, pp. 8-9).

Topical Antimicrobial and Antiseptic Products

NOTE: These products are recommended for use in surgical settings.
The primary actions of topical antimicrobial and antiseptic products include both the mechanical removal and the killing or inhibition of both transient and resident flora (9, p. 253; 8, p. 11). These products usually have a chemical composition and concentration that allow safe application to skin, wounds, and mucous membranes. They also have the ability to bind with the stratum corneum, resulting in persistent chemical activity (8, p. 11). Topical antiseptic or antimicrobial hand products should be used before engaging in the following:
- Invasive procedures such as surgery or the placement and care of intravascular catheters, indwelling catheters, or other invasive devices (9, pp. 253-254).

- Contact with patients who are immunocompromised such as those with burns, pressure ulcers, wounds, and those undergoing chemotherapy (2, p. 12).
- Care of patients with extremes of age (9, pp. 253-254)

Antimicrobial-containing foams or rinses that do not require water can be used when sinks are not available (3, p. 10; 20, p. 261).

Alcohol or alcohol-based products

These products have excellent bactericidal activity against most vegetative gram-positive and gram-negative microorganisms and effective activity against the tubercle bacillus. They are not sporicidal, but they do act against many fungi and viruses such as respiratory syncytial virus, hepatitis B virus, and human immunodeficiency virus (HIV) (9, p. 254; 19, p. 207; 1, p. 17).

- Alcohol denatures microbial proteins but can be inactivated by organic materials such as blood, mucus, and sputum (6, p. 14).
- Application of ethyl alcohol (50% to 70%) or isopropyl alcohol (70% to 99%) to contaminated hands has been found to reduce microorganism counts more rapidly than some other products (6, p. 14; 9, p. 253; 11, pp. 382-385; 16, p. 697).
- The bacterial count on alcohol-scrubbed hands continues to drop for several hours after gloving, probably as a result of the continued deaths of damaged microorganisms (9, p. 254; 11, pp. 382-385).
- A vigorous 1-minute hand rubbing with enough alcohol to get the hands wet has been shown to be the most effective method for hand antisepsis by providing the greatest and most rapid reduction in microbial counts on the skin (9, p. 254).
- Alcohol combined with other antimicrobials or plain soap has been found to be very effective against microorganisms. The most effective product regimen from both an overall microorganism reduction profile and a skin irritation potential, is the combination of alcohol gel with either an antimicrobial soap or a plain lotion soap. Both of these configurations produce microbicidal properties (14, p. 337).
- Alcohols have a rapid antimicrobial effect and, in contrast to chlorhexidine, are equally effective against gram-positive and gram-negative microorganisms (19, p. 207).
- The disadvantage of using alcohol or alcohol-based products is the drying effect on the skin (6, p. 14).
- A disadvantage of pure alcohol is its drying effect on the skin and the absence of residual antimicrobial activity. These

problems are resolved in modern alcoholic hand disinfection products containing different alcohols, additional antimicrobial compounds with residual activity, and refattening agents (19, p. 207).

Chlorhexidine gluconate

Chlorhexidine gluconate (CHG) attains its level of antimicrobial action by causing a disruption of microbial cell plasma membranes and precipitation of cell contents. CHG has a persistent effect that is independent of its cumulative action, allowing it to be chemically active for 5 to 6 hours.

CHG is more effective against gram-positive than gram-negative bacteria, has minimal action against the tubercle bacillus, and is only a fair inhibitor of fungi. In vitro studies have demonstrated activity against viruses including HIV, herpes simplex, cytomegalovirus, and influenza (9, p. 255). Absorption of CHG from intact skin is negligible, but it should be kept out of eyes and ears. Repeated regular application of CHG results in an enhanced effect of residual action (6, p. 14; 1, p. 17).

Iodine/iodophor agents

These products produce their antimicrobial effect by penetrating cell walls. They are highly bactericidal, fungicidal, and virucidal. There is some activity against bacterial spores and effective activity against the tubercle bacillus. Iodophors contain water-soluble organic iodine that breaks down on skin or mucous membranes to release free iodine. They have rapid initial antimicrobial activity after application, but minimal residual effect. Their effectiveness is reduced by the presence of organic materials such as blood and sputum (6, p. 15; 1, p. 17). Concentrations as low as 0.05% have good antimicrobial activity (1, p. 17).

Parachlorometaxylenol

Parachlorometaxylenol (PCMX) disrupts cell walls and inactivates cell enzymes. It is active against gram-positive microorganisms and is fairly active against gram-negative microorganisms, viruses, and tubercle bacilli. The action of PCMX is fairly rapid, and residual effects last for a few hours. However, it is less effective than CHG or the iodophors in reducing skin flora (6, p. 15). PCMX is minimally affected by organic matter (1, p. 17).

Triclosan

Triclosan is an organic ether that disrupts microbial cell walls. It produces a broad spectrum of activity against gram-positive bacteria and most gram-negative bacteria, except perhaps *Pseudomonas*. Triclosan produces some activity against the tubercle bacillus but produces poor activity against viruses. Triclosan has slow initial action but good substantivity and is only minimally affected by organic matter (6, p. 15). A product containing 1% triclosan has been found to be efficacious against methicillin-resistant *Staphylococcus aureus* (5, p. 326). Triclosan is minimally affected by organic matter (1, p. 17).

Hexachlorophene

Hexachlorophene is a phenol preparation that disrupts the cell wall by altering and denaturing the cell protein. It is more effective against gram-positive bacteria than gram-negative bacteria, has a potent bactericidal effect against *S. aureus,* but has little or no effect on either the tubercle bacillus or viruses (6, p. 15). Its activity is reduced by the presence of organic material and blood.

Hexachlorophene is inactivated by alcohol and nonmedicated soaps. It is used only in special circumstances because it can be absorbed through the skin and has been known to cause neurotoxicity (6, p. 15). Hexachlorophene exhibits slow to intermediate antimicrobial activity (1, p. 17).

Topical antimicrobial soap and detergent products

These combination products have been developed to increase foam production, heighten the effectiveness of handwashing, and improve overall skin care. They appear to be aesthetically pleasing to use as well (8, p. 16).

Other Hand Products
Hand rubs

The hygienic hand rub procedure is a more effective and less time-consuming process than standard handwashing. Hand rubs use an antiseptic or topical antimicrobial agent to reduce a substantial part of the transient flora by killing rather than removing the flora (1, p. 16; 16, pp. 695-696). Hygienic hand rub products, especially those containing alcohol, are better suited than soap and water to render hands safe after known or suspected contamination with potentially pathogenic microorganisms. Inference can be made that alcohol-treated hands are less likely to transmit microorganisms than hands washed with plain soap (16, pp. 696-697).

The hand rub technique calls for rubbing 3 to 5 ml of a fast-acting antiseptic on both hands until dry, or for a preset duration recommended by the manufacturer—usually 30 seconds to 1 minute. All areas of the hands should be covered, and the subungual spaces cleaned by rubbing the fingertips on the antiseptic-covered palms. Depending on the microbial species and the antimicrobial agent used, a bacterial reduction of up to more than 5 logs is possible within 1 minute (16, pp. 695-696).

Antimicrobial foams

Well-formulated alcohol emollient preparations cause less dryness and irritation than traditional soap and water washing (1, p. 16). In antimicrobial foams alcohol is added to a specific antimicrobial agent, usually CHG or hexachlorophene. The foam is dispensed from an aerosol container and is rubbed on the skin surface and allowed to air dry. Foams are generally nonirritating to the skin and are effective against both transient and resident microorganisms (8, p. 16).

Hand wipes

Hand wipes are tissues that are impregnated with alcohol, a combination of benzalkonium chloride and alcohol, or tincture of iodine and alcohol. The moistened tissue is rubbed over the soiled skin surface, and the skin is allowed to dry. Alcohol is the preferred ingredient. Wipes are only satisfactory if large enough to wet hands completely with sufficient amounts of alcohol to keep the hands wet for approximately 30 seconds (16, p. 698; 8, p. 16).

Hand rinses

Hand rinses may contain a variety of antimicrobial agents such as CHG or alcohol. The rinse is poured over hands while friction is applied to the skin surface. Hands are allowed to dry before the start of an activity so the antimicrobial agent has full effect (8, p. 17).

Summary

New products are frequently being introduced and advertised as more effective against microorganisms and less harsh on skin. It is important to ascertain whether the ingredients contained in a product are antimicrobial and to compare the manufacturer's educational information with the results of the many studies of these antimicrobial agents. If they pass the scrutiny of the infection control officer for infection control requirements and cost, they should be evaluated by the staff for usability and aesthetic appeal (18, p. 28).

SKIN CARE

Handwashing and hand antisepsis have the potential to cause skin to be dry and irritated, even when associated with proper use of cleansing agents and complete drying.

- Damaged skin is associated with changes in the composition of microbial flora of the hands, such as colonization with more species and increased prevalence of certain significant microorganisms. Skin care products should be made available to personnel following testing by the infection control officer and evaluation by healthcare personnel (10, p. 519).

- Lotions that are aqueous are preferred over those that are oil-based. Oil-based lotions will break down latex gloves and interfere with their barrier properties. In addition, some oil-based lotions are not compatible with CHG products and will negate their persistent activity (13, p. 62).
- Use of two skin care regimens that included oil- and non–oil-containing barrier skin creams showed marked improvement in the overall condition of the hands (1, pp. 16-18).
- Barrier creams are marketed as aids in managing contact dermatitis. However, these creams can be irritating or sensitizing. Most have little positive effect, and some products even worsen skin damage. The safety of barrier creams depends on proper use. These products are not intended to replace gloving or hand care. And since these products do not give any visible signs that they are deteriorating or diminishing in effectiveness, the potential for continued or even intermittent exposure to an irritant is significant (15, p. 24).
- Barrier creams are often intended for use under a glove. This combination can occlude the skin surface and concentrate exposure to the sensitizing agents contained in either the glove or cream. Since HCWs often wear gloves for a prolonged period, the combination of such creams containing oils or petroleum products and latex gloves may well contribute to premature glove failure and are specifically contraindicated by the Occupational Safety and Health Administration (OSHA) (1, p. 18; 15, p. 24).

References

1. Alvarado CJ, Farr BM, McCormick RD: *The science of hand hygiene: self-study monograph for physicians, nurses and other health care professionals,* Cincinnati, 2000, Sci-Health Communications and the University of Wisconsin Medical School.
2. Buck K: Handwashing and glove use for infection control, *Infection Control Today* 2(6):12-18, 1998.
3. Centers for Disease Control: *Guideline for handwashing and hospital environmental control,* Washington, DC, 1985, U.S. Department of Health and Human Services, Public Health Service.
4. Donowitz L: *Infection control for the healthcare worker,* Boston, 1994, Williams & Wilkins.
5. Faoagali JL et al: Comparison of the antibacterial efficacy of 4% chlorhexidine gluconate and 1% triclosan handwash products in an acute clinical ward, *Am J Infect Control* 27(4):320-326, 1999.
6. Gruendemann BJ: *Hand hygiene: a manual for health care professionals,* Arlington, Tex, 1992, Johnson & Johnson Medical.

7. Jennings J, Manian FA, editors: *APIC handbook of infection control,* ed 2, Washington, DC, 1999, Association for Professionals in Infection Control and Epidemiology.

8. Johnson & Johnson Medical: *Hand hygiene II: a self-instructional module,* Arlington, Tex, 1994, Author.

9. Larson EL and APIC Guidelines Committee: APIC guideline for handwashing and hand antisepsis in health care settings, *Am J Infect Control* 23(4):251-269, 1995.

10. Larson EL et al: Changes in bacterial flora associated with skin damage on hands of health care personnel, *Am J Infect Control* 26(5):513-521, 1998.

11. Lily HA et al: Limits to progressive reduction of resident skin bacteria by disinfection, *J Clin Pathol* 31:382-385, 1979.

12. Maley MP: Handwashing and potential contamination of boxes of gloves, *Infection Control Today* 27(2):36, 1999.

13. Manz EA, Gardner D: Hand hygiene and hand health: important links to infection prevention, *Infection Control Today* 3(7):59-62,1999.

14. Paulson DS et al: A close look at alcohol gel as an antimicrobial sanitizing agent, *Am J Infect Control* 27(4):332-338, 1999.

15. Rodgers PA, Sullivan KM, Hamann CP: Skin care: maintaining your best defense, *Infection Control Today* 2(6):20-24, 1998.

16. Rotter ML: Hand washing, hand disinfection and skin disinfection. In Wenzel RP, editor: *Prevention and control of nosocomial infections,* ed 3, Baltimore, 1997, Williams & Wilkins, pp. 691-709.

17. Springthorpe S, Sattar S: Handwashing: what can we learn from recent research? *Infection Control Today* 2(4):20-25, 1998.

18. Stout G: Handwashing agents, *Infection Control Today* 2(4):28, 1998.

19. Voss A, Widmer A: No time for handwashing!? Handwashing versus alcoholic rub: can we afford 100% compliance? *Infect Control Hosp Epidemiol* 18(3):205-208, 1997.

20. Zaragoza M et al: Handwashing with soap or alcoholic solutions? A randomized clinical trial of its effectiveness, *Am J Infect Control* 27(3):258-261, 1999.

Suggested Reading

1. Boyce JM: Using alcohol for hand antisepsis: dispelling old myths, *Infect Control Hosp Epidemiol* 21(7):438-447, 2000.

2. Boyce JM, Kelliher S, Vallende N: Skin irritation and dryness associated with two hand-hygiene regimens: soap and water handwashing versus hand antisepsis with an alcohol gel, *Infect Control Hosp Epidemiol* 21(7):442-448, 2000.

3. Cohen ML: Proper hand washing protocols: critical for preventing nosocomial infections, *Surgical Services Management* 6(3):21-28, 2000.

4. Dyer DL: Handwashing: problems and solutions, part 1, *Infection Control Today* 4(4):34-39, 2000.

5. Gruendemann BJ, Larson EL: Antisepsis in current practice. In Rutala WA, editor: *Disinfection, sterilization and antisepsis in health care,* Champlain, NY, Polyscience; Washington, DC, Association for Professionals in Infection Control and Epidemiology, 1998, pp. 183-195.

6. Jacobsen G et al: Handwashing: ring wearing and the numbers of organisms, *Nurs Res* 31:186-188, 1985.

7. Metules TJ: Tips for nurses who wash too much, *RN* 63(3):34-37, 2000.

8. McGuckin M et al: Patient education model for increasing handwashing compliance, *Am J Infect Control* 27(4):309-314, 1999.
9. Newman JL, Jampani HB: Waterless antimicrobial disinfection, *Surgical Services Management* 6(3):36-39, 2000.
10. Stone P: Handwashing products to control emerging pathogens, *Infection Control Today* 4(2):46-47, 2000.
11. Tydell P: The fundamentals of handwashing, *Infection Control Today* 2(6):54-57, 1998.

D. Surgical Scrubbing

Scrubbing, along with gowning and gloving, creates a protective system that deters microbial, body fluid, and liquid contamination during a surgical procedure.

This protective system uses (1) the sterile boundaries provided by gowns and gloves and (2) scrubbing of hands and arms by the surgical team, which creates a reinforcement, or back-up system, for the sterile gowns and gloves should there be a break in the integrity of these shields. Even though skin cannot be made sterile, it can be rendered extremely clean (surgically clean) (5, p. 2).

Members of the surgical team who have direct contact with the sterile operating field or sterile instruments or supplies used in the field wash their hands and forearms by performing a traditional procedure known as scrubbing immediately before donning a sterile gown and gloves (13, p. 258).

The surgical scrub is analogous to preoperative preparation—ꞓrepping—of the patient's skin.

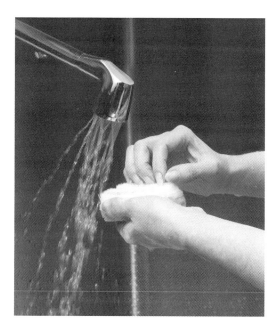

PURPOSE

The purposes of scrubbing are to:
- Remove debris and transient organisms from the nails, hands, and forearms (10, p. 258).
- Reduce the resident microbial count to a minimum (4, p. 244).
- Inhibit rapid rebound growth of microorganisms (2, p. 271).
- Minimize regrowth of microorganisms for the length of the procedure, or as long as possible (7, p. 185).
- Reduce the numbers of microorganisms on hands and reduce contamination of the operative site by recognized or unrecognized breaks in surgical gloves (18, p. 161).

PREPARATION

- All personnel should be in surgical attire before beginning the surgical scrub (2, p. 271).
- All jewelry on fingers, hands, and forearms must be removed and other jewelry removed or confined because jewelry harbors microorganisms (4, p. 245; 6, p. 195; 13, p. 267).
- Fingernails must be short, clean, and healthy. The relationship between nail length and surgical site infection (SSI) is unknown, but long nails—artificial or natural—may be associated with tears in surgical gloves (2, p. 271; 13, p. 258).
- Artificial nails should not be worn, and artificial devices must not cover natural fingernails (2, p. 271; 4, p. 245).
- A surgical team member who wears artificial nails may have increased bacterial and fungal colonization of the hands, despite performing an adequate hand scrub. Hand carriage of gram-negative organisms has been shown to be greater among wearers of artificial nails than among nonwearers (13, p. 258).
- Artificial or acrylic nails on healthy hands have not been proven to increase the risk of SSI, but artificial nails may harbor organisms and prevent effective handwashing. Numerous state cosmetology boards have reported that fungal growth occurs frequently under artificial nails as a result of moisture becoming trapped between the natural and artificial nail (2, pp. 271-272).
- Freshly applied nail polish on well-manicured nails may be acceptable. Nails with polish that is obviously chipped or that has been worn for more than 4 days have been found to harbor greater numbers of bacteria than unpolished nails. Nails should be well manicured (2, p. 271).
- Freshly applied polish may be worn if permitted by facility policy. Individuals who choose to wear nail polish in the surgical setting should be guided by surgical conscience (2, p. 271; 4, p. 245).

- The relationship between the wearing of nail polish or jewelry by surgical team members and the risk of SSI has not been adequately studied (13, p. 258).

CHOICE OF AGENT
Desired Characteristics
- Should significantly reduce microorganisms on intact skin (17, p. 528).
- Must be broad spectrum, fast acting, and have a residual effect (7, p. 186).
- Should contain a nonirritating antimicrobial agent (2, p. 272).

Agents
- Antiseptic (antimicrobial) agents commercially available in the United States contain alcohol, chlorhexidine gluconate (CHG), iodine/iodophors, parachlorometaxylenol, or triclosan. Povidone-iodine and CHG are the current preferred agents of choice for most surgical team members in the United States (13, p. 258).
- Alcohol is considered the gold standard for surgical hand preparation in several European countries. Alcohol-containing products are used less frequently in the United States than in Europe, possibly because of concerns about flammability and skin irritation. In a study, alcoholic chlorhexidine was found to have greater residual antimicrobial activity than povidone-iodine or CHG alone. No agent is ideal for every situation, and a major factor, aside from product efficacy, is its acceptability by operating room personnel after repeated use. Most studies have focused on measuring hand bacterial colony counts. No clinical trials have evaluated the impact of scrub agent choice on SSI risk (13 p. 258).
- If an alcohol-based preparation specific for surgical hand scrubs is used, the manufacturer's written instructions should prevail because scrub procedures may differ (2, p. 273).
- Foams, gels, and other antimicrobial agents should be used for surgical scrubs only with specific instructions from the manufacturer for that use and after consultation with infection control professionals. AORN has taken no position on the use of foam products for the surgical scrub and is unaware of any studies on the efficacy of substituting foam products for the more traditional surgical scrub (1).
- The high potential of hexachlorophene for neurotoxicity makes it unsuitable for routine use. Hexachlorophene is available by prescription only (4, p. 245).

- Persons sensitive to antimicrobial agents may use a non-medicated soap scrub followed by an alcohol-based hand cleanser (2, p. 272).
- Hand scrubbing agents should be stored in clean, closed containers; reusable containers should be washed and dried thoroughly before refilling. Reusable containers should not be "topped off." Disposable containers are discarded after use (2, p. 273).
- Manufacturers' instructions should be followed for all scrubbing agents.

TRADITIONAL SCRUBBING
Scrubbing with a Brush

An anatomic timed scrub is used most commonly. Although mentioned in the literature, the counted stroke method is seldom used, except perhaps in instruction of novices (5, p. 1).

Preparation

The process begins with washing hands and forearms to remove dirt and transient bacteria (10, p. 258). Cleaning underneath each fingernail is done before performing the first scrub of the day (13, p. 267). Single-use disposable nail cleaning products are available. Reusable nail cleaners are terminally cleaned and sterilized between uses. Orangewood sticks are not to be used to clean under fingernails because the wood may splinter and harbor *Pseudomonas* organisms (4, p. 244).

Scrub

The surgical scrub includes hand and forearms up to and including the elbows. The scrub is done before gowning and gloving and before the sterile field, sterile instruments, or the patient's prepped skin is touched, after gowning and gloving (6, pp. 195-196; 2, p. 273).

Antimicrobial agent is applied, and friction is used. Four sides of the fingers, hands, and arms are visualized and scrubbed. Hands are held higher than elbows. The spilling of water onto surgical attire is avoided (2, p. 273). The direction of the scrubbing procedure is from the hands to the arms, without returning to the cleaned hands (5, p. 8).

The scrubbing sequence is as follows: After the initial cleaning of the hands, nails, and forearms, the scrub begins, with the majority of time spent on the hands, especially the nails, fingertips, and palms. (In a 3-minute timed scrub, 1 minute would be spent on each hand, and ½ minute on each arm.) Each finger is scrubbed. Each forearm can then be visually divided into two sections: the first section adjoining the wrist, and the second section including the elbow. The first sections will be scrubbed before progressing to the second sections. The brush is transferred between hands as the scrub progresses toward the elbow. The scrub is completed at the elbow; the brush is discarded (5, pp. 6-12).

After performing the scrub, the hands are kept up and away from the body, elbows in flexed position, so that water runs from the tips of the fingers toward the elbows. The water is turned off; hands and arms are dried with a sterile towel; sterile gown and gloves are donned (13, p. 267).

Throughout the entire procedure, contact with unclean areas must be avoided. If there is any contact of clean hands with unclean surfaces during scrubbing, the procedure must be restarted using a fresh brush (5, pp. 5, 12).

Reusable Versus Disposable Brushes

The choice of reusable versus disposable brushes should be based on realistic considerations of effectiveness and economy. Studies show no significant differences in scrub effectiveness between the two types of brushes (2, p. 273).

Duration

- No study has determined the ideal duration for the traditional surgical scrub (17, p. 528).
- The Association for Professionals in Infection Control and Epidemiology (APIC) guidelines state that the optimum duration of a surgical scrub is unclear, although research indicates that it may be agent dependent. Also unclear is whether scrubs for subsequent consecutive procedures may be shorter than for the first procedure (10, p. 258).
- The American College of Surgeons (ACS) guidelines are for 2 minutes (14, pp. 1-8).
- AORN states that research from the United States indicates that 2- to 3-minute scrubs are clinically effective. European and Australian studies generally show that 3- to 4-minute scrubs are as effective as 5-minute scrubs. Procedures for subsequent hand scrubs should be the same as for initial scrubs because this reduces confusion and increases compliance by providing clear, easily followed guidelines (2, p. 274).
- The Centers for Disease Control and Prevention (CDC) SSI guideline: Recent studies suggest that scrubbing for at least 2 minutes is as effective as the traditional 10-minute scrub in reducing hand bacterial colony counts but that the optimum duration of scrubbing is not known. However, recommendations are for a 2- to 5-minute surgical scrub using an appropriate antiseptic (13, pp. 258, 267).

- Prolonged scrubbing raises resident microbes from deep dermal layers and is therefore counterproductive. Care should be taken not to abrade the skin during the scrub process (4, p. 245).

BRUSHLESS SCRUBBING

NOTE: The idea of "scrubbing" without the use of either a brush or sponge is receiving added attention now for two reasons: (1) the introduction of increasingly efficacious products designed to be used without a brush or sponge, and (2) the gradual shift in perception away from thinking of the brush as the hallowed tool of the surgical scrub. At the same time, there is a growing acceptance in the United States of new agents, especially the proven alcohol-based formulations that combine rapid antimicrobial action with improved emollient and moisturizing additives. These new agents cause less damage to skin and produce better antimicrobial reductions, even without the use of a brush.

- Loeb's study (12) of brushless scrubbing showed that washing for 5 minutes with an antimicrobial agent alone (4% CHG soap with isopropyl alcohol without a brush) is as effective as washing for 5 minutes with 4% CHG with isopropyl alcohol using an inert surgical scrub brush. Two conclusions were drawn: (1) the effect of using soap alone in reducing hand bacterial counts at 45 minutes is similar to that of using soap plus a brush, and (2) soap can safely be used alone with the SSI rate prospectively monitored.
- Jones and colleagues conducted a surgical scrub test, using brushless, waterless applications of 2- to 5-ml doses of a 60% ethyl alcohol hand gel that was rubbed vigorously over the hands and lower forearms of subjects until dry (45 to 75 seconds, with total application times of 2 to 4 minutes). Use of the hand gel demonstrated dramatically enhanced, immediate, cumulative, and persistent antimicrobial activity when compared with a traditional 6-minute scrub with a brush using a 2% CHG scrub solution. Nondrying skin moisturization qualities were also present in the waterless, alcohol-based formulation (9).
- Hobson and others found that a surgical hand "scrub" formulation consisting of 70% alcohol, along with a unique blend of surfactants, emollients, and preservatives, produced greater initial and persistent hand antisepsis improvements than both 4% CHG and 7.5% povidone-iodine. The alcohol formulation also demonstrated similar antimicrobial efficacy when used in a brushless 3-minute scrub procedure. The

protocol included two 1.5-minute applications to the hands, without a brush, with a concentrated focus on the subungual and interdigital spaces. Brushless applications yielded results similar to those from applications of the product with either a brush or a sponge (8).

- Newman and Jampani (15) discussed the benefits of waterless antimicrobial hand disinfection, particularly with the use of alcohol, stating that new-formulation technology has overcome some earlier shortcomings. Newer alcohol-based formulations have lotion-like characteristics, providing hands with moisture and skin conditioning instead of having a drying effect. The generally accepted view of antimicrobial agents is that increased efficacy is accompanied by decreased mildness to the skin. The authors state that incorporating lotion-like characteristics balances efficacy and mildness, even in surgical hand preparation.

- Dr. Elaine Larson advocated the use of waterless alcohol formulations for brushless surgical scrubbing during a recent AORN Congress presentation (11). She cited studies (8, 12, 16) that note heightened skin damage and increased microbial counts with prolonged brush scrub times, show advantages of alcohol-based formulations that contain emollients and moisturizers for overall protection of the skin, and suggest the superiority in efficacy of alcohol products when compared with CHG and povidone-iodine. One final comment was that a brush for surgical scrubbing is probably unnecessary and is a ritual that we should consider discarding. On the topic of surgical scrubbing, Dr. Larson also discussed a study (3) that showed a significant increase in gram-negative organisms on hands with artificial fingernails compared with polished, natural nails; excessively long natural nails were also implicated.

NOTE: When using topical antimicrobials, including alcohol preparations, manufacturers' written instructions should always be followed. Alcohol is flammable; therefore caution must be used, and alcohol preparations must be completely dried before donning gowns and gloves. Because alcohol preparations are not generally effective on organic matter, arms and hands, particularly subungual areas, must be thoroughly cleansed of dirt and debris and thoroughly dried before applying alcohol-based scrubbing products. For additional information on topical antimicrobials and skin care, see the chapters "Handwashing" and "Preparing the Patient's Skin."

References

1. AORN Online Clinical Practice FAQ Database, www.aorn.org/_results, 2000.
2. AORN: Recommended practices for surgical hand scrubs. In *Standards, recommended practices and guidelines,* Denver, 2000, Author, pp 271-276.
3. Edel E et al: Impact of a 5-minute scrub on the microbial flora found on artificial, polished, or natural fingernails of operating room staff, *Nurs Res* 47:54-59, 1998.
4. Fortunato N: *Berry & Kohn's operating room technique,* ed 9, St Louis, 2000, Mosby.
5. Gruendemann BJ: *Illustrated guide to surgical scrubbing, gowning, and gloving,* ed 1, Arlington, Tex, 1990, Johnson & Johnson Medical.
6. Gruendemann BJ, Fernsebner B: *Comprehensive perioperative nursing,* vol 1, *Principles,* Boston, 1995, Jones & Bartlett.
7. Gruendemann BJ, Larson EL: Antisepsis in current practice. In Rutala WA, editor: *Disinfection, sterilization and antisepsis in health care,* Champlain, NY, Polyscience; Washington, DC, Association for Professionals in Infection Control and Epidemiology, 1998, pp 183-195.
8. Hobson DW et al: Development and evaluation of a new alcohol-based surgical hand scrub formulation with persistent antimicrobial characteristics and brushless application, *Am J Infect Control* 26(5):507-512, 1998.
9. Jones RD et al: Moisturizing alcohol hand gels for surgical hand preparation, *AORN J* 71(3):584-599, 2000.
10. Larson EL and APIC Guidelines Committee: APIC guideline for handwashing and hand antisepsis in health care settings, *Am J Infect Control* 23(4):251-269, 1995.
11. Larson E, O'Boyle C: Hot topics in skin microbial control: the art and science of hand hygiene and health. Presentation, AORN Congress, New Orleans, April 5, 2000.
12. Loeb MB et al: A randomized trial of surgical scrubbing with a brush compared to antiseptic soap alone, *Am J Infect Control* 25(1):11-15, 1997.
13. Mangram AJ, Hospital Infection Control Practices Advisory Committee (HICPAC), Centers for Disease Control and Prevention: Guideline for prevention of surgical site infection, 1999, *Infect Control Hosp Epidemiol* 24(4):247-278, 1999. (Reprinted, in part, in Appendix B.)
14. Materson BJ: Skin preparation. In Wilmore DW et al, editors: *Care of the surgical patient,* vol 2, New York, 1990, Scientific American Books, pp 1-8.
15. Newman JL, Jampani HB: Waterless antimicrobial hand disinfection, *Surgical Services Management* 6(3):36-39, 2000.
16. Pereira LJ, Lee GM, Wade KJ: An evaluation of five protocols for surgical handwashing in relation to skin condition and microbial counts, *J Hosp Infect* 36:49-65, 1997.
17. Roy MC: The operating theater: a special environmental area. In Wenzel RP, editor: *Prevention and control of nosocomial infections,* ed 3, Baltimore, 1997, Williams & Wilkins, pp 515-538.
18. Wong ES: Surgical site infections. In Mayhall CG, editor: *Hospital epidemiology and infection control,* Baltimore, 1996, Williams & Wilkins, pp 154-175.

Suggested Reading

1. Baumgardner CA et al: Effects of nail polish on microbial growth on fingernails, *AORN J* 58(1):84-88, 1993.

2. Fogg DM: Clinical issues, *AORN J* 69(5):1014, 1017-1018, 1999.
3. Hagen KS, Treston-Aurand J: A comparison of two skin preps used in cardiac surgical procedures, *AORN J* 62:393-402, 1995.
4. Hingst V et al: Evaluation of the efficacy of surgical hand disinfection following a reduced application time of 3 instead of 5 minutes, *J Hosp Infect* 20:79-86, 1992.
5. Larson E: Handwashing: it's essential—even when you use gloves, *Am J Nurs* 89:934-937, 1989.
6. Larson EL et al: Alcohol for surgical scrubbing, *Infect Control Hosp Epidemiol* 11:139-143, 1990.
7. Larson E et al: Effects of a protective foam on scrubbing and gloving, *Am J Infect Control* 21:297-301, 1993.
8. McNeil SA, Foster CL, Kauffman CA: The effect of hand cleansing with antimicrobial soap or gel on microbial colonization of artificial nails. Presentation, Society for Healthcare Epidemiology of America (SHEA), 8th Annual Meeting, April 1998. From University of Michigan and VA Medical Center, Ann Arbor, Mich. (Information available from Dr. C. Kauffman, University of Michigan Medical Center.)
9. Paulson DS: Comparative evaluation of five surgical hand scrub preparations, *AORN J* 60:246-256, 1994.
10. Paulson DS et al: A close look at alcohol gel as an antimicrobial sanitizing agent, *Am J Infect Control* 27(4):332-338, 1999.
11. Salisbury DM et al: The effect of rings on microbial load of health care workers' hands, *Am J Infect Control* 25(1):24-27, 1997.
12. Wheelock SM, Lookinland S: Effect of surgical hand scrub time on subsequent bacterial growth, *AORN J* 65(6):1087-1098, 1997.
13. Wynd CA, Samstag DE, Lapp AM: Bacterial carriage on the fingernails of OR nurses, *AORN J* 60(5):796, 799-805, 1994.

E. Gowning

Gowning is an integral part of the scrubbing, gowning, and gloving procedures that take place each day in an operating room (OR). All of these preparations and procedures have one common goal: to ensure a safe, protective, and aseptic environment for the patient and the surgical team.

The purpose of scrubbing, gowning, and gloving is to create a system of shielding that deters microbial, body fluid, and liquid contamination during a surgical procedure. This protective system uses the sterile boundaries provided by gowns and gloves (8, p. 2).

Knowledge and practice of aseptic techniques and donning of appropriate surgical attire are prerequisites to understanding and carrying out the gowning procedures that are outlined in this chapter. This chapter also contains discussions on gown usage in surgical settings and gown characteristics that should be considered when choosing materials and products.

NOTE: Since similar materials and testing methods are used for both gowns and drapes, to avoid redundancy between chapters, the reader should refer to the chapter "Draping" for drape and gown materials (single-use and multiple-use), materials testing, and desired

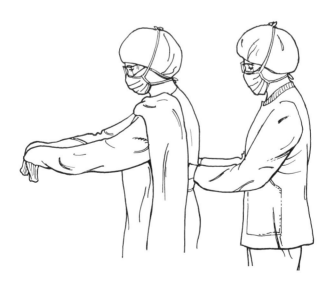

drape and gown characteristics. Choosing reusables or disposables is discussed in this chapter.

GOWN USAGE

· A gown should be worn to protect skin and clothing during procedures that are likely to generate splashes of blood, body fluids, secretions, and excretions. Gowns are required under Standard Precautions to provide barrier protection and to reduce opportunities for transmission of microorganisms in the hospital. If large-volume splashes or large quantities of infective material are anticipated, wearing a gown that is impermeable to liquids—as well as leg coverings and boots or shoe covers—provides greater protection to the skin than wearing a "regular" gown (6, pp. 79, 81).

· Gowns should provide a protective barrier from strike-through. A sterile gown prevents intercontamination between the wearer and the field and differentiates sterile (scrubbed) from nonsterile (unscrubbed) team members (7, p. 242).

· The use of gowns and drapes to prevent surgical site contamination and infection is logical, and their value is implied but not proven in clinical studies. One of the most important roles for surgical gowns is protection of the operative team from contamination by blood and body fluids (18, p. 163).

GOWN CHARACTERISTICS

· Gowns should be resistant to penetration by fluids and blood and should be comfortable without producing excessive heat buildup (7, p. 242).

· The choice of gowns as personal protective equipment (PPE) should be based on the procedure or task being performed and the degree of exposure that is anticipated, according to the Occupational Safety and Health Administration (OSHA). Protective garments are made with varying degrees of resistance to liquid penetration. The key to decision-making is to select a material that will not allow blood or other potentially infectious materials to pass through or reach the employee's work clothes, street clothes, undergarments, skin, eyes, mouth, or other mucous membranes under normal use conditions and for the duration of time that the protective equipment will be used. For example, eye surgery usually provides little exposure to blood in sufficient quantities to create strike-through; therefore a regular gown or one with minimal reinforcement would be adequate. On the other hand, a vascular procedure during which blood loss is expected would require a gown that is reinforced in areas where penetration is likely or one that is made entirely of reinforced barrier materials (15, p. 64177; 10, pp. 248, 250).

- Sterile team members may not need a reinforced barrier gown for every procedure; the scrub person usually can safely wear a single-layer impervious gown. The surgeon and first assistant are at greatest risk during procedures within the abdomen or chest cavity, when blood loss will be more than 200 ml, or when the procedure will exceed 2 hours. Bloodborne pathogens can penetrate fabric without visible strike-through. The forearms are the most frequently contaminated areas. Therefore the surgeon and first assistant should wear a gown with at least reinforced or plastic-coated sleeves for these procedures (7, p. 242).
- Gowns and drapes function as barriers and thus prevent transmission of microorganisms from nonsterile to sterile areas. A critical factor in choosing materials for gowns and drapes is impermeability to moisture (strike-through). Manufacturers have developed many types of impermeable and semipermeable materials for use in either single-use or reusable barriers (10, p. 258).

GOWN SELECTION

Surgical gowns and drapes should:
- Provide appropriate barriers to microorganisms, particulate matter, and fluids
- Be safe and comfortable
- Permit sterilization while maintaining integrity and durability
- Resist tears, punctures, fiber strains, and abrasions
- Be low linting and without toxic ingredients
- Have acceptable quality levels (e.g., freedom from holes and defects)
- Have a positive cost/benefit ratio
- Follow OSHA guidelines for PPE (4, p, 267)

Product selection should be guided by the anticipated use of the product, the performance attributes of the product in relation to the anticipated use, the cost of the product, and the quality systems built into the manufacture and supply of the product. The Association for the Advancement of Medical Instrumentation (AAMI) recommends that gowns and drapes be evaluated on the following performance attributes:
- Liquid barrier effectiveness
- Microbial barrier effectiveness
- Abrasion resistance
- Strength
- Comfort

- Shrinkage
- Toxicity
- Flammability
- Linting propensity (5)

Koch (11, p. 28) reviewed research studies that led to six factors that should be considered when selecting surgical attire for OR team members exposed to significant amounts of blood and fluids:

1. Length of procedure
2. Estimated blood loss
3. Procedure type
4. Blood exposure record
5. Staff members' desired level of comfort
6. Cost

Stull and Pournoor (16) provide tables that apply Telford and Quebbeman's research (17) to suggested procedures according to the following exposure levels for surgeons and assistants:

Substantial exposure: >500 ml of potentially infectious material; exposure time of >2 hours; exposure likely limited to thorax and extremities. Examples: total joint replacements, trauma surgeries, cesarean sections and vaginal deliveries, coronary artery bypass grafts, peripheral vascular procedures, organ transplants, nephrectomies, craniotomies, and breast reductions.

Moderate exposure: <500 ml of potentially infectious material; exposure time of <2 hours; exposure likely to hands and forearms; possibility of endoscopic procedure to become emergent. Examples: laminectomy, hand/foot procedures, dilatation and curettage (D & C), mastectomy, angiography, chest tube insertion.

Minimal exposure: exposure time of <2 hours; exposure limited to hands. Examples: carpal tunnel release, laceration repairs, debridement, cataract extractions, excision of lesions.

Recommendations for gowns:

Category A: liquid or microbial barrier (or zoned); liquid-proof for majority of gown.

Category B: liquid or microbial barrier (or zoned) for limited portions of gown.

Category C: zoned liquid-resistant, or liquid-resistant (16, p. 22)

The choice of which gown to use for which procedure is not an easy one because there are no "standard" surgical procedures. Each facility must develop a knowledge base of criteria that are meaningful to their particular setting (11, p. 28). For readers who are in the process of choosing gown and drape materials, obtaining the AAMI Technical Information Report (TIR) (5) is a *must.*

REUSABLES VERSUS DISPOSABLES
Overview
- Gowns and drapes are classified as disposable (single-use, nonwoven) or reusable (multiple-use, woven). Regardless of the material used in manufacturing, gown and drape fabrics should be impermeable to liquids and viruses. In general, only gowns reinforced with films, coatings, or membranes appear to meet standards developed by the American Society for Testing Materials (ASTM). However, such "liquid-proof" gowns may be uncomfortable because they also inhibit heat loss and the evaporation of sweat from the wearer's body. These factors should be considered when selecting gowns (12, pp. 262-263; 13; 1; 2). NOTE: See the chapter "Draping" for materials testing for both drapes and gowns.
- Most single-use disposable gowns are made of spunlace fiber or nonwoven, moisture-repellent fabrics. Some of these gowns are reinforced on the forearms and front (7, p. 242).
- The two most widely used disposable gown and drape fabrics are made of a spunlace, wet-laid wood pulp and polyester fiber blend and a spun-bonded, meltblown polyethylene. Both of these fabrics have polyethylene film laminated beneath the nonwoven fabric in critical areas. Disposables reduce setup time and provide barriers with less material (14, pp. 86-87).
- Gowns are made of fabrics that are either fluid proof or fluid resistant. *Fluid-proof* fabrics provide impervious barriers, thereby preventing the gown from becoming soaked with blood or other potentially infectious fluids. *Fluid-resistant* fabrics provide an effective barrier and should be worn if there is a possibility that blood or other potentially infectious fluids may be splashed or sprayed (14, p. 71).
- Reusable (woven) gowns should be made of a densely woven fabric. Loosely woven, 140-thread count, all carded cotton muslin or similar-quality permeable fabric is not a barrier to microbial migration. Some 180-thread-count cotton gowns have insets of 270-thread-count fluid-resistant fabric or plastic film to reinforce sleeves from the cuffs to the elbows, and the front from the midchest to below the waist. Pima cotton with a 270- to 280-thread-count per square inch, reinforced with a moisture-repellent finish, is an acceptable woven textile. Some reusable gowns are a cotton-polyester blend. Tightly woven 100% polyester gowns are impervious to moisture. Gown seams should be constructed to prevent fluid penetration (7, p. 242).
- A recent development in reusable fabrics is Gore-Tex, a barrier fabric laminate bonded between two layers of lightweight

polyester. The fabric is liquid proof, durable, breathable, and prevents strike-through (14, p. 86).

- Reusable (woven) fabrics should maintain a protective barrier through multiple laundering and sterilization processes (4, p. 267).
- Woven textile gowns withstand about 75 launderings and sterilizing cycles before appreciable deterioration of the finish occurs. An additional rinse cycle when laundering may be necessary to remove residual detergent. Woven gowns must be monitored for number of uses and removed from use at the sterile field when they are no longer an effective barrier (7, p. 242).
- Textile gowns can be patched only with heat-applied vulcanized mending fabrics (7, p. 242).
- Unused single-use (disposable, nonwoven) surgical gowns and drapes should not be resterilized unless manufacturers provide written instructions for reprocessing (4, p. 268).
- Manufacturers should provide data to verify that fabrics for gowns and drapes are protective barriers against microorganisms, particulates, and fluids and that they can maintain their ability to withstand potential tears, punctures, fiber stains, and abrasions (4, p. 268).
- All woven (reusable) and some nonwoven (single-use) gowns are not flame resistant. Flame-resistant gowns should be worn for laser surgery and are preferred when electrosurgery is performed (7, p. 242).
- Barrier materials should resist combustion. Care should be taken when barrier materials are exposed to light and heat sources, electrosurgical devices, lasers, and other power equipment. Even fabrics said to be flame resistant may burn or melt when subjected to intense heat or an oxygen-rich environment (4, pp. 268-269).
- Gowns or aprons made of fluid-resistant fabric protect the wearer from splashes with blood and body fluids. Impervious gowns offer better protection. Disposable (single-use) impervious gowns are preferred (7, p. 228).
- For orthopedic surgery, a fluid-impervious gown should be worn, and a waterproof apron should be worn under the gown. Copious irrigation is often used (7, p. 713).

   NOTE: See the chapter "Draping" for more information on gown and drape materials and desired gown and drape characteristics.

Criteria for Choosing

Infection control concerns are paramount and are inherent in the use of both reusables and disposables. With the advent of harmful multidrug-resistant microorganisms, more attention is paid to decreasing risks of disease transmission, both to patients and staff. Cleaning, reprocessing, decontamination, disinfection, and sterilization processes are under close scrutiny. This emphasis on prevention and control of infectious diseases will only increase (9, pp. 24-25).

Basic requirements are generally the same for gown and drape fabrics as they are for packaging materials. The materials must meet a high standard of safety and effectiveness and be free of any inherent dangers to both staff and patients. All materials must be of a barrier quality that meets standard requirements, such as those of AORN, AAMI, and ASTM and must be able to withstand sterilization and quality assurance parameters. The materials, especially gown materials, must also meet the requirements of different types of invasive surgical procedures (dependent on length of procedure, amount of expected blood loss, area of body entered, and risk to surgical team members), with no compromise to aseptic technique (9, p. 25).

Approximately 80% of U.S. hospitals use single-use drapes and gowns, particularly in ORs. Of the remaining 20% that use reusable systems, some have migrated to "high-tech" synthetic materials and composites that possess vastly improved longevity and barrier qualities compared with previous reusable systems. Although the materials have advanced, handling of reusable gowns and drapes soiled with body fluids remains problematic because they must be treated as potentially infectious materials. Single-use products, on the other hand, are more convenient because of their ready availability, guarantee of consistent barrier quality and performance, and ease of disposal (9, pp. 25-26).

Although single-use products add to landfills and consume more energy and materials to produce than reusables, the cleaning of reusables consumes water and chemicals and adds pollutants to both water and air (9, p. 26).

There are many excellent gown and drape systems in use today, both single-use and reusable. Answering the following questions can help readers make decisions about which products, single-use or reusable, are best for each surgical setting, resulting in the most cost-effective and safe patient care while also considering waste management issues.

For any system (yes or no)
- Consistency of materials and products?
- Compatibility with infection control mandates (e.g., barrier qualities, effectiveness in preventing occupational exposures to blood and body fluids, aseptic handling qualities, meet professional organization guidelines, clinical studies available)?
- Good drapability?
- Reasonable time spent in opening packages?

- Adherence to aseptic technique by requiring the opening of the least number of items possible?
- Comfortable?
- Meets needs of surgeons and nurses?
- Convenient and easy to use?
- Alternate delivery systems available, such as customized procedure packs?
- Opportunities for reduction in total waste by use of custom packs?
- Design features that enhance product usage (e.g., built-in fluid pouches; fasteners that hold tubings in place)?
- Meets requirements of different procedures (e.g., amount of blood loss; length of procedure; resistance to abrasion)?
- Presence of stitching that could allow penetration of microorganisms or liquids?
- Environmental and waste disposal concerns?
- Quality control of production and sterilization by manufacturers that is consistent with requirements for performance?
- Quality variations over time?
- High loss and damage rates?
- Satisfactory cost/benefit ratio?

For reusables (yes or no)
- Verifiable laundry standards?
- Chance of wear and tear defects in materials?
- Resterilization process verified by quality assurance standards?
- Potential for presence of pyrogens in resterilized materials, particles trapped in interstices, detrimental effects on barrier qualities by procedures used in laundering?
- Consistency in performance over the product's lifetime?
- Accurate method in place for calculating number of launderings?
- Able to use in custom kits and packs?
- Adequate storage space?
- Reliable just in time (JIT) deliveries?

For reusables (other considerations)
- Costs of laundry, energy, chemicals and detergents, labor, sterilization.
- Quantity needed to provide a consistent supply.
- Contribution of laundry wastes to the water supply and environmental issues of pollution (9, pp. 30-31).

Choosing between single-use and reusable gowns and drapes is a complex exercise. Because there are advantages and disadvantages to both systems, there are no simple formulas for weighing the trade-offs. When making decisions, it is most important to balance the considerations of barrier properties and effectiveness, safety for patients and personnel, infection prevention issues, and the environment. Decision makers in healthcare facilities must continually evaluate priorities, ask questions, and then decide which products are best for each situation and each facility (9, pp. 26-27).

ASSISTED GOWNING
Drying of Hands after Scrubbing
The scrub person opens the sterile towel and places it in the surgical team member's hands. The scrub person's hands should not touch the surgical team member's scrubbed hands (7, p. 252). The scrubbed hands are nested in the sterile absorbent towel to avoid contact with less clean arm areas. Movement of the towel is from hands to elbows. The towel is discarded (8, p. 13).

Gowning
The gown is unfolded carefully by the scrub person, holding the gown at the neckline. The scrub person offers the gown to the surgical team member, forming a protective cuff of the neck and shoulder area of the gown (7, p. 252). The hands of the surgical team member are extended into and through the opened gown. Arms are kept above waist level. Ungloved, nonsterile hands must not touch the sterile outside of the front of the gown. The gown is closed in back by the nonscrubbed circulating nurse. The scrub person assists the gowned surgical team member in gloving, or the gowned person gloves himself or herself. Gloved hands are held above waist level. If required, closure of gown ties is now completed (8, pp. 14-15).

- Gowns are only considered sterile from the operative area upward to within 1 to 2 inches of the neckline and around the sleeves; in other words, the areas that the gowned and gloved person can see himself or herself. The backs and armpits of gowns are not considered sterile even if the gown is a wraparound type (8, p. 18).
- Gowns are considered sterile only from the chest to the level of the sterile field in the front and from 2 inches above the elbows to the cuffs on the sleeve. Only the area that can be seen in front down to the level of the sterile field is considered sterile. The back of the gown is not under constant observation and therefore must be considered contaminated (7, pp. 230-231).

NONASSISTED GOWNING
Drying of Hands after Scrubbing
The gown, towel, and gloves should be opened on a separate sterile field, away from the back table and operative area. After scrubbing, the surgical team member picks up the sterile towel from the gown

table, taking care not to drip water onto the sterile gown, gloves, or wrapper. A slight bending forward will prevent the towel from touching the nonsterile attire of the surgical team member. Hands and arms are sequentially dried, using a fresh area of the towel for each arm and using oscillating motions of the arms. Motions are from hands to elbows, without bringing the towel back down over the already-dried hands (8, pp. 19-20; 7, p. 247).

Gowning

The gown is picked up and unfolded by touching only the inside. Scrubbed clean hands must not touch the sterile outer side of the gown, gloves, or wrapper. Arms and hands are extended into the gown to the cuff level only for closed gloving or through the cuffs for open gloving. The stockinette cuffs will be enclosed beneath sterile gloves. The stockinette is absorbent and retains moisture; therefore this part of the gown does not provide a microbial barrier. Also, the cuffs are areas of friction and can cause microbial contamination. Once the gown is on, the initial back closure is done by the circulating nurse, the gloving takes place, and closure of the gown is completed (8, pp. 21, 28; 7, p. 230).

CHANGING LEVELS AT THE STERILE FIELD

- Sterile persons are aware of the height of team members in relation to each other and the sterile field. Changing levels at the sterile field is avoided. The gown is considered sterile only down to the highest level of the sterile tables. If a sterile person must stand on a platform to reach the surgical site, the standing platform should be positioned before this person steps up to the draped area. Sterile persons should sit only when the entire procedure will be performed at a seated level. If one person on the team sits, the entire team should be seated (7, p. 231).
- Scrubbed persons should avoid changing levels and should be seated only when the entire surgical procedure will be performed at that level (3, p. 344).

CHANGING GOWNS DURING A PROCEDURE

Occasionally a contaminated gown must be changed during a surgical procedure. The neck and waist portions of the gown should be unfastened by the circulating nurse. The gown is always removed before the gloves. Grasped at the shoulders, the gown is pulled off inside out. The gloves are removed using a glove-to-glove and then a skin-to-skin technique. If only a sleeve is contaminated, a sterile sleeve may be put on over the contaminated one (7, p. 252).

REMOVING USED GOWNS

- At the end of the procedure, used gowns are untied by the circulating nurse and removed inside out. The outside of the used gown and gloves are considered contaminated and should not come in contact with clean scrub apparel or hands (8, pp. 35-36).
- Gowns are always removed before the gloves at the end of the surgical procedure (7, p. 252).
- Used gloves are also removed inside out, using the dirty-to-dirty and clean-to-clean technique. Gown and gloves are discarded before leaving the room (8, pp. 37-38).

References

1. American Society of Testing Materials (ASTM): *Standard test method for resistance of materials used in protective clothing to penetration by synthetic blood, F1670-98,* West Conshohocken, Penn, 1998, Author.
2. American Society of Testing Materials (ASTM): *Standard test method for resistance of materials used in protective clothing to penetration by bloodborne pathogens using Phi-X174 bacteriophage penetration as a test system, F1671-976,* West Conshohocken, Penn, 1997, Author.
3. AORN: Recommended practices for maintaining a sterile field. In *Standards, recommended practices and guidelines,* Denver, 2000, Author, pp 341-346.
4. AORN: Recommended practices for use and selection of barrier materials for surgical gowns and drapes. In *Standards, recommended practices and guidelines,* Denver, 2000, Author, pp 267-270.
5. Association for the Advancement of Medical Instrumentation (AAMI): *Selection of surgical gowns and drapes in health care facilities,* AAMI Technical Information Report (TIR), No 11-1994, Arlington, Va, 1994, Author.
6. Beekman SE, Henderson DK: Controversies in isolation policies and practices. In Wenzel RP, editor: *Prevention and control of nosocomial infections,* ed 3, Baltimore, 1997, Williams & Wilkins, pp 71-84.
7. Fortunato N: *Berry & Kohn's operating room technique,* ed 9, St Louis, 2000, Mosby.
8. Gruendemann BJ: *Illustrated guide to surgical scrubbing, gowning, and gloving,* ed 1, Arlington, Tex, 1990, Johnson & Johnson Medical.
9. Gruendemann BJ: Reusables versus disposables. In *Healthcare waste management: a template for action,* Cary, NC, 1999, INDA, Association of the Nonwoven Fabrics Industry, pp 24-31.
10. Gruendemann BJ, Fernsebner B: *Comprehensive perioperative nursing,* vol 1, *Principles,* Boston, 1995, Jones & Bartlett.
11. Koch F: Surgical gowns and drapes: selecting the best fit for your facility, *Surgical Services Management* 4(2):25-28, 1998.
12. Mangram AJ, Hospital Infection Control Practices Advisory Committee (HICPAC), Centers for Disease Control and Prevention: Guideline for prevention of surgical site infection, 1999, *Infect Control Hosp Epidemiol* 24(4):247-278, 1999. (Reprinted, in part, in Appendix B.)
13. McCullough EA: Methods for determining the barrier efficacy of surgical gowns, *Am J Infect Control* 21:368-374, 1993.

14. Mews PA: Establishing and maintaining a sterile field. In Phippen ML, Wells, MP: *Patient care during operative and invasive procedures,* Philadelphia, 2000, WB Saunders, pp 61-93.

15. Occupational Safety and Health Administration: Occupational exposure to bloodborne pathogens: final rule, *Federal Register* 56(235):64175-64182, 1991.

16. Stull JO, Pournoor KJ: Using the ASTM test methods to select surgical gowns and drapes, *Surgical Services Management* 4(2):13-15, 19-22, 1998.

17. Telford GL, Quebbeman EJ: Assessing the risk of blood exposure in the operating room, *Am J Infect Control* 21(12):351-356, 1993.

18. Wong ES: Surgical site infections. In Mayhall CG, editor: *Hospital epidemiology and infection control,* Baltimore, 1996, Williams & Wilkins, pp 154-175.

Suggested Reading

1. Beck WC: Aseptic barriers in surgery: their present status, *Arch Surg* 116:240-244, 1981.

2. Beck WC, Collette TA: False faith in the surgeon's gown and surgical drape, *Am J Surg* 85:125-126, 1952.

3. Belkin NL: Are "impervious" surgical gowns really liquid-proof? *Bull Am Coll Surg* 84(8):19-21, 36, 1999.

4. Granzow JW et al: Evaluation of the protective value of hospital gowns against blood strike-through and methicillin-resistant *Staphylococcus aureus* penetration, *Am J Infect Control* 26:85-93, 1998.

5. Herwaldt LA et al: Infection control guidelines for the operating suite. In Abrutyn E, Goldmann DA, Scheckler WE, editors: *Saunders infection control reference service,* Philadelphia, 1998, WB Saunders, pp 551-582.

6. Laufman HA, Eudy WW, Vandermoot AM: Strike-through of moist contamination by woven and nonwoven surgical materials, *Ann Surg* 181:857-862, 1975.

7. Leonas KK: Effect of laundering on the barrier properties of reusable surgical gown fabrics, *Am J Infect Control* 26(5):495-501, 1998.

8. Leonas KK, Jinkins RS: The relationship of selected fabric characteristics and the barrier effectiveness of surgical gown fabrics, *Am J Infect Control* 25(1):16-23, 1997.

9. Lewis JA, Brown PL: Breaking the comfort barrier in impervious gowns, *Surgical Services Management* 4(2):29-38, 1998.

10. Pournoor J: New scientific tools to expand the understanding of aseptic practices, *Surgical Services Management* 6(4):28, 31-32, 2000.

11. Ritter MA, Marmion P: The exogenous sources and controls of microorganisms in the operating room, *Orthop Nurs* 7(4):23-28, 1988.

12. Roy MC: The operating theater: a special environmental area. In Wenzel RP, editor: *Prevention and control of nosocomial infections,* ed 3, Baltimore, 1997, Williams & Wilkins, pp 515-538.

13. Smith JC, Nichols RJ: Barrier efficacy of surgical gowns, *Arch Surg* 26:756-761, 1991.

F. Gloving

Gloving is the final step in the scrubbing, gowning, and gloving process. Sterile gloves are worn to permit the wearer to handle sterile supplies or tissues of the operative wound. Sterile gloves establish a shield that protects the patient from contamination by flora from the hands of healthcare workers (HCWs). Nonsterile gloves are used to protect the hands of nonsterile personnel from contamination (13, p. 10).

GLOVE CHOICE

Strength, durability, and glove thickness are primary factors to consider when choosing a glove for barrier protection. The tensile strength of gloves (measured in megapascals) is the amount of stretch or pull required to rupture the glove material. Elongation, expressed as a percentage of the original length at the time the glove ruptures, is the length a glove material can be stretched before it breaks (21, p. 408). Other tests (e.g., protein and powder levels) may be performed as well (21, pp. 407-408).

The minimum requirements of the American Society of Testing Materials differ for strength and durability for each glove material because the chemical composition and molecular structure of glove materials differ (21, p. 408).

Latex

Latex gloves are made of natural rubber latex (NRL) and comprise approximately 98% of the gloves used in surgical settings. Latex gloves

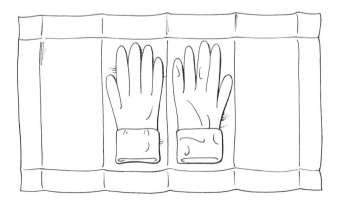

are thin, fit tightly, provide excellent tactility, and are minimally fatiguing to the wearer's hands (16, p. 660).

- The microporosity of many latex gloves allows some air and water to permeate across the latex membrane. For this reason, the wearer may feel that latex gloves are cooler to wear than synthetic gloves (16, p. 660).
- The inherent material properties of NRL gloves include softness, porosity, variable thickness, composition of the glove membrane, sensitivity to material fatigue, and chemical deterioration. The softness of NRL makes the glove vulnerable to sharp and pointed objects. However, the flexibility of NRL somewhat diminishes the probability that sharp objects will pierce the glove membrane (16, p. 662).
- When tested in a simulated use situation, latex gloves had failure rates of 0% to 1%. They should be used when there is a potential for blood and body fluid exposure (21, p. 410).

Synthetic Nonlatex

Synthetic nonlatex gloves do not contain latex proteins but may contain additives similar to those found in latex gloves. They are made of nitrile, neoprene, styrene, or butyl. These gloves are more expensive than latex gloves. They generally provide an effective barrier and a better tactile sensitivity than vinyl gloves (3, p. 25).

- Nitrile provides protection while affording the latex-sensitive person a necessary synthetic alternative (21, p. 409).
- Presently several types of non-NRL gloves, including synthetic rubber, are available. These are significantly improved in quality and can be a good substitute for NRL-sensitized individuals (27, p. 7).
- When tested in simulated use conditions, nitrile gloves had failure rates of 3% to 4%. Nitrile gloves are comparable to NRL gloves in barrier performance, both unused and in simulated patient care procedures (21, p. 409).

Vinyl

The barrier properties of vinyl gloves generally have been found to be inferior to those of NRL gloves (14, p. 146).

- Vinyl gloves, which are made of polyvinyl chloride, do not contain NRL proteins or chemicals. They allow as much tactile sensitivity as latex gloves but are not considered as good a barrier (3, p. 25).
- Different vinyl gloves vary in performance, but all degrade quickly with use (21, p. 409).

- No difference in the failure rates of NRL and vinyl gloves was detected when gloves were tested straight out of the box with no manipulation. However, after manipulation intended to simulate in-use conditions, vinyl gloves failed 12% to 61% of the time (21, p. 409).

Vinyl is an appropriate barrier for nonrigorous, low-risk procedures of short duration. However, latex should be the glove of choice for high-risk situations involving potential exposure to bloodborne pathogens (21, p. 410).

The awareness of surgical staff of proper glove usage needs to be increased. Information, including technical measures and infection control indications, should be obtained on available products so that surgical staff members have the opportunity to make informed choices. Having the information on technical data and clinical issues helps the user to be better prepared to make a selection (11, p. 26; 10, pp. 28-29; 9, pp. 22-28).

CLOSED GLOVING

Closed gloving is defined as the method of donning sterile gloves whereby the scrubbed hands remain inside the cuffs and sleeves of the gown until the cuffs of the gloves are secured outside of the gown's sleeves and cuffs. The bare hands are not exposed outside the gown's sleeves and cuffs (13, p. 11). The closed gloving method is preferred over other gloving methods, except when changing a glove during a surgical procedure or when donning gloves for procedures not requiring a gown. Properly executed, the closed gloving method affords assurance against contamination when gloving oneself because no skin is exposed in the process (5, p. 247).

Gloves are packaged in pairs with an everted cuff on each to protect the outside of the sterile glove during donning. In closed gloving the gloves are handled through the fabric of the gown sleeves. The hands are not extended through the cuffs until the gloves are being pulled into place (13, pp. 10-11).

The closed gloving procedure is as follows: The glove wrapper is opened, and sterile gloves are exposed. This is accomplished by working inside the cuffs of the gown and leaning forward to avoid contact with unsterile surfaces or wrapper edges hanging below a sterile zone. If right-handed, it may be best to don the left glove first, using the dominant right hand to begin the procedure. The palm of the left hand inside the gown sleeve is open and facing up. The left glove is grasped at the cuff, lifted up from the wrapper and placed over the palm area, thumb down. The cuff edges are grasped by both hands through the gown sleeves. With a broad sweeping motion, the glove

134 SECTION THREE Preparation of Personnel

is placed over the cuff of the gown. During this motion, the left hand begins advancing through the cuff of the gown. The glove is advanced by grasping both gown and glove and then positioned so it extends above the cuff and the cuff seam all the way around. The second glove is donned using the same steps (7, pp. 22-26).

OPEN GLOVING

The open gloving technique is used for changing a glove or the gown and gloves during a surgical procedure. This technique is also used for procedures not requiring a gown, when only sterile gloves are worn, such as for intravenous cutdown or suturing lacerations. This method uses a skin-to-skin, glove-to-glove technique. The hands, although scrubbed, are not sterile and must not touch the outside of the gloves (5, p. 250).

The open gloving procedure is as follows: The right glove is grasped with the left hand on the fold. The glove is picked up as the person donning the glove steps back from the sterile area. The right hand is inserted into the glove. The glove is pulled on. The cuff is left still folded as it was in the glove wrapper. The fingers of the gloved right hand are slipped under the folded cuff of the left glove. The glove is picked up. The left hand is inserted in the left glove and pulled on by the gloved hand. The fingers of the left hand are slipped under the cuff of the right glove. The glove is pulled upward while avoiding inward rolling of the cuff edge (5, p. 251; 19, p. 76).

ASSISTED GLOVING

The assisted gloving procedure is as follows: The right hand is usually donned first. The scrub person grasps the glove under the inverted cuff. The glove cuff is stretched open with both hands. The palm side is toward the person being gloved. The hand of the team member is assisted into the glove by gently pulling the glove upward as the hand is inserted. The cuff of the gown is covered completely. Care should be taken not to pull the glove too high on the sleeve, causing the person being gloved to pull the gown sleeve partially out of the glove. Since the hand has touched the inside of the glove and the gown sleeve has had contact with the inside of the glove, the gown cuff is considered contaminated. The process is repeated for the other hand. The person being gloved may assist by stretching the glove cuff outward at the same time the scrubbed person is opening the glove (19, p. 77).

REGLOVING

• If the integrity of the glove is compromised (e.g., punctured), it should be changed as promptly as safety permits (18, p. 262).

- If a glove becomes contaminated or torn during a procedure, it must be replaced. One method of replacement is to place a sterile glove over the contaminated one. This procedure can be done quickly, uses the open gloving technique, and avoids exposure of the inside of the gloves and ungloved hands near the sterile field (19, p. 77).
- A common method for removing a contaminated glove is to have a nonsterile person, wearing nonsterile gloves, remove the glove, touching only the glove and not the gown. The cuff of the gown, not considered sterile at this point, is not brought over the hand when using this method (7, p. 31; 23, p. 687; 1, p. 342). Then for regloving, the preferred method is for one member of the sterile team to glove another. If this is not possible, the new sterile glove should be applied by the open gloving method (1, p. 342).

GLOVE REMOVAL

- Used gloves are removed inside out, using the dirty-to-dirty and clean-to-clean technique (7, p. 37).
- The cuffs usually turn down as the gown is pulled off the arms. The glove cuff of the left hand is then grasped by the right hand, and the glove is pulled off inside out. The scrubbed person slips the ungloved fingers of the left hand under the cuff of the remaining glove and pulls it off while turning it inside out (5, p. 253).
- Hands should be washed following glove removal (5, p. 253).

DOUBLE GLOVING

Double gloving is beneficial for protecting the wearer from blood exposures; thus wearing two pair of gloves may be indicated for some procedures (e.g., orthopedics, vascular procedures). In a clinical study the overall glove failure rate was 51% when a single pair of gloves was worn. When a second pair was added, the failure rate dropped to 7%. The probability of glove failure increased with surgical exposure time (4, p. 501).

- Double gloving has been shown to reduce hand contact with patients' blood and body fluids when compared with wearing only a single pair of gloves (18, p. 262).
- Double gloving is recommended for procedures in which the patient is known to be infected with a transmissible virus and for major procedures lasting more than 2 hours or having a blood loss of greater than 100 ml. For people who choose not to double glove, frequent monitoring of the hands to check whether they are contaminated by blood is recommended.

Changing gloves at regular intervals is also recommended (4, p. 501).

• Surgical team members may perceive double gloving as a problem for comfort as well as for decreased dexterity, which may in turn increase the likelihood of injury. However, surgical site infections have been linked to glove puncture and tears (22, p. 529).

• Because gloves are more permeable to blood than to water, double gloves are suggested in situations in which the HCWs will be in contact with a large amount of blood or body fluids. In situations in which punctures are likely such as during orthopedic surgery, extra strength gloves or glove liners are suggested (8, p. 200).

SPECIAL CONSIDERATIONS
Latex Allergy

Latex allergy is a reaction to certain proteins in latex rubber. Exposure can also occur through direct contact with the NRL material and by latex particles carried on glove powder in the air. Airborne latex proteins bound to this powder become inhaled antigens and also can inoculate surgical tissues and contaminate suture materials, instruments, drapes, and sponges (2, p. 605).

Increasing the exposure to latex proteins increases the risk of developing allergic symptoms. The three most often cited reactions to latex are irritation, type IV allergic contact dermatitis (chemical allergy), and type I hypersensitivity (protein allergy) (2, p. 605).

1. *Irritation* is a nonallergenic condition to which all individuals are susceptible. The first symptoms are usually redness, itching, or burning of the affected area. More intense symptoms appear where the glove is tight or where it imparts repetitive friction such as at the knuckles, on the back of the hands, or at the wrists. Irritation can be caused by either synthetic or NRL gloves, which may contain the same additives (28, pp. 48, 52).

2. *Type IV* is a delayed hypersensitivity or allergic contact dermatitis. The wearer is allergic to contact sensitizers in the gloves. Only genetically programmed individuals who respond to these chemicals will experience this type of reaction. Repeated exposure to the specific chemical sensitizer increases the asymptomatic level of sensitization until a critical threshold level is reached. Subsequent exposure will elicit a reaction (28, p. 52).

3. *Type I* immediate and anaphylactic reaction is an allergy caused by proteins such as those in NRL. Repeated exposures

to these allergens increases the asymptomatic level of sensitization in genetically susceptible individuals until a threshold is reached. Additional exposure may result in itching, tingling, swelling of lips or eyelids, runny nose, watery eyes, and hives. Symptoms may progress to tightening of the throat, abdominal cramping, asthma, tachycardia, and shock. These symptoms may occur within seconds to an hour after exposure (28, p. 52).

Body sweat inside latex gloves may make latex proteins more soluble. The proteins are absorbed through the skin and can sensitize the wearer to the foreign particles (2, p. 605).

To reduce the incidence of allergic reactions to latex, the amount of contact with NRL products should be reduced.

- Nonlatex gloves should be used for activities that are not likely to involve contact with infectious materials (e.g., damp dusting of operating room furniture). However, appropriate barrier protection is necessary when handling infectious materials. Powder-free gloves with reduced protein content may reduce the risk of latex allergy (20, p. 2).
- Appropriate work practices can be used to reduce the risk of a reaction to latex. These include not using oil-based hand creams or lotions that can cause glove deterioration, washing hands with a mild soap following removal of gloves, and drying hands thoroughly (20, p. 2; 24, p. 24).
- The use of latex gloves for barrier protection may need to be reevaluated in light of the increasing number of individuals who are sensitive to latex (15, p. 1037). With the increase in numbers of HCWs experiencing type I hypersensitivity to latex, synthetic alternatives are being developed that exhibit barrier protection comparable to latex without the accompanying latex proteins (21, p. 406; 6, pp. 30-33; 17, pp. 20-28).
- Persons with type I hypersensitivty to NRL must use latex-free alternatives and need to be aware of the potential for barrier integrity limitations with the various synthetic choices (21, p. 406).
- Individuals who must wear gloves routinely should be given low-protein gloves as early as possible in their careers to avoid becoming sensitized to latex. HCWs who are latex sensitive should wear synthetic gloves, and all HCWs must wear powder-free products (28, p. 52).
- HCWs should use nonlatex gloves when caring for patients with known sensitivity to latex (15, p. 1037).
- Using latex avoidance for sensitized patients is critical. Equally important is a powder-free environment. If the environment is

contaminated with latex proteins, no intervention can effectively eliminate exposures. The knowledge that a small amount of latex (0.6 ng/m^3 is the threshold for sensitization) is all that is needed to trigger reactions in some sensitized individuals makes a powder-free environment imperative to prevent sensitization and eliminate reactions in sensitized patients and HCWs (26, p. 30).

- Principles of risk management support the use of latex allergy precautions for patients who have a definite latex allergy and those who have experienced a contact dermatitis suspected to have been caused by latex (25, pp. 475-493).

Glove Failure

Any time the barrier effectiveness of a surgical glove is compromised, it is considered glove failure. A surgical glove fails the instant it ceases to be an effective barrier against microorganisms, body fluids, or toxic substances (16, p. 662).

- Although perioperative staff members depend on surgical gloves to provide adequate barrier effectiveness, studies report that surgical gloves fail more than 50% of the time during operative procedures. Gloves develop holes, cuts, tears, or punctures under normal work conditions. These are often not detected until hands are inspected at the conclusion of the operative procedure (16, p. 660).
- During clinical use, latex surgical gloves undergo a series of chemical and physical stresses that change their composition and properties. Pulling, twisting, or pinching, as well as exposure to fluids, fat, and chemical substances, change barrier effectiveness (16, p. 662).
- Operative procedures that require high degrees of dexterity and use a variety of surgical instruments (e.g., saws, drills, other sharp instruments), as well as longer durations of glove usage, tend to decrease the barrier properties of latex gloves (16, p. 662).
- As a surgical procedure lengthens, transient flora removed by scrubbing quickly reestablishes itself on the hands because of the accumulation of moisture and sweat. As a result, a punctured glove on scrubbed hands will allow resident flora to contaminate the wound. A surgical team member who realizes that a glove has been punctured should change it as quickly as safety permits (22, pp. 528-529).

Puncture-Resistant Gloves

The potential benefits of wearing puncture- or laceration-resistant gloves or finger guards to prevent percutaneous injuries to the hands should be assessed. The acceptance of this approach in the surgical setting remains low because of the loss of tactile sensation and the less-than-total puncture resistance of most available barrier materials. Nevertheless, given the predictable distribution of percutaneous injuries to the hands, puncture-resistant gloves or finger guards should be evaluated for selective use under circumstances in which the risk of injury to the hands is greatest and in a manner that interferes least with tactile sensation (e.g., worn selectively on the nondominant hand) (12, pp. 992-993).

References

1. AORN: Recommended practices for maintaining a sterile field. In *Standards, recommended practices and guidelines,* Denver, 2000, Author, pp 341-346.
2. Beezhold DH, Kostyal DA, Wiseman J: The transfer of protein allergens from latex gloves, *AORN J* 59(3):605-613, 1994.
3. Burt S: What you need to know about latex allergy, *Nurs Manage* 30(8):20-25, 1999.
4. Fogg D: Clinical issues, *AORN J* 70(3):501, 1999.
5. Fortunato N: *Berry & Kohn's operating room technique,* ed 9, St Louis, 2000, Mosby.
6. Glove Manufacturers' Product Index, *Infection Control Today* 4(4):30-33, 2000.
7. Gruendemann BJ: *Illustrated guide to surgical scrubbing, gowning, and gloving,* ed 1, Arlington, Tex, 1990, Johnson & Johnson Medical.
8. Gruendemann BJ, Fernsebner B: *Comprehensive perioperative nursing,* vol 1, *Principles,* Boston, 1995, Jones & Bartlett.
9. Hamann C, Long T, Rodgers P: Cost effective glove selection, *Infection Control Today* 4(4):22-28, 2000.
10. Higa L: Glove manufacturers' product matrix, *Infection Control Today* 3(2):28-29, 1999.
11. Huggins KA: A hand in the glove: lessons learned about glove selection, *Infection Control Today* 3(2):20-26, 1999.
12. Jagger J, Bentley M, Tereskerz P: A study of patterns and prevention of blood exposures in OR personnel, *AORN J* 67(5):979-996, 1998.
13. Johnson & Johnson Medical: *Study guide: surgical scrubbing, gowning and gloving,* Arlington, Tex, 1996, Author.
14. Korniewicz DM et al: Integrity of vinyl and latex procedure gloves, *Nurs Res* 38(3):144-146, 1989.
15. Korniewicz DM, Kelly KJ: Barrier protection and latex allergy associated with surgical gloves, *AORN J* 61(6):1037-1040, 1995.
16. Korniewicz DM, Rabussay D: Surgical glove failures in clinical practice settings, *AORN J* 66(4):660-668, 1997.
17. Korniewicz DM: Glove technology for a new millennium, *Infection Control Today* 3(9):20-28, 1999.
18. Mangram AJ, Hospital Infection Control Practices Advisory Committee (HICPAC), Centers for Disease Control and Prevention: Guideline for prevention of surgical site infection, 1999, *Infect Control Hosp Epidemiol* 24(4):247-278, 1999. (Reprinted, in part, in Appendix B.)
19. Mews PA: Establishing and maintaining a sterile field. In Phippen ML, Wells, MP: *Patient care during operative and invasive procedures,* Philadelphia, 2000, WB Saunders, pp 61-93.

20. National Institute for Occupational Safety and Health (NIOSH): *Latex allergy: a prevention guide,* 2000, www.cdc.gov/niosh (accessed 2000).

21. Rego A, Roley L: In-use barrier integrity of gloves: latex and nitrile superior to vinyl, *Am J Infect Control* 27(5):405-410, 1999.

22. Roy M: The operating theater: a special environmental area. In Wenzel RP, editor: *Prevention and control of nosocomial infections,* Baltimore, 1997, Williams & Wilkins, pp 515-538.

23. Smith CD: Clinical issues, *AORN J* 59(3):687, 1994.

24. Springthorpe S, Sattar S: Handwashing: what can we learn from recent research? *Infection Control Today* 2(4):20-25, 1998.

25. Steelman VM: Latex allergy precautions: a research-based protocol, *Nurs Clin North Am* 30(3):475-493, 1995.

26. Steelman VM: Is it really necessary to go powder free? *Infection Control Today* 2(5):32-39, 1998.

27. Tomazic VJ: Glove quality and selection criteria, *Food and Drug Admin User Facility Reporting Bull* Issue 19, p. 7, 1997.

28. Truscott W: Examination glove selection criteria, *Infection Control Today* 2(5):40-56, 1998.

Suggested Reading

1. Association for Professionals in Infection Control and Epidemiology (APIC): *Glove use for healthcare providers: hand covering and barrier protection,* Washington, DC, 2000, Author (pamphlet).

2. Donaldson K: Creating a latex-safe environment: converting to powder-free gloves, *Infection Control Today* 4(2):32-34, 2000.

3. icanPREVENT (www.icanPREVENT.com): A description of surgeons' gloves and patient examination gloves (Product Information, Synopsis). Updated 6/27/00, accessed 6/30/00.

4. Yassin MS et al: Latex allergy in hospital employees, *Ann Allergy* 72(3):245-259, 1994.

Surgical Practices

A. Sterile Techniques and Practices

Surgical asepsis (sterile techniques and practices) forms the foundation of most procedures carried out in surgical settings. Perioperative personnel use their knowledge of surgical asepsis every day in clinical practice. Most perioperative nursing courses and textbooks begin by educating students and new perioperative nurses about the thought processes and behaviors that are referred to as sterile technique or surgical asepsis. These practices are so ingrained in perioperative personnel that they can almost be likened to a unique culture that exists "behind the closed doors of the operating room (OR)." The fact is, asepsis is truly at the heart of infection prevention and control in surgical settings.

Regardless of whether a surgical procedure is being performed in the OR or another surgical setting, all personnel involved have responsibilities for adhering to aseptic practices. Principles of asepsis are applicable to practices in clinical areas other than an OR, but they are practiced in their "purest" form in a surgical (OR) environment.

This chapter examines surgical asepsis and also its rituals. Principles of asepsis that guide practice are discussed and explained. Controversial practices that are related to asepsis (e.g., using a "skin knife," having food and chewing gum in the OR) are also examined.

SURGICAL ASEPSIS

Surgical asepsis is often thought of as rules, infractions, and shoulds. It is assumed sometimes that surgical site infection (SSI) rates and trends are directly and causally related to aseptic practices. This is an oversimplification since the causes of SSIs are multifactorial and of-

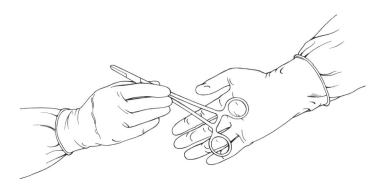

ten difficult to describe or study. Nonetheless, sterile techniques are highly important in the care of surgical patients and do make a difference in eventual outcomes of surgical procedures.

Rigorous adherence to the principles of surgical asepsis by all scrubbed personnel is the foundation of SSI prevention. Others who work in close proximity to the sterile surgical field, such as circulating nurses and anesthesia personnel who are separated from the field only by a drape barrier, also must abide by these principles (10, p. 263).

PROTECTIVE SURGICAL ASEPSIS

The term *protective asepsis* is applicable to the surgical environment. It clearly defines the fundamental principles of infection control that have their origins in good hygiene, sanitation, and asepsis. Protective asepsis focuses defensive measures on both patients and personnel (8, p. 11). Both Standard Precautions and Universal Precautions provide guidelines for protective practices.

Protective measures are a mainstay of aseptic practices in surgical settings and have received renewed interest, especially with the advent of bloodborne pathogens and the growing significance of antibiotic-resistant organisms. As Lister admonished, protective surgical asepsis requires that "we see sepsis with our mental eye" and furthermore that we understand and believe in the principles of microbiology, epidemiology, and protection (8, p. 11).

Protective surgical asepsis can be condensed into five basic do's:

1. *First, do no harm.* First stated by Florence Nightingale, "First, do no harm" directs personnel to ensure that no additional bioburden or contaminants are introduced at the time of surgery. The surgical site is protected by all means possible.

2. *Remove contaminants and harmful microorganisms.* The protective practices of simple handwashing, proper decontamination of instruments and equipment, appropriate attire, and thorough sanitation and cleaning of surgical areas and surfaces go far in the removal of contaminants.

3. *Destroy harmful microorganisms.* Destruction processes include cleansing and scrubbing with antimicrobial agents, use of high-level disinfectants, and sterilization.

4. *Shield and separate when removal or destruction is not possible.* Shielding and separation are necessary when contact with potentially harmful agents is inevitable. Personal protective equipment serves as a barrier to contact by touch. Separation of clean from contaminated can be accomplished by physical space and distance and by barriers such as walls, traffic patterns, protective clothing, handwashing, and decontamina-

tion and reprocessing of instruments and equipment. Isolation of instruments used in nonsterile body parts (e.g., stomach, intestines, vaginal cuff) is an another example of separation of clean from contaminated items.

5. *Dispose of contaminants properly.* Proper containment and disposal of contaminated items, materials, sharps, and waste complete the protective asepsis cycle. Scientific rationale; factual data; and local, state, and federal regulations should dictate the promulgation of waste disposal policies (8, pp. 11-12).

Surgical asepsis, along with its protective aspects, consists of judicious use of rituals, a sense of surgical conscience—integrity, honesty, and outspokenness concerning shortcomings regarding a sterile field—and the ability to blend these into effective everyday practices (8, p. 13). A surgical conscience, the motivating internal value system, guides the daily aseptic practices of personnel in a surgical setting (9, p. 189).

RITUALS

Knowledge of surgical practices is important for internalizing surgical aseptic principles, but it is not enough. These principles must be organized into meaningful learning units. Rituals—established procedures that are performed in a set manner—have a place in perioperative practice and do help to organize information into easy-to-understand learning units (8, p. 12).

Rituals define boundaries, act as rules, set limits on behavior, and assist healthcare workers (HCWs) to label actions as right or wrong. Most rituals in perioperative practice concern avoiding contamination of the patient from the outside, and they express beliefs and values as symbolized by the words *clean, dirty,* and *contaminated.* Rituals categorize and help to clarify unclear boundaries (8, p. 12).

Rituals in the OR assist in communicating asepsis by providing guidelines; most of these guidelines are embedded in logic. Rituals not only define and maintain sterility but also assist OR team members to "see within the mind's eye." For example, the top of a table covered by a sterile table cover is considered to be sterile, and anything falling over the edge of that table is considered to be nonsterile. This assumption cannot be substantiated by bacteriological studies. Moreover, common sense tells us that microbes do not know to stop at a table's edge. But by defining, through aseptic principles, where sterility begins and ends, we are more equipped to "see areas of sterility with the mind's eye," and therefore can apply the principles to all surgical practices (6, p. 6).

Rituals also provide freedom in the OR. To the patient's benefit, certain traditions become so much a part of the OR team's practice that attention can then be focused on the surgical procedure (6, p. 6).

Relying solely on data collection to determine practices limits patient care. Perioperative nursing, like all other patient care, is not just a science but also an art. Until clinical data are available that support or disclaim established traditions, it may be wise to hold onto some customs that we believe have kept patients safe. Not all aseptic practices in the OR have been—and many probably cannot ever be—scientifically validated (6, pp. 6, 8). But all personnel must be involved in studies that continue to test the validity of practices that can be scientifically observed and measured.

Rituals may or may not affect SSI rates. Although the efficacy of many rituals has not been established, even though increasingly being studied, these procedures *do protect the patient* from environmental sources of infection and *are worth following for reasons of improved and disciplined OR personnel behavior* (8, p. 12).

Rituals have their greatest use in teaching surgical personnel. Grouped together, surgical asepsis procedures create order, consistency, and an aura of cleanliness and sterility. They also facilitate teaching and learning. An inherent danger with rituals, however, is that HCWs might believe that the ritualistic acts are ends in themselves rather than the means of achieving optimal and safe patient outcomes. Nevertheless, rituals may both aid efficiency and enable team members to function in circumstances of ambiguity. And rituals do, perhaps, perpetuate the mystical component of surgery, especially as perceived by the public (8, p. 12).

PRINCIPLES OF ASEPSIS

Sterile technique is the basis of modern surgery. The patient is the center of the sterile field, which includes personnel wearing sterile attire and the areas of the patient, OR bed, and furniture that are covered with sterile drapes (7, p. 230). All individuals involved in surgical interventions have a responsibility to provide and maintain a safe environment. Adherence to aseptic practices aids in fulfilling this responsibility. Preoperative, intraoperative, and postoperative aseptic practices are implemented to minimize wound contamination (2, p. 341).

Scrubbed Personnel
- Personnel in the sterile area must remain in that area throughout the procedure (8, p. 13).
- Scrubbed persons function within a sterile field (2, p. 341).
- Sterile persons are gowned and gloved. Sterile persons touch only sterile items or areas; nonsterile persons touch only nonsterile

items or areas. Sterile team members maintain contact with the sterile field by means of sterile gowns and gloves (7, p. 231).

- Once gowned and gloved, sterile team members may not lower forearms below waist level. When passing each other, scrubbed persons always pass front to front or back to back (8, p. 13).
- Scrubbed personnel should keep their arms and hands within the sterile field at all times. Contamination of hands and arms may occur when they are moved below the level of or outside of the sterile field (2, p. 344).
- Scrubbed persons should avoid changing levels and should be seated only when the entire surgical procedure will be performed at that level. If levels are changed, exposure of the nonsterile portion of the surgical gown is likely (2, p. 344).
- If one person on the team sits, the entire team should be seated (7, p. 231). NOTE: This is not always feasible or reasonable (e.g., a vaginal hysterectomy in which a surgeon is seated and a scrub person stands to hold retractors).
- When wearing a gown, only the area that can be seen in front down to the level of the sterile field should be considered sterile; usually this does not extend below waist level. Hands are never placed under the upper arms because of perspiration in the axillary region (7, pp. 230-231).
- Walking outside the periphery of the sterile field or leaving and returning to the OR in sterile attire increases the potential for contamination (2, p. 344).
- Talking is kept to a minimum in the surgical area (8, p. 13).
- Talking is kept to a minimum in the presence of a sterile field to reduce the spread of moisture droplets (2, p. 344).
- Movement and air currents around a sterile area are kept to a minimum to avoid contamination (8, p. 13).

Nonscrubbed (Nonsterile) Personnel

- Personnel who are not scrubbed must stay in areas at the periphery of the OR, a distance away from sterile areas (8, p. 12).
- Nonscrubbed personnel should face sterile fields on approach, should not walk between two sterile fields, and should be aware of the need for distance from the sterile field (2, pp. 344-345).
- Nonsterile personnel should not lean or reach over a sterile field (8, p. 12).

Margin of Safety

- A margin of safety, that small extra distance or space, is useful as a guide to movement and adherence to aseptic principles (8, p. 12).

- The boundaries between sterile and nonsterile areas are not always rigidly defined (e.g., the edges of wrappers on sterile packages and caps on solution bottles). But when opening sterile packages, a margin of safety is always maintained. The inside of a wrapper is considered sterile to within 1 inch of the edges (7, p. 232).
- The flaps on peel-open packages should be pulled back, not torn, to expose the sterile contents. The contents should not be permitted to slide over the edge. The inner edge of the heat seal is considered the line of demarcation between sterile and nonsterile. The sterile item should be presented to the scrub person; "flipping" can cause air turbulence, and the item may miss its mark and fall to a nonsterile area (7, p. 232). NOTE: For a reference on the acceptability of flipping, see the section on opening sterile items in the chapter "Opening and Setting Up Rooms."
- Sterile persons allow a wide margin of safety when passing nonsterile areas, and nonsterile persons allow a wide margin of safety when passing sterile areas (7, p. 233).
- Nonsterile persons should maintain a distance of at least 1 foot (30 cm) from any area of the sterile field. Nonsterile persons never walk between two sterile areas (e.g., between sterile instrument tables). The circulator restricts to a minimum all activity near the sterile field (7, p. 234).

Sterile Items in the Sterile Field

- Sterile fluids, equipment, and supplies are opened and delivered to the sterile surface without contacting the edges of the wrapper or container; only sterile articles may touch sterile surfaces (8, p. 12).
- Items used within a sterile field should be sterile. These items should be opened, dispensed, and transferred to the sterile field by methods that maintain sterility and integrity (2, pp. 342-343).
- When opening wrapped supplies, nonscrubbed personnel should open the wrapper flap farthest away from them first, and the nearest wrapper flap last. All wrapper edges should be secured when presenting supplies to the sterile field (2, p. 343).
- Sterile items should be presented to the scrub person or placed securely on the sterile field (2, p. 343).
- When dispensing solutions to the sterile field, the solution receptacle should be held by the scrub person or placed near the table edge. Solutions should be poured slowly, and any remaining fluids discarded; reuse of opened containers may contaminate the solutions. Edges of containers are considered contaminated after the cap has been removed (2, p. 343).

- The edges of anything that encloses sterile contents are considered nonsterile (7, p. 232).
- The sterile field is created as close as possible to the time of use (7, p. 233; 10, p. 268).
- The sterile field should be maintained and monitored constantly (2, p. 343).

Tables and Sterility

- Tables are sterile only at and above table level (8, p. 12).
- Only the top of a sterile, draped table is considered sterile. The edges and sides of a drape extending below table level are considered nonsterile. Anything falling or extending over the table edge, such as a piece of suture, is nonsterile. Cords, tubings, and other materials are secured on the sterile (operative) field with a nonperforating clip to prevent them from sliding over the edge (7, p. 231).

Sterile Drapes

- Sterile drapes should be used to establish a sterile field and should be handled as little as possible, avoiding rapid movements of draping material that create air currents on which dust, lint, and droplet nuclei can migrate (2, p. 342).
- Sterile drapes, towels, and covers are folded in such a way that a generous cuff is provided for handling by personnel in the sterile area (8, pp. 12-13). The gloved hands are therefore protected by cuffing the draping material over the gloved hand to avoid contamination (2, p. 342).
- A sterile person first covers the near side of any nonsterile surface with sterile drapes and then covers the far side (8, p. 13).
- The placement of sterile drapes from the prepped incision to unprepped areas minimizes the risk of contamination of the sterile field (2, p. 342).
- Once placed in position, sterile drapes are never moved or shifted (8, p. 13).

   For more information, the reader is referred to the chapter "Draping."

Doubtful Sterility

- If there is any doubt about the sterility of an item, it is considered contaminated (8, p. 13).
- There is no compromise with sterility. In clinical practice an item is considered either sterile or nonsterile. OR personnel must maintain the high standards of sterile technique that they know

are essential. Every individual is accountable for his or her own role in infection control (7, p. 235).

OTHER PRACTICES

Various practices that relate to asepsis are controversial but are frequent topics of discussion among perioperative personnel. Some practices have been studied and the results are referenced, some need more analysis and research, and perhaps some can never be studied in depth.

Use of a Skin Knife

A *skin knife* is defined as the traditional first scalpel or knife blade used to make the initial skin incision in a surgical procedure. If a skin knife is used, it is discarded after the skin incision is made and a second, new blade is used for the deeper layers. The skin knife is usually not used again, except perhaps only to lengthen the original skin opening or to make a stab wound through the skin for insertion of a drain. Is the use of a skin knife effective in reducing bacterial counts, especially in deeper tissues, and is its use justified?

- Instruments used in contact with skin are discarded and not reused (7, p. 234).
- Because skin cannot be sterilized, the initial skin knife is considered contaminated regardless of whether the surgeon has cut through an adhering plastic skin drape. The skin incision exposes deep skin flora of the hair follicles and sebaceous gland ducts (7, p. 467). This probably will not bring microbes from skin into deep tissues, however (4, p. 415).
- One study evaluated knife blades used in clean surgeries (no clean-contaminated or contaminated procedures) performed in both conventional and laminar airflow ORs. There was no statistical difference in the amount of contamination on skin knives versus deep knives, but there was a definite statistical difference in numbers of knife blades contaminated in conventional versus laminar airflow ORs (13, p. 25).
- Some European studies have indicated that pathogenic organisms are not carried into the wound by the skin knife; therefore the use of a separate skin knife is unnecessary. Other studies demonstrated that separate skin knives do not affect the rate of surgical wound infections (12, p. 234).
- Removing the skin knife after the initial incision remains an acceptable technique in many institutions. However, the final decision on the use of a separate skin knife, is the surgeon's preference (12, p. 234).

Food in the Operating Room

• Work practice controls should include prohibition of eating, drinking, smoking, applying cosmetics or lip balm, and handling contact lenses in work areas where there is reasonable likelihood of occupational exposure to bloodborne pathogens. Activities involving hand-to-nose, hand-to-mouth, or hand-to-eye action can contribute to indirect transmission (1; 3, p. 336; 11, p. 64176).

• Eating should *never* be allowed in the OR during a surgical procedure. Eating and drinking are prohibited in areas where contact with blood or other potentially hazardous material is possible (7, p. 197; 11, p. 64176).

Chewing Gum in the Operating Room

• AORN believes that chewing gum in the OR setting should be avoided. Jaw movement beneath the surgical mask causes friction between skin and the mask, leading to shedding of the epidermis, known as scurf. Scurf can become airborne, can be transported to any area of the surgical field, and can fall into the open wound (5, p. 693).

• A surgical mask collects bacteria from the nasopharyngeal airway of the wearer. With chewing motion and excessive talking, exhaled droplets containing bacteria are more likely to be expelled into the environment (5, p. 693).

References

1. AORN Online Clinical Practice FAQ Database, 1999: www.aorn.org/_results/clinical.asp (accessed 2000).
2. AORN: Recommended practices for maintaining a sterile field. In *Standards, recommended practices and guidelines,* Denver, 2000, Author, pp 341-346.
3. AORN: Recommended practices for Standard and Transmission-Based Precautions in the perioperative practice setting. In *Standards, recommended practices and guidelines,* Denver, 2000, Author, pp 335-340.
4. Atkinson LJ, Fortunato NH: *Berry & Kohn's operating room technique,* ed 8, St Louis, 1996, Mosby.
5. Conner R: Clinical issues, *AORN J* 71(3):688-694, 2000.
6. Crow S: It's second nature to me now, *Today's OR Nurse* 12(10):6-8, 1990.
7. Fortunato N: *Berry & Kohn's operating room technique,* ed 9, St Louis, 2000, Mosby.
8. Gruendemann BJ: Surgical asepsis revisited, *Today's OR Nurse* 12(10):10-13, 1990.
9. Gruendemann BJ, Fernsebner B: *Comprehensive perioperative nursing,* vol 1, *Principles,* Boston, 1995, Jones & Bartlett.
10. Mangram AJ, Hospital Infection Control Practices Advisory Committee (HICPAC), Centers for Disease Control and Prevention: Guideline for prevention of surgical site infection, 1999, *Infect Control Hosp Epidemiol* 24(4):247-278, 1999. (Reprinted, in part, in Appendix B.)
11. Occupational Health and Safety Administration: Occupational exposure to bloodborne pathogens: final rule, *Federal Register* 56(235):64175-64182, 1991.

12. Petersen C: Clinical issues, *AORN J* 71(1):234, 237-239, 2000.
13. Ritter MA, Marmion P: The exogenous sources and controls of microorganisms in the operating room, *Orthop Nurs* 7(4):23-28, 1988.

Suggested Reading

1. Fogg DM: Clinical issues, *AORN J* 71(6):1270-1277, 2000.
2. Hagen L, Lane C: The sterile field, *Infection Control Today* 3(8):46, 48, 1999.
3. Hasselgren PO et al: One instead of two knives for surgical incisions: does it increase the risk of postoperative wound infection? *Arch Surg* 119(8):917-920, 1984.
4. Laufman H: Environmental concerns in surgery in the 1990s, *Today's OR Nurse* 12(10):41-48, 1990.
5. Laufman H: What's happened to aseptic discipline in the OR? *Today's OR Nurse* 12(10):15-19, 1990.

B. Cleaning and Decontamination of Surgical Instruments

All surgical instruments and other items used for surgical procedures must be meticulously cleaned and decontaminated in preparation for storage or packaging or for a disinfection or sterilization process. This chapter applies to most surgical instruments, although cleaning of endoscopes is covered in the chapter "Disinfection." The cleaning of powered equipment is discussed in this chapter.

Cleaning is the removal of visible dirt, soil, organic matter, or any other foreign material from an instrument or object. *Cleaning* and *precleaning* are terms that generally mean the removal rather than the killing of microorganisms. Cleaning precedes disinfection or sterilization.

Cleaning is normally accomplished with water, mechanical action, and detergents or enzymatic products. Failure to remove foreign material (e.g., lubricants, soils) from an object is likely to render disinfection or sterilization ineffective. For example, studies have shown that manual and mechanical cleaning of endoscopes achieves approximately a 4-log reduction of contaminating organisms. Thus cleaning alone is very effective in reducing the number of microorganisms present on contaminated equipment (4, p. 315). It is the single most important step in making a medical device ready for reuse (5, p. 15).

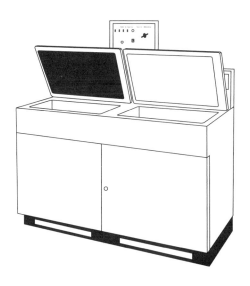

Decontamination is a process (physical, chemical, or both) that renders an inanimate object safe for handling by removing or reducing contamination from infectious organisms or other harmful substances. *Cleaning* and *decontamination* are terms that are often used synonymously. If soil, organic material, and microorganisms are removed from an item, cleaning and decontamination have both taken place, rendering an item safe to handle. Cleaning and decontamination can take place by thorough manual cleaning or by the use of a automated system, such as a washer/decontaminator.

Sometimes enzymatic products are used during the cleaning and decontamination process. *Enzymatic detergents or products* are catalysts that enhance and help to loosen dried or hard-to-remove debris that cannot be rinsed or wiped off the object. These enzymatic products are usually added to the water or cleaning solution. Manufacturers' instructions should be followed.

Whenever possible, cleaning by machine is preferable to hand cleaning because it offers greater protection for the worker. Hand cleaning requires manipulation of devices, which offers opportunity for glove and skin punctures and the possibility of disease transmission. However, some devices cannot tolerate automated cleaning, and some facilities may not have mechanical processes available in all areas where they could be used (5, p. 15). Because of the processes involved, the cleaning and decontamination area must be separated from the area where instrument sets are reassembled, wrapped, and sterilized (2, pp. 228-229).

CLEANING AND DECONTAMINATION PROCESS

- Instruments should be kept free of gross soil during the surgical procedure. Wiping instruments with sterile water-moistened sponges helps to eliminate gross soil. Irrigating cannulated or lumened instruments with sterile water during the surgical procedure removes residues and prevents tissue damage. Saline must not be used since it causes deterioration of instrument surfaces (1, p. 283).
- Stainless steel or other metal devices must never be soaked in saline or bleach (sodium hypochlorite) solutions because the chloride ions in these two substances will cause rapid metal corrosion (5, p. 15).
- Before leaving an operating room (OR), used instruments should be wiped clean of gross blood and debris. Soaking instruments in a basin with sterile water and enzymatic detergents may begin in the OR at the end of the procedure. All instruments are opened and placed in a carrier for transportation to the processing area.

Reusable sharps are placed in a separate puncture-resistant container (2, pp. 228-229).

- Initial decontamination of instruments should begin immediately after the completion of any invasive procedure; automated or manual methods of equal effectiveness should be used for the initial step in the decontamination of instruments after use (1, p. 283).

MANUAL CLEANING

Manual cleaning may be recommended by the instrument manufacturers or by facility policy for delicate or other hard-to-clean instruments, or for instruments that may not withstand automated processes. During manual cleaning personnel should wear protective attire and be protected from aerosolization, splashing of infectious materials, and injuries from sharp objects (1, p. 284).

Personal Protective Attire

- Scrub suits are worn under a moisture-impervious gown or jumpsuit. A mask and goggles or a full-face shield is worn to prevent contamination from splashes and aerosolization. Heavy-duty, long-cuffed gloves are worn during all decontamination activities. Clothing worn in the decontamination area is removed before leaving the area for another part of the hospital. Employers should provide healthcare workers (HCWs) with an environment that minimizes their exposure to body fluids (2, p. 229).
- The instruments should be submerged in warm water, with appropriate detergent, and be cleaned and rinsed while submerged (1, p. 284).

Selection of a Cleaner/Detergent

- Detergents should facilitate loosening of debris and not be damaging to instruments; enzymatic cleaners are frequently used.
- Detergents should be low sudsing and rinse off without leaving a residue.
- Detergents with a pH less than 7, on the acid side, are best for inorganic debris such as urine or hard water scale. Detergents with a pH of more than 7, on the alkaline side, are best suited for organic soil such as blood, fat, and feces.
- Manufacturers of stainless steel instruments generally recommend using detergents that have a slightly alkaline pH (between 7 and 10 on a 14-point pH scale).
- Manufacturers' instructions should be followed (5, p. 15).

NOTE: Topical antimicrobials intended for skin antisepsis should not be used for cleaning instruments.

AUTOMATED WASHERS
Washer-Decontaminators

Washer-decontaminators may be used, processing instruments through several cycles. Prerinsing in an enzymatic detergent solution effectively removes all visible debris except ointment, thus proving to be an acceptable alternative to manual cleaning (1, pp. 283-284).

Washer-Decontaminators/Disinfectors

Both single-chamber and multi-chamber tunnel units are relatively new in the U.S. decontamination market. Cycles vary but usually include prerinse, wash, and rinse processes. The last rinse is with very hot water (180° to 195° F [70° to 76° C]). Other cycle options may be ultrasonic cleaning or chemical disinfectant rinses. Manufacturers' instructions must be followed.

- Instruments should be taken apart at the point of use and arranged in an orderly fashion in mesh-bottom trays so that all surfaces are exposed to the action of the automatic cleaner (1, p. 284).
- This washer-decontamination process renders items clean and at least disinfected at an intermediate level, making them safe for handling but not immediately ready for reuse (5, pp. 16-17).
- Total hands-off processing is possible with these units. Most machines can also be used for reprocessing sterilization container system components and utensils such as basins and bedpans.

ULTRASONIC CLEANERS

Ultrasonic cleaners use high-intensity sound waves produced by ultrasonic transducers (cavitation) to remove microorganisms and organic debris from soiled instruments (3, p. 48). Ultrasonic cleaners provide a cleaning process and *not* a thermal or chemical *biocidal* (disinfection or sterilization) process. Instruments are not considered safe to handle after ultrasonic cleaning alone (2, p. 230).

- Instruments must be free of gross debris before being placed in an ultrasonic cleaner (5, p. 16).
- Ultrasonic cleaners facilitate the removal of small particles and debris from instrument crevices (1, p. 284).
- Dissimilar metals should not be combined in this cleaner (1, p. 284).

- A detergent can be added to the water to enhance the cleaning process. The water may also be heated. Wash water should be changed when visibly dirty and at least every 8 hours to minimize microbial growth (5, p. 16).
- Instruments should be rinsed and dried after ultrasonic cleaning (1, p. 284).
- If washer-decontaminators are used to process instruments, ultrasonic processes may not be necessary (1, p. 284).
- The concept of when to use the ultrasonic cleaner is controversial. Some facilities use the process for every instrument after initial rinse and before mechanical cleaning, others use it for hinged instruments before mechanical cleaning, and others use it after mechanical washing and sterilization (e.g., after the use of washer-sterilizers). However, debris that remains on items after sterilization is very difficult to clean. Also, aerosols created by ultrasonic processing may possibly pose a hazard to HCWs (2, p. 230).

POWERED EQUIPMENT

- Powered equipment must be cleaned and decontaminated after use, since debris left on the instruments hinders the sterilization process, rendering the equipment nonsterile after processing, and may interfere with proper functioning.
- Powered equipment and air hoses should not be immersed in water or placed in automated or ultrasonic cleaners because permanent damage may result from water entering the internal mechanisms.
- Air hoses and power cords must be inspected for damage or wear; hoses should remain attached to hand pieces during cleaning.
- Manufacturers' instructions should be followed for cleaning; all traces of detergent solution should be rinsed from equipment.
- Air hoses should be wiped with clean, damp cloths; excess water should be removed from equipment. The outside of equipment should be dried with lint-free towels (1, pp. 285-286).

PREPARATION OF CLEANED AND DECONTAMINATED INSTRUMENTS

- Instruments should be inspected for cleanliness, proper functioning and alignment, defects, sharpness of cutting edges, looseness of pins, and chipping of plated surfaces.
- Instruments with moving parts must be lubricated with water-soluble lubricants after being cleaned, according to manufacturers' instructions.

- Instruments are dried before being stored. Delicate and sharp instruments should be protected according to manufacturers' written instructions (1, p. 285).

Properly cleaned and decontaminated instruments are safe to handle and ready for storage or packaging, or for disinfection or sterilization.

References

1. AORN: Recommended practices for the care and cleaning of surgical instruments and powered equipment. In *Standards, recommended practices and guidelines,* Denver, 2000, Author, pp 283-288.
2. Gruendemann BJ, Fernsebner B: *Comprehensive perioperative nursing,* vol 1, *Principles,* Boston, 1995, Jones & Bartlett.
3. Muscarella LF: Ultrasonic cleaning, *Surgical Services Management* 5(6):48-54, 1999.
4. Rutala WA: APIC guidelines for selection and use of disinfectants, *Am J Infect Control* 24(4):313-342, 1996.
5. Schultz JK: Decontamination: recommended practices. In Reichert M, Young JH: *Sterilization technology for the health care facility,* ed 2, Gaithersburg, Md, 1997, Aspen, pp 10-20.

Suggested Reading

1. Finkelstein LE, Mendelson MH: Infection control: how to safely clean surgical instruments, *Am J Nurs* 97(6):59, 1997.
2. Gassel M: Too clean or not too clean, *Infection Control Today* 4(1):36, 38, 77, 2000.
3. Higa LS: Cleaning the impossible: success with difficult-to-clean instruments, *Infection Control Today* 3(8)16, 18, 1999.
4. Jennings J, Manian FA, editors: *APIC handbook of infection control and epidemiology,* ed 2, Washington, DC, 1999, Association for Professionals in Infection Control and Epidemiology.
5. Lind N: Cleaning by hand, *Infection Control Today* 4(1):64-65, 2000.

C. Disinfection

Disinfection is a process that eliminates many or all pathogenic microorganisms, with the exception of bacterial spores, from inanimate objects and surfaces. In contrast, *sterilization* is a process that destroys all forms of microbial life, including spores, from inanimate objects and surfaces. (See the chapter "Sterilization.")

Factors shown to affect disinfection effectiveness are:
- Previous cleaning of the object
- Type and level of microbial contamination
- Concentration and exposure time to the germicide
- Physical configuration of the object (e.g., contains crevices, hinges, lumens)
- Temperature and pH of the disinfection process

Bacterial spores are the most resistant pathogens to germicides, followed, in descending order, by *mycobacteria, nonlipid or small viruses, fungi, vegetative bacteria,* and *lipid or medium-sized viruses.* The last category, lipid viruses, is the least resistant—in other words, the most susceptible—to the action of chemical germicides and therefore these viruses are the easiest on this list to kill. The diagram on p. 160 represents the general susceptibility of groups of microorganisms to disinfectants, from most to least resistant.

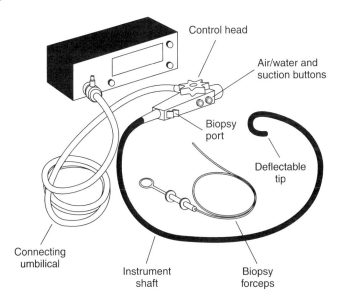

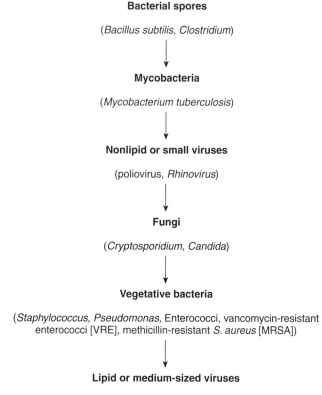

Bacterial spores

(*Bacillus subtilis, Clostridium*)

Mycobacteria

(*Mycobacterium tuberculosis*)

Nonlipid or small viruses

(poliovirus, *Rhinovirus*)

Fungi

(*Cryptosporidium, Candida*)

Vegetative bacteria

(*Staphylococcus, Pseudomonas,* Enterococci, vancomycin-resistant
enterococci [VRE], methicillin-resistant *S. aureus* [MRSA])

Lipid or medium-sized viruses

(hepatitis B virus, hepatitis C virus, human immunodeficiency virus, herpes
simplex, *Cytomegalovirus,* respiratory syncytial virus, Ebola virus) (21, p. 314)

ITEM CLASSIFICATION

The Spaulding classification system, devised in 1968, divides patient
care items into three categories according to the nature of the items,
the manner in which they are to be used, and the degree of risk of
infection involved in their use.

Critical Items

Critical items present a high risk of infection if contaminated with
any microorganisms, including bacterial spores. These items enter
the sterile tissues or vascular system of the body or will have blood
flowing through them. *Sterilization is required for critical items*
(21, pp. 315-316). Examples of critical items are surgical instruments, implants, needles, some endoscopy accessories (biopsy forceps, cytology brushes), catheters (vascular and urinary), laparoscopes and arthroscopes, and some dental instruments.

Semicritical Items

Semicritical items are those that contact mucous membranes or non-intact skin. These items should *minimally receive high-level disinfection* (HLD) before use. Semicritical devices contaminated with the hepatitis B virus (HBV), human immunodeficiency virus (HIV), or *Mycobacterium tuberculosis* should receive a minimum of HLD. *Semicritical items may also be sterilized* (6, p. 221). Some semicritical items (hydrotherapy tanks and thermometers) may require only *intermediate-level disinfection* (ILD), which inactivates *M. tuberculosis,* vegetative bacteria, and most viruses and fungi but not necessarily bacterial spores (21, p. 316). Examples of semicritical items are gastrointestinal (G-I) endoscopes, bronchoscopes, laryngoscopes, endotracheal tubes, respiratory and reusable anesthesia equipment, dialyzers, transducers, diaphragm-fitting rings, tonometers, thermometers, and hydrotherapy tanks if used on patients with nonintact skin (e.g., burn patients).

Noncritical Items

Noncritical items come in contact with intact skin (not mucous membranes). Sterility is not critical because intact skin is an effective barrier to most microorganisms. *Noncritical items should receive* ILD *or low-level disinfection* (LLD) *or cleaning* (21, pp. 315-316; 6, p. 222). Examples of noncritical items are stethoscopes; blood pressure and tourniquet cuffs; electrocardiogram leads; bedpans; linens; and environmental surfaces such as tabletops, bedside stands, furniture, and floors.

LEVELS OF DISINFECTION
High-Level Disinfection

HLD is a process that eliminates all microorganisms except large populations of bacterial endospores (15, pp. 212-213). HLD is achieved by immersing an item for a specified period in a chemical agent that has been cleared by the U.S. Food and Drug Administration (FDA) as a disinfectant or sterilant (6, p. 223). Some high-level disinfectants can, with prolonged contact, be classified as sterilants. HLD is used with semicritical and some critical items (15, pp. 212-213). Thermal HLD is accomplished with pasteurization (discussed later in this chapter).

Intermediate-Level Disinfection

ILD inactivates vegetative bacteria, including mycobacteria, most viruses, and fungi, but not necessarily bacterial spores. ILD is used for some semicritical items, such as thermometers, and hydrotherapy tanks that are used for patients with nonintact skin, and also some noncritical items (21, pp. 315-317). ILD is achieved by immersion in a specified chemical agent or by surface disinfection.

Low-Level Disinfection

LLD, used on noncritical items, kills most vegetative bacteria and some viruses and fungi, but not tubercle bacilli or bacterial spores (15, pp. 212-213). LLD is accomplished by surface cleaning or disinfection or by washing or cleaning an item using specific chemical agents.

Table 4-1 summarizes the disinfection and sterilization processes for each Spaulding classification category.

CHEMICAL DISINFECTANT AGENTS

Liquid chemical germicides (chemical disinfectants and sterilants), products used to reprocess critical and semicritical devices, are regulated by the FDA. General purpose disinfectants for low-level and general purpose disinfection are regulated by the U.S. Environmental Protection Agency (EPA) (1, p. 2). Information on FDA clearance is included in the chapter "Sterilization."

Chemical Disinfectants/Sterilants Used Primarily for HLD

Exposure time = ≥20 minutes; 12 minutes for Cidex OPA.
- 2% to 3.4% glutaraldehyde (Cidex, Metricide, Omnicide, Wavicide, Procide, Cetylcide-G, MedSci)
- 0.08% peroxyacetic acid and 1% hydrogen peroxide (Peract)
- 7.5% hydrogen peroxide/0.85% phosphoric acid (Sporox)
- 0.95% glutaraldehyde/1.64% phenol/phenate (Sporicidin)
- 0.2% peracetic acid (Steris 20) (only cleared for use with Steris 1 Processor)
- 0.55% orthophthalaldehyde (Cidex OPA—is FDA cleared as a high-level disinfectant only and not as a sterilant)
- Demand-release chlorine dioxide (limited use)

Intermediate-Level Disinfectants

Exposure time = ≤10 minutes.
- Ethyl or isopropyl alcohol (70% to 90%)
- Phenolic germicidal detergent solution
- Iodophor germicidal detergent solution
- Sodium hypochlorite (5.25% household bleach) 1:50 dilution (1000 ppm)

Low-Level Disinfectants

Exposure time = ≤10 minutes.
- Ethyl or isopropyl alcohol (70% to 90%)
- Phenolic germicidal detergent solution
- Iodophor germicidal detergent solution

TABLE 4-1	Summary of Disinfection and Sterilization Processes		
Definition	**Items and Devices**	**Processes Used***	**Products Used**
Critical items		*Sterilization*	*Liquid chemical, sporicidal sterilants*
Enter vascular systems or sterile tissues, or have blood flowing through them	Surgical instruments Implants Needles Catheters (vascular and urinary) Laparoscopes and arthroscopes (if sterilization is not feasible, should receive at least high-level disinfection) Endoscopy accessories (e.g., biopsy forceps, cytology brushes) Some dental instruments (e.g., scalers, burs, forceps, scalpels)	Heat (steam, dry) Chemical gas, vapor, plasma Radiation	Aldehydes (e.g., glutaraldehyde) Hydrogen peroxide Peracetic acid Peracetic acid with hydrogen peroxide NOTE: longer exposure times required for sterilization than disinfection

Continued

EPA, Environmental Protection Agency; *FDA*, U.S. Food and Drug Administration; *ppm*, parts per million.
*Using FDA- and EPA-approved products and following manufacturers' instructions.

TABLE 4-1 Summary of Disinfection and Sterilization Processes—cont'd

Definition	Items and Devices	Processes Used*	Products Used
Semicritical items			
Contact with mucous membranes or nonintact skin	Gastrointestinal endoscopes Laryngoscopes Bronchoscopes Endotracheal tubes Respiratory therapy and anesthesia equipment Dialyzers Diaphragm-fitting rings Cryosurgical probes Some dental instruments (e.g., amalgam, condensers, air/water syringes)	*High-level disinfection* ≥20-min minimum required; 12 min for orthophthalaldehyde (Cidex OPA) NOTE: sterilization may be preferred	*Wet pasteurization or liquid chemicals* Aldehydes (e.g., glutaraldehyde) Cidex OPA Hydrogen peroxide Peracetic acid Peracetic acid with hydrogen peroxide Chlorines (sodium hypochlorite, 1000 ppm, 1:50 dilution)
	Hydrotherapy tanks (if used for patients with intact skin) Tonometers (recommend 5-min immersion) Thermometers (alcohols preferred)	*Intermediate-level disinfection* ≤10-min immersion NOTE: with label claim for tuberculocidal activity	Alcohols (70%-90%) Iodophors Phenolics Chlorines

Noncritical items

Category	Items	Level of disinfection	Agents*
Contact with intact skin (not mucous membranes)	Stethoscopes Blood pressure and tourniquet cuffs Electrocardiogram leads Bedpans Linens	*Intermediate-level disinfection* NOTE: required if contamination is heavy or there is significant blood contamination	Alcohols (70%-90%) Iodophors Phenolics Chlorines
	Environmental surfaces (e.g., tabletops, bedside stands, furniture, floors)	*Low-level disinfection* NOTE: adequate for most noncritical items and surfaces	Alcohols (70%-90%) Iodophors Phenolics Chlorines (sodium hypochlorite, 100 ppm, 1:500 dilution) Quaternary ammonium compounds ("quats")

EPA, Environmental Protection Agency; *FDA*, U.S. Food and Drug Administration; *ppm*, parts per million.
*Using FDA- and EPA-approved products and following manufacturers' instructions.

- Sodium hypochlorite (5.25% household bleach) 1:500 dilution (100 ppm)
- Quaternary ammonium germicidal detergent solution (disinfectant, not antiseptic, concentration) (21; 24; 10; 11)

Readers are highly encouraged to seek out the cited references for further information on selection and use of these disinfectants.

Disinfectants That Inactivate Hepatitis B Virus

- 2% glutaraldehyde; 0.55% orthophthalaldehyde
- Iodophor (80 ppm)
- 70% isopropyl alcohol
- 80% ethyl alcohol
- 0.3% hydrogen peroxide
- Sodium hypochlorite 1:100 dilution (500 ppm)

Disinfectants That Inactivate Human Immunodeficiency Virus

- 2% glutaraldehyde; 0.55% orthophthalaldehyde
- 0.3% hydrogen peroxide
- 50% ethyl alcohol
- 70% isopropyl alcohol
- Phenolics
- Sodium hypochlorite 1:1000 dilution (50 ppm)

Environmental surfaces in rooms of patients with HBV or HIV infection can be cleaned with any EPA-approved hospital disinfectant, including quaternary ammonium germicidal disinfectants (16, p. 165)

CONTROVERSIES AND GRAY AREAS

Except for some well-defined inclusions in the previous lists, there are several gray areas (e.g., endoscopes could be included either in the list of critical items or semicritical items). Many discussions have centered on the reasons for their inclusion in one or the other categories. There are also controversies regarding the appropriate chemicals/disinfectants for each category of items.

A case in point involves the Occupational Safety and Health Administration (OSHA) Bloodborne Pathogen Rule and the recommendations for disinfectants. Although the OSHA standard does not specify types of disinfectants or procedures for their use, an OSHA compliance document suggested that a tuberculocidal agent (phenolic, chlorine) was necessary to clean blood spills on noncritical surfaces (e.g., to kill the HBV and HIV organisms). It is known that nontuberculocidal disinfectants such as quaternary ammonium compounds inactivate HBV. Thus this directive was clearly overkill and caused consternation among manufacturers and housekeeping personnel (21, p. 323).

Questions regarding this issue came from the manufacturers of disinfectants approved by the EPA as disinfectants for HIV and HBV. These companies had asked whether EPA-registered products would be "appropriate disinfectants" under OSHA's bloodborne pathogens standard. An earlier compliance memo stated that the products could be used under limited conditions, when HIV and HBV were the only pathogens of concern.

Following receipt of information offering further support for use of these products, OSHA reconsidered and decided that the compliance document that requires the use of EPA-registered tuberculocidal disinfectants and/or a diluted bleach solution to decontaminate work surfaces would be expanded to include EPA-registered disinfectants that are labeled as effective against HIV and HBV, provided such surfaces have not become contaminated with agents or volumes or concentrations of agents for which higher levels of disinfection are recommended.

Furthermore, the 1997 OSHA directive states that all blood must be removed and the surface cleaned thoroughly before applying the disinfectant *and* that the surface must be left wet with the disinfectant for 30 seconds for HIV and 10 *minutes* for HBV! It is virtually impossible to wet a surface for 10 minutes when doing surface disinfection; therefore, even though this OSHA directive does give more latitude in choice of products for decontaminating noncritical surfaces, the contact times required are not reasonable and in many ways cause more confusion than previously envisioned (18; 19).

Because of the inherent dilemmas involved in choosing and using disinfectants wisely, it is of supreme importance for the clinician to read labels and label claims carefully, be familiar with regulations that set parameters for use, and obtain results of clinical studies that support manufacturers' claims. Written instructions for use from the manufacturer must be carefully followed.

PROCESS

The infection control department should provide input into selection of disinfectants for surgical settings (15, p. 213).

Items should be thoroughly cleaned and decontaminated before disinfection.

Types of chemical cleaners chosen should be appropriate to the cleaning/decontamination procedure being used. Chemical cleaners include enzymatic cleaners, manual detergent cleaners, ultrasonic cleaning compounds, and cleaners for washers/decontaminators. Manufacturers' recommendations for use of chemical cleaners should always be followed. After the cleaning process, instruments should be rinsed and dried before being subjected to the HLD process (6, pp. 222-223). NOTE: The importance of adequate cleaning before disinfection cannot be overestimated. With all forms of disinfection, the condition of the items before disinfection is perhaps the most important determinant of the outcome of the process. Items must be *thoroughly* cleaned before being subjected to a disinfection process. Failure to remove soil, organic material, and microorganisms from an object will render disinfection ineffective. Therefore inadequate cleaning before disinfection can pose serious problems to the disinfection process. The reader is encouraged to review the chapter "Cleaning and Decontamination of Surgical Instruments" in this text before beginning any disinfection process.

CHEMICAL HIGH-LEVEL DISINFECTION

A chemical agent cleared by the FDA as a disinfectant/sterilant should be used (6, p. 223). NOTE: If contact time is long enough—usually 10 hours—a disinfectant could be used as a sterilant, if approved for that purpose. Contact time is one of the most important variables differentiating sterilization from HLD with a specific chemical.

Factors that influence efficacy of chemical agents include the following:

- Organic load present on the items to be disinfected
- Type and level of microbial contamination
- Precleaning, rinsing, and drying processes used on the item before disinfection
- Active ingredients of the chemical agents
- Concentration of the chemical agents
- Exposure time to the chemical agents
- Physical configuration of the item (e.g., crevices, hinges, lumens)
- Temperature and pH of the chemical agent
- Hardness of the water
- Presence of surfactants (6, pp. 223-224)

Immersion Recommendations

- Items should be completely immersed in the disinfectant solution according to recommendations of established infection control practice and/or the product manufacturer. Lumens of endoscopes should be flushed with the germicide and the entire item completely immersed for the designated exposure time (6, p. 224).
- Recommendations for immersion (exposure) times range from 12 to 45 minutes. Exposure time to achieve HLD in 2% activated

glutaraldehyde is a minimum of 20 minutes at 68° F (20° C) when used on meticulously cleaned devices (21, p. 318; 25).

Vapor Exposure

- Personnel should use protective apparel when using chemical disinfectants, including those with vapors. Apparel can include eyewear (to prevent splashing to eyes), gloves specific to handling chemicals, masks (fumes may still be inhaled), and moisture-repellent or splash-proof skin protection (6, p. 225).
- Chemical disinfectant vapors may be toxic, even those scented for aesthetic reasons. Covered containers and adequate ventilation reduce personnel exposure to fumes (6, p. 225).
- Glutaraldehyde fumes may be irritating to eyes, nose, and throat. The permissible exposure limit is 0.2 ppm per exposure (or a ceiling level of 0.05 ppm); a dosimeter can determine the airborne concentration of fumes. Glutaraldehyde should be used only in closed containers and well-ventilated areas (14, p. 196; 24, p. 71).

HOSPITALS AT RISK?

Are hospitals at risk of being cited or penalized if they do not follow FDA label claims for extended immersion times of, for example, 2% glutaraldehyde (Cidex)? Hospitals are not under the purview of the FDA; therefore labeling information, including use instructions, are matters that are usually discussed only between the FDA and manufacturers. The consensus of a committee of the American Public Health Association was that if hospitals wish, they can follow the Association for Professionals in Infection Control and Epidemiology (APIC) guideline (20 minutes at room temperature, 68° F [20° C]) for HLD of semicritical devices (e.g., endoscopes) with glutaraldehyde and that there is no justification for penalties by a federal or accreditation agency. Exposure times for solutions other than 2% glutaraldehyde should be based on recommendations of manufacturers and/or established infection control practice regarding HLD (22; 20).

On another note, there is no evidence that HLD of endoscopes such as laparoscopes and arthroscopes increases the risk of infection compared with sterilization of these devices (22, p. 378).

ENDOSCOPES

Both endogenous and exogenous microbes cause infections related to endoscopic procedures. Infections caused by *endogenous* microbes occur when the microflora colonizing the mucosal surfaces of the G-I or respiratory tracts gain access to the bloodstream or other normally sterile body sites as a consequence of the procedure. *Exogenous* microorganisms most frequently associated with transmission during endoscopy have been gram-negative bacteria or mycobacteria, transferred from previous patients or the inanimate environment via contaminated endoscopes or accessories. Common factors associated with transmission have been inadequate manual cleaning, inadequate exposure of surfaces to disinfectant, inadequate rinsing and drying, and use of automated endoscope reprocessors (AERs) (2, pp. 138-139). Failure to follow recommended cleaning and disinfection procedures is often the reason for transmission of disease from contaminated endoscopes. Improperly disinfected endoscopes have been implicated in multiple nosocomial outbreaks (23, p. 545; 28).

Troubling concerns about endoscope-related infections include the ability of bacteria to form *biofilms* that adhere to internal channels of endoscopes, resulting in ineffective disinfection. Another issue relates to nontuberculous mycobacteria and other microorganisms growing in tap water and causing nosocomial infections, especially in immunocompromised persons; inactivation of these microorganisms is of great importance. Although concern has been raised, there are no reported cases of HIV, *Clostridium difficile, Cryptosporidium,* or Creutzfeldt-Jakob disease cross-transmission from endoscopic equipment (2, pp. 140-141).

Endoscopes are complex devices with narrow, long lumens; crevices; channels; ports; cords; controls; and accessories that present challenges for cleaning and reprocessing. Acute angles and rough, porous, occluded surfaces allow for collection of organic material. This potential for sequestered organic material poses the greatest risk of cross-contamination for patients undergoing endoscopic procedures. If parts and accessories such as valves, forceps, brushes, snares, tubing, and water bottles cannot be adequately cleaned before further processing, sterile, disposable items should be used. Also, nonimmersible endoscopes should be phased out immediately or removed from use (2, pp. 142-143, 152; 29, p. 27). The remainder of this chapter focuses primarily on the HLD of endoscopes.

General Information

- Personal protective equipment (e.g., gloves, eyewear, respiratory protective devices) should be readily available and used by healthcare workers to protect themselves from exposure to infectious agents (e.g., HIV, HBV, and *M. tuberculosis*) and toxic chemicals (2, p. 153).
- Detailed, written reprocessing protocols for endoscopes should follow guidelines published by professional associations and endoscope manufacturers (29, p. 26).

Cleaning

- Endoscopes, endoscopic accessories, and related equipment should be disassembled and cleaned manually. Flexible endoscopes that have crevices, joints, and internal channels are more difficult to clean and disinfect than rigid endoscopes that have flat surfaces (7, p. 244).

- With use, flexible endoscopes become more contaminated microbiologically than rigid endoscopes because flexible endoscopes are used on heavily colonized body sites (24, p. 70).

- Immediately after removing the endoscope from the patient, the insertion tube should be wiped with a wet cloth or sponge soaked in a freshly prepared enzymatic solution. Used endoscopes should be transported to the reprocessing area in an enclosed container (27, pp. 3-4).

- Meticulous cleaning of endoscopes and accessories should be performed with nonabrasive, manufacturer-recommended enzymatic detergents immediately after use to prevent drying of secretions. Before mechanical cleaning, all channels should be irrigated with copious amounts of detergent and tap water to moisten, soften, and dilute the organic debris, and the air-water channel should be cleared with forced air. Irrigation adaptors should be used to facilitate cleaning of all channels; detachable parts must be thoroughly cleaned with a detergent cleaner. The insertion tube should be washed with detergent and rinsed, and the endoscope tip must be gently wiped or brushed to remove debris or tissue lodged in or around the air and water nozzle. All immersible parts of the endoscope, including the lumens, are then rinsed with water and dried with forced air. Detergent solutions should be discarded after each use (2, pp. 144-145, 152; 7, p. 244).

- Equipment should be inspected for damage at all stages of reprocessing, and a leak (pressure) test should be performed before submerging the entire instrument. If damage is detected, the endoscope should be removed from service and the manufacturer notified (2, pp. 144-145, 152; 7, p. 244).

- Reusable accessories that penetrate mucosal barriers (e.g., invasive devices such as biopsy forceps and cytology brushes) should be mechanically cleaned by ultrasonics and then steam sterilized between uses, or, if disposable, used once and discarded. Single-use disposable accessories may be safer, more efficient, and more economical (2, p. 152; 7, p. 244).

- Sterile water should be used to fill the irrigation water bottle. The water bottle and its connecting tubing should be sterilized or high-level disinfected at least daily (2, p. 152).

Disinfection Versus Sterilization

- When developing infection control procedures for endoscopic equipment, it is useful to have a well-established classification system for making decisions about whether to use sterilization or HLD between each patient use (2, p. 145).
- Laparoscopes, arthroscopes, and other scopes that enter normally sterile tissue should be subjected to a sterilization process before each use; if this is not feasible, they should receive at least HLD (21, pp. 320, 334).
- Endoscopes that come in contact with mucous membranes are classified as semicritical items and should receive at least HLD. An FDA-cleared disinfectant/sterilant should be used for HLD or sterilization (2, p. 152).
- The only circumstance in which sterilization of the endoscope is required is for use in a sterile, operative field (27, p. 6).
- After meticulous cleaning HLD is achievable with a 20-minute soak at room temperature, using a 2% glutaraldehyde solution that tests above its minimum effective concentration (27, p. 6).
- For manual disinfection the disinfectant should be injected into all channels of the endoscope until it can be seen exiting the opposite end of each channel. Care should be taken that all channels are filled with the chemical and that no air pockets remain within the channels (27, p. 6).
- The soaking basin should be covered with a tight-fitting lid to minimize vapor exposure. The endoscope should be soaked in the high-level disinfectant/sterilant for the time and temperature required to achieve HLD. A timer should be used to verify soaking time (27, p. 7).
- Agents *recommended* by APIC for HLD of endoscopes include glutaraldehydes, hydrogen peroxide, peracetic acid, peracetic acid and hydrogen peroxide, and orthophthalaldehyde. Agents *not recommended* for chemical disinfection of endoscopes are products not FDA-cleared for use on semicritical or critical medical devices, skin antiseptics (products formulated only for skin antisepsis), hypochlorites, quaternary ammonium products, and phenolics (2, p. 148).

Rinsing and Drying

- HLD should be followed by a rinse with sterile water that prevents contamination with tap water microorganisms. After rinsing, the scopes must be dried according to a method that does not recontaminate the items (21, pp. 320, 334).
- If sterile water is not used for rinsing, a 70% to 90% alcohol rinse followed by complete drying is essential. Drying can be facilitated

by directing compressed air through the damp lumens. These steps greatly reduce the possibility of recontamination of the endoscope by waterborne organisms (2, pp. 148-149, 152).
- Alcohol flushes for drying should be used even when sterile water is used for rinsing (27, p. 7). NOTE: In contrast to the previous item, this directive implies that alcohol be used for rinsing with either sterile or nonsterile water.
- Routine testing of high-level disinfectants and sterilants should be performed to ensure minimal effective concentration of the active ingredient (2, p. 153).

Storage

If not used immediately, the endoscope should be stored to prevent contamination (23, p. 545). Endoscopes should not be coiled or stored in cases that cannot be properly cleaned (2, p. 152). Instead they should be hung vertically with the distal tip hanging freely in a well-ventilated, dust-free area. This prevents undue moisture buildup and thus discourages microbial contamination. Correct storage also prevents damage to the exterior of the instrument by protecting it from physical impact. Padding the lower portion of the storage area with nonporous material may prevent damage to the distal end of the endoscope (27, p. 8).

Terminal Disinfection

If HLD is used for critical items, these items should be processed immediately before use. The safest practice is to terminally disinfect endoscopes at the end of each day's use and again before the first and each subsequent use throughout the next day. Many infections have been caused by endoscopes that were cleaned, disinfected, and stored but nevertheless were colonized with pathogenic microorganisms. Fatalities have occurred (7, p. 245; 12, pp. 402-403). NOTE: This practice is controversial. The pros and cons are being discussed by several professional organizations.

AUTOMATED REPROCESSING

AERs standardize the disinfection process and decrease personnel exposure to disinfectants. However, *no currently available AERs provide adequate cleaning of endoscopes.* It is therefore necessary to follow all steps for the mechanical cleaning of the endoscope *before* using an AER (27, pp. 8-9; 29, p. 27).

An AER should have the following features:
- The ability to circulate fluids through all endoscope channels at an equal pressure without trapping air
- Thorough rinse cycles and forced air to remove all used solutions following detergent and disinfectant cycles

- The ability to prevent the disinfectant from being diluted with any fluids
- The ability to self-disinfect
- No residual water remaining in hoses and reservoirs
- Cycles for alcohol flushing and forced air drying (desirable) (27, p. 8)

The FDA and the Centers for Disease Control and Prevention (CDC) recently issued an advisory regarding reports of serious infections resulting from the use of endoscopes inadequately reprocessed by an AER system. Investigation of the reported incidents revealed two scenarios for inadequate reprocessing: (1) inconsistencies between the reprocessing instructions provided by the manufacturer of the bronchoscope and the manufacturer of the AER, and (2) the use of inappropriate channel connectors when reprocessing bronchoscopes. Eight recommendations covering manufacturer instructions, endoscope preparation, and staff training accompany the advisory (13; 9).

DOUBLE STANDARDS IN PROCESSING PATIENT CARE EQUIPMENT?

First, does a double standard exist if some semicritical equipment is *sterilized* after use on patients with certain infectious diseases (e.g., HIV, HBV, tuberculosis [TB]) but the same equipment is only *high-level disinfected* after it is used for other patients? Under these circumstances, sterilization should not be performed in the belief that it is providing a greater margin of safety. However, it is not a double standard to sterilize endoscopes in one hospital area (e.g., the operating room [OR]) and high-level disinfect them in another area (e.g., the G-I lab) because the outcome is equivalent from an infectious disease transmission perspective (21, p. 325). Furthermore, the results of a literature review show that HLD of thoroughly cleaned flexible and rigid endoscopes does not contribute to higher infection rates and is not less safe than sterilization (17).

Endoscope reprocessing guidelines should not be interpreted to mean that HLD is inferior to sterilization because significant clinical differences have not been demonstrated. Therefore performing either of the two processes on a thoroughly cleaned instrument does not constitute two standards of care. Although there may be a theoretical distinction between the highest level of disinfection and sterilization, thorough cleaning eliminates clinical differences between the two (17).

A low-temperature sterilization process for an endoscope should be considered only if it is comparable in cost to disinfection or if it offers advantages without damaging the instrument (17).

ENDOSCOPY AND GASTROINTESTINAL LABORATORIES

NOTE: G-I procedures performed outside of the sterile environment of the OR are considered clean, and most of the equipment therefore need not be sterile. Patient condition, risk of infection, and the nature of the procedures being performed all determine the policies and procedures followed: clean versus sterile and HLD versus sterilization.

To prevent cross-contamination in an endoscopic procedure room, most areas of the room should be designated as clean areas. Contaminated areas where accessories and specimens are handled should be separated from clean counter areas. All contaminated areas must be cleaned and decontaminated between patients with an EPA-registered hospital grade disinfectant. Negative pressure rooms or rooms with air circulated through high-efficiency particulate air (HEPA) filters are recommended when endoscopy is performed on patients with known or suspected TB (27, p. 2).

ANESTHESIA EQUIPMENT

- Reusable anesthesia equipment that comes in contact with mucous membranes, blood, or body fluid is considered semicritical and should be cleaned and then processed by HLD, pasteurization, or sterilization between each patient use. Examples are reusable laryngeal mask airways, masks, breathing circuits, connectors, self-inflating bags, airways, forceps, and laryngoscope blades (5, p. 195).
- Reusable temperature and esophageal probes, laryngoscope handles and blades, fiberoptic laryngoscope systems, Magill forceps, stylets, and any other items that make direct contact with a patient's mucous membranes should be decontaminated with a detergent and water solution and subjected to a HLD process or sterilized before reuse (3, p. 19).
- Semicritical items such as laryngoscope blades, oral and nasal airways, face masks, breathing circuits and connectors, self-inflating resuscitation bags, esophageal stethoscopes, and esophageal/nasopharyngeal/rectal temperature probes should receive HLD (4, pp. 6-7).
- Single-use items such as suction catheters, breathing circuits, endotracheal tubes, and stylets should be used once and discarded according to facility policies and applicable local, state, and federal regulations (5, p. 195).

Internal Components

- Routine disinfection or sterilization of the internal components of the anesthesia machine (gas outlets, gas valves, pressure regulators,

flow meters, and vaporizers) is not necessary or reasonably feasible. Unidirectional valves and carbon dioxide absorber chambers should be cleaned and disinfected periodically (4, p. 7).
• Internal components of the anesthesia machine breathing circuit (e.g., absorbers, valves, and vent bellows) should be cleaned regularly (5, p. 196).

Bacterial Filters

NOTE: There is inconsistency among the experts regarding use of bacterial filters.
• Anesthesia ventilator bellows and the bellows base are part of the patient circuit and should be sterilized after every procedure unless bacterial filters are used to protect the inspiratory, expiratory, and ventilator limbs of the circuit (3, p. 18).
• Using a bacterial filter between the breathing circuit of the disposable absorber and the mask of endotracheal tube is recommended to prevent potential infectious airborne organisms from contaminating the ventilator (3, p. 16).
• Controversy and debate continue to cloud the issue of whether bacterial filtration is useful and effective for anesthesia applications. However, the literature does report the finding of *Pseudomonas aeruginosa, Klebsiella pneumonie, Escherichia coli, Staphylococcus,* TB bacilli, and other organisms growing inside absorber and patient circuit components (3, p. 20).
• There are insufficient clinical outcome data to support the routine use of bacterial filters for breathing circuits or anesthesia ventilators at this time. However, a filter should be used on the anesthesia breathing circuit between the patient's airway and the Y-connector before contacting a patient with or at high risk for having pulmonary TB (4, p. 7).
• Ventilator tubing and bellows should be cleaned and disinfected at regular intervals. In contrast to respiratory therapy equipment, anesthesia ventilators are thought to represent a low risk for infection transmission and need not undergo cleaning and disinfection after each use (4, p. 7).
• Ventilator bellows represent a low risk for transmission of infection and do not require cleaning and disinfection after each use (5, p. 196).

External Components

• As a general rule, only the components between the common gas outlet and the patient require sterilization. All other components, surfaces, and compartments require HLD (3, p. 16).

- Changes of breathing circuits and rebreathing bags are necessary to prevent the transfer of bacteria from one patient to another (3, p. 20).
- Equipment such as anesthesia machine surfaces, blood pressure cuffs, carts, and monitors not in contact with mucous membranes, sterile areas of the body, or nonintact skin should be cleaned/decontaminated when contamination or visible soiling occurs and at the end of the day (5, p. 196).
- Anesthesia equipment should be processed in the same manner in all areas of the practice setting. All patients are entitled to the same standard of care, according to the Joint Commission on Accreditation of Healthcare Organizations (JCAHO) (5, p. 196).

PASTEURIZATION

- A pasteurization process may be used to achieve *thermal* HLD.
- Pasteurization is suitable for HLD of some anesthesia, respiratory therapy, and other semicritical equipment.
- In a pasteurization unit, all surfaces of the item to be disinfected are exposed to a hot water bath, heated to 160° to 180° F (60° to 70° C) for a minimum of 30 minutes. Pasteurization destroys all microorganisms with the exception of bacterial spores (6, p. 223).

PNEUMATIC TOURNIQUETS

- Disposable tourniquets should be discarded after use unless the manufacturer recommends that they can be resterilized (8, p. 305).
- Reusable cuffs and bladders should be washed according to the manufacturers' instructions. An enzymatic detergent should be used if blood or body fluids came in contact with the cuff. A disposable cuff cover facilitates cleaning (14, p. 529).
- Reusable cuffs and bladders should be cleaned, rinsed, and dried according to the level of contamination and manufacturers' instructions. If the bladder is removable, care must be taken to prevent introducing water into the bladder through the ports. All connecting tubing should be wiped with a hospital-grade chemical germicide and dried before storage (8, p. 305).
- The tourniquet cuff should be adequately protected from contamination during surgery by padding and other protective materials; therefore washing is the only decontamination procedure indicated. However, if blood or other body fluids come in contact with tourniquet components, more intensive cleaning with an enzymatic detergent is necessary (8, p. 306).

MICROBIAL RESISTANCE TO DISINFECTANTS

Since the advent of antibiotic-resistant microorganisms, the question of possible resistance to disinfectants has also been raised. A recent study (26), one of very few, examined the germicidal activity of two hospital disinfectants (a phenolic and a quaternary ammonium compound) and evaluated whether hospital strains of antibiotic-resistant bacteria exhibited altered susceptibility to these disinfectants. In 3 of the 20 trials, the more antibiotic-resistant strain was statistically more susceptible to the germicide. In only one comparative trial was the more antibiotic-resistant strain significantly more resistant to the germicide. Nonpaired isolates of *Enterococcus* and *Salmonella cholerae-suis* demonstrated susceptibility to the tested disinfectants. Data from this study demonstrate that the development of antibiotic resistance does not appear to be correlated with increased resistance to disinfectants. Furthermore, the authors (of reference 26) do not recommend any alterations in current routine disinfection and housekeeping protocols. (NOTE: As long as these protocols meet national professional organization and regulatory guidelines.) Routine monitoring of antibiotic-resistant bacteria for susceptibility to disinfectants is unnecessary (26).

References

1. Alvarado C: Current label claims for liquid chemical sterilants/high level disinfectants, *APIC News* 13(6):2, 1994, pp 22-23.
2. Alvarado CJ, Reichelderfer M, APIC Guidelines Committee: APIC guideline for infection prevention and control in flexible endoscopy, *Am J Infect Control* 28(2):138-155, 2000.
3. American Association of Nurse Anesthetists: *Infection control guide,* Park Ridge, Ill, 1997, Author.
4. American Society of Anesthesiologists: *Recommendations for infection control for the practice of anesthesiology,* ed 2, Park Ridge, Ill, 1998, Author.
5. AORN: Recommended practices for cleaning and processing anesthesia equipment. In *Standards, recommended practices and guidelines,* Denver, 2000, Author, pp 195-198.
6. AORN: Recommended practices for high-level disinfection. In *Standards, recommended practices and guidelines,* Denver, 2000, Author, pp 221-227.
7. AORN: Recommended practices for use and care of endoscopes. In *Standards, recommended practices and guidelines,* Denver, 2000, Author, pp 243-247.
8. AORN: Recommended practices for use of the pneumatic tourniquet. In *Standards, recommended practices and guidelines,* Denver, 2000, Author, pp 305-309.
9. Centers for Disease Control and Prevention (CDC): Bronchoscope-related infections and pseudoinfections: New York, 1996 and 1998, *MMWR* 48(26):557-560, 1999. Online: www2.cdc.gov/mmwr
10. FDA approves new sterilants, *Infect Control Hosp Epidemiol* 19(3):217, 1998.
11. FDA clears 3 more germicides, *The Q-Net Monthly* 5(10):1-3, 1999.

12. Fogg DM: Clinical issues, *AORN J* 71(2):398, 401-403, 2000.
13. Food and Drug Administration (FDA): *FDA and CDC public health advisory: infections from endoscopes inadequately reprocessed by an automated endoscope reprocessing system,* Rockville, Md, Sept 10, 1999, Author. Online: www.fda.gov/cdrh/safety/endoreprocess.html
14. Fortunato N: *Berry & Kohn's operating room technique,* ed 9, St Louis, 2000, Mosby.
15. Gruendemann BJ, Fernsebner B: *Comprehensive perioperative nursing,* vol 1, *Principles,* Boston, 1995, Jones & Bartlett.
16. Jennings J, Manian FA, editors: *APIC handbook of infection control,* ed 2, Washington, DC, 1999, Association for Professionals in Infection Control and Epidemiology.
17. Muscarella LF: High-level disinfection or "sterilization" of endoscopes? *Infect Control Hosp Epidemiol* 17(3):183-187, 1996.
18. Occupational Safety and Health Administration (OSHA): Occupational exposure to bloodborne pathogens: final rule, *Federal Register* 56(235):64175-64182, 1991.
19. Occupational Safety and Health Administration: Memorandum to OSHA regional directors and bloodborne coordinators regarding EPA-registered disinfectants for HIV/HBV, February 28, 1997.
20. Pugliese G, Favero MS: APHA challenges glutaraldehyde instructions, *Infect Control Hosp Epidemiol* 17(7):422, 1996.
21. Rutala WA: APIC guidelines for selection and use of disinfectants, *Am J Infect Control* 24(4):313-342, 1996.
22. Rutala WA: Disinfection and sterilization of patient-care items, *Infect Control Hosp Epidemiol* 17(6):377-384, 1996.
23. Rutala WA: Disinfection, sterilization, and waste disposal. In Wenzel RP, editor: *Prevention and control of nosocomial infections,* ed 3, Baltimore, 1997, Williams & Wilkins, pp 538-593.
24. Rutala WA, Weber DJ: Disinfection of endoscopes: review of new chemical sterilants used for high-level disinfection, *Infect Control Hosp Epidemiol* 20(6):69-76, 1999.
25. Rutala WA, Weber DJ: FDA labeling requirements for disinfection of endoscopes: a counterpoint, *Infect Control Hosp Epidemiol* 16(4):231-235, 1995.
26. Rutala WA et al: Susceptibility of antibiotic-susceptible and antibiotic-resistant hospital bacteria to disinfectants, *Infect Control Hosp Epidemiol* 18(6):417-421, 1997.
27. Society of Gastroenterology Nurses and Associates: *Standards of infection control in reprocessing of flexible gastrointestinal endoscopes,* Chicago, 2000, Author.
28. Spach DH, Silverstein FE, Stamm WE: Transmission of infection by gastrointestinal endoscopy and bronchoscopy, *Ann Intern Med* 118:117-128, 1993.
29. Walker SB: Caring for flexible gastrointestinal endoscopes, *Surgical Services Management* 5(6):26-29, 1999.

Suggested Reading

1. Alfa MJ, Sitter DL: In-hospital evaluation of orthophthalaldehyde as a high-level disinfectant for flexible endoscopes, *J Hosp Infect* 26:15-26, 1994.
2. American Society for Gastrointestinal Endoscopy: Reprocessing of flexible gastrointestinal endoscopes, *Gasterointerol Nurs* 19:109-112, 1996.

3. American Society of Testing Materials (ASTM): F1518-94 Standard practice for cleaning and disinfection of flexible fiberoptic and video endoscopes used in the examination of the hollow viscera. In *Annual Book of ASTM Standards,* West Conshohocken, Penn, 1998, Author, pp 834-839.

4. Assadian O et al: The stethoscope as a potential source of transmission of bacteria, *Infect Control Hosp Epidemiol* 19(5):298-299, 1998 (letter to the editor).

5. Blanc DS et al: Nosocomial infections and pseudoinfections from contaminated bronchoscopes: two-year follow-up using molecular markers, *Infect Control Hosp Epidemiol* 18:134-136, 1997.

6. Bronowicki JP et al: Patient-to-patient transmission of hepatitis C virus during colonoscopy, *N Engl J Med* 337(4):237-240, 1999.

7. Davis R: Endoscopes can transmit infection, *USA Today* Feb 18, 1999.

8. ECRI: Recommended protocol for reprocessing immersible flexible endoscopes, *Health Devices* 28:178, 1999.

9. Finkelstein LE, coordinator: Infection control: infection risk from contaminated endoscopes, *Am J Nurs* 97(2):56, 1997.

10. Goldstine S: Processing flexible endoscopes, *Infection Control Today* 3(3):30, 32, 34, 36, 1998.

11. Health advisory targets reprocessing endoscopes, *Same Day Surg* 24(1):9-11, 2000.

12. Hilgren J: The exposure time dilemma: how long to use disinfectants on environmental surfaces, *Infection Control Today* 2:12, 16-18, 1998.

13. icanPREVENT (www.icanPREVENT.com): Agents for disinfection. Infection control topics: Disinfection (synopsis). Updated 5/8/00, accessed 5/10/00.

14. icanPREVENT (www.icanPREVENT.com): Outbreaks associated with cleaning, disinfection, and sterilization. Infection control topics: Disinfection (synopsis). Updated 3/5/00, accessed 5/1/00.

15. Kovacs BJ: High-level disinfection of gastrointestinal endoscopes: are current guidelines adequate? *Am J Gastroenterol* 94:1546-1550, 1999.

16. Marinella MA: The stethoscope and potential nosocomial infection, *Infect Control Hosp Epidemiol* 19(7):477-478, 1998.

17. Mayhall CG: Proper use of aqueous quaternary ammonium compounds, *Disease Prevention News,* Texas Department of Health, 60(2):1-2, 2000.

18. Rutala WA et al: Stability and bactericidal activity of chlorine solutions, *Infect Control Hosp Epidemiol* 19(5):323-327, 1998.

19. Rutala WA et al: Antimicrobial activity of home disinfectants and natural products against potential human pathogens, *Infect Control Hosp Epidemiol* 21(1):33-38, 2000.

20. Underwood A: Do scopes spread sickness? *Newsweek* pp 72-73, March 1, 1999.

D. Sterilization

Sterilization is a process that destroys all forms of microbial life, including spores, on inanimate surfaces or in fluids. Sterilization and sterility are absolute, not relative, terms. Items cannot be partially sterilized (5, p. 212).

In reality, the concept of what constitutes *sterile* is measured as a probability of sterility for each item to be sterilized. This probability is commonly referred to as the sterility assurance level (SAL) of the item. SAL is defined as the $\log_{10}$ number of the probability of a survivor on a single item. For example, a SAL of 6 indicates a 1 in 1 million probability of a spore or microorganism's survival (8, p. 568).

Sterilization can be accomplished by physical or chemical agents. *Physical sterilization* can take place, for example, with dry or moist heat, in a gravity or prevacuum sterilizer. *Chemical sterilization* involves chemicals, such as ethylene oxide, gas plasma, and hydrogen peroxide (5, p. 211).

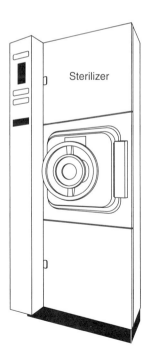

Sterilizer

When chemicals are used for the purpose of destroying all forms of microbial life, including fungal and bacterial spores, they may be called chemical sterilants. These same chemical germicides used for shorter exposure times also may be used for the disinfection process (7, p. 377). (See the chapter "Disinfection.")

NOTE: As with all forms of disinfection and sterilization, the condition of the items is perhaps the most important determinant of the outcome of the process (e.g., items must be *thoroughly* cleaned and decontaminated before being subjected to sterilization). This precleaning cannot be ignored nor treated lightly; the importance of this preparation phase cannot be overestimated. Failure to remove soil, organic material, and microorganisms from an object will render disinfection or sterilization ineffective. Therefore, inadequate precleaning can be hazardous and will pose serious risks of infection to both patients and staff. The reader is encouraged to review the chapter "Cleaning and Decontamination of Surgical Instruments" in this text before embarking on any sterilization process.

Decontamination/cleaning is universally recommended as a key component of disinfection and sterilization processes (13, p. 145).

FOOD AND DRUG ADMINISTRATION CLEARANCE

All sterilization processes must be approved by the U.S. Food and Drug Administration (FDA). Sterilizer microbiocidal performance must be tested under simulated use conditions (10, p. 397).

FDA clearance requires that the process eliminate 10^6 colony-forming units (CFU) of an organism highly resistant to the process; the most resistant spore-forming organisms are used (10, p. 397). For ethylene oxide (EtO) technologies and hydrogen peroxide gas plasma, the recommended test organism is *Bacillus subtilis;* for peracetic acid immersion and steam sterilizers, the recommended test organism is *Bacillus stearothermophilus* (2, p. 354; 8, p. 568). (See the chapter "Monitoring of Sterilization Processes" in this text.)

In addition to the use of the most resistant organism, a design configuration (e.g., lumens) that provides the greatest barrier for penetration of the sterilant is also used and tested before FDA clearance is achieved (10, p. 397).

STEAM STERILIZATION (AUTOCLAVES)

Saturated steam under pressure—moist heat—is the preferred method to sterilize heat- and moisture-stable items (2, p. 348).

The two most common steam-sterilizing temperatures are 250° F (121° C) and 270° F (132° C). Recognized exposure periods for sterilization of wrapped supplies are 30 minutes at 250° F (121° C) in a gravity-displacement sterilizer, and 4 minutes at 270° F (132° C) in a prevacuum sterilizer. Sterilization times may vary, depending on the type of item, whether it is wrapped or unwrapped, and the type of sterilizer (8, p. 568).

- This process carries the greatest margin of safety of all sterilizing processes.
- Moist heat is an efficient and cost-effective means of sterilization; it is the most reliable and common mode of sterilization in use today.
- All surfaces to be sterilized must come into contact with saturated steam.
- Time, temperature, and pressure parameters are significant. Time relates to the type of load and type of sterilizer, gravity or prevacuum, used (5, pp. 216, 218).
- Supplies to be sterilized should be wrapped loosely in a permeable material. Basins, jars, and glassware should not be packed with gowns or dressings because this almost always results in the development of air pockets, the single greatest deterrent to sterilization (5, p. 218).
- Packs should be prepared so that all folds are parallel to each other, and packs should be placed in the sterilizer so that the folds are perpendicular to the bottom of the sterilizer to allow free flow of air and steam (primarily for gravity sterilization loads). Also, items should be dry before wrapping and placing in the sterilizer. Wrappers must be single-use nonwoven, or reusable linen that has been hydrated by washing. A common error is to use reusable linen that has not been freshly rewashed but only sterilized (5, p. 218).
- Basins and instrument sets should be kept low in the sterilizer to prevent condensation from wetting materials beneath them. They should be positioned on their sides or open at the end to allow air and moisture to escape. Packs should not touch each other or the walls of the sterilizer (5, p. 218).
- It is important to remove the loading cart from the sterilizer and place it in an area away from traffic and air vents. Items should be inspected for wet spots and allowed to return to room temperature without being touched. This may take up to 1 hour (5, p. 218).
- All sterilizing methods in which humidity, usually steam, is a factor carry the possibility of producing wet packs. Unless a package wrapper is completely impermeable to water, a pack should be considered unsterile and unacceptable for use if any part of its contents is wet (4, p. 277).
- A stain on a wrapper may indicate that moisture was present and has dried. The cause of the wet pack should be investi-

gated and promptly corrected. Reprocessing is necessary for a wet package or a load with one or more wet or suspect packages (4, p. 277).

· At the end of the sterilization cycle, even after appropriate drying times, items may still contain some steam vapor. Touching items at this vulnerable stage could result in compromise to the barrier properties of some packaging material. Condensation, both inside and outside of the package, can occur if hot items come in contact with cold surfaces. As a result, packages will become damp and their contents contaminated. Therefore, if the packaging material is breached by this liquid condensate, items inside the package are considered contaminated (2, p. 348).

· If impermeable materials (e.g., closed-bottom containers, plastic-reinforced wrappers) are used, contact contamination is prevented, but the condensate inside the package may damage the item if contact is prolonged. The practitioner should question the acceptability of this item for use (2, p. 348).

Common types of steam sterilizers are gravity displacement, pre-vacuum (high-vacuum), and steam-flush/pressure pulse.

Gravity Displacement

· Air is displaced downward and out through a drain at the bottom of the sterilizer chamber. A steam jacket, if present, prevents excess condensation of steam during heat-up of the chamber and thus affords faster drying of packs.

· Gravity displacement sterilizers have low initial cost, but the following limitations decrease their usefulness in many central processing and operating room departments:

    · Somewhat inefficient for heavy, dense loads
    · Long sterilization and drying times; insufficient drying may contribute to contamination
    · Difficult to determine if all parts of a load have received contact with saturated steam for appropriate amount of time at proper temperature
    · Excess moisture and heat are generated in working area around the sterilizer (5, p. 218)

· Gravity-displacement autoclaves are primarily used to process laboratory media, water, pharmaceutical products, infectious waste, and nonporous articles whose surfaces have direct steam contact (8, p. 568).

· Parameters for gravity-displacement sterilization are temperatures of 250° to 254° F (121° to 132°, C), with exposure times (usually 15 to 30 minutes) that are dependent on load, number of instruments, and written manufacturers' instructions (2, p. 348). Parameters for flash sterilization are discussed in the chapter "Flash Sterilization."

Prevacuum (High-Vacuum)

• Free air in the sterilizer chamber and load is removed, and the load is brought to sterilization temperature before the exposure timing begins.
• This process is quite efficient, but the possibility of excessive air leaks exists. The process may be inefficient for small loads relative to chamber size because of the potential for air pocket formation (a small load in a small sterilizer is not a problem) (5, p. 218).
• Prevacuum steam sterilization is generally fast, causes minimal damage from overheating, and does not heat up the surrounding area (5, p. 218).
• High-speed prevacuum sterilizers are different than gravity-displacement types in that they are fitted with a vacuum pump to remove air from the sterilizing chamber and load before the steam is admitted; thus almost instantaneous steam penetration occurs (8, pp. 568-569).
• Either the Bowie-Dick test (using 100% cotton surgical towels) or small disposable test packs are used daily in the first cycle of all vacuum-type autoclaves to evaluate the efficacy of air removal. Air removal is critical because, if not removed, air will interfere with the steam penetration of items to be sterilized (8, pp. 568-569).
• Parameters for prevacuum sterilization include temperatures of 270° to 272° F (132° to 135° C), with exposure time dependent on load, instruments, and written manufacturers' instructions (2, p. 348).

Steam-Flush/Pressure Pulse Sterilizers

Parameters for steam-flush/pressure pulse sterilizers range from 250° to 270° F (121° to 122° C) with exposure times of 3 to 20 minutes, depending on load, number of instruments, and manufacturers' instructions (2, p. 348).

DRY-HEAT STERILIZATION

Dry heat (high-temperature ovens) is the sterilization process of choice for certain items and materials. Dry-heat sterilizers may not always be available. This method is infrequently used in healthcare settings in the United States today.

• Dry heat in the form of hot air is used primarily to sterilize anhydrous oils, petrolatum products, and talcum powder, which steam and EtO gas cannot penetrate. Higher temperatures are required in the absence of moisture because the microorganisms are destroyed through a very slow process of heat absorption by conduction (4, p. 268). NOTE: Commercially presterilized versions of infrequently used items should be purchased when available.

- Dry-heat sterilization can be used for powders, anhydrous oils, and glass. Dry heat also reaches surfaces of instruments that cannot be disassembled, and has no corrosive or rusting effect on instruments (11, p. 15-11).

- During dry-heat sterilization, products in jars and canisters take longer to sterilize than those in peel pouches, because the container must be fully heated before the heat is transferred to the product inside (5, p. 216).

- Dry heat penetrates material slowly and unevenly; therefore, long exposure times are required. Exposure times of 4 to 6 hours or longer are not unusual, depending on the amount of product being sterilized and the properties of the container (5, p. 216).

- Dry heat penetrates certain substances that cannot be sterilized by steam or other methods. Dry heat is also a protective method of sterilizing some delicate, sharp, or cutting-edge instruments. Instruments that cannot be disassembled may be sterilized by this method. Steam may erode or corrode cutting edges of instruments (4, p. 268).

- Exposure times for dry-heat sterilization vary depending on the characteristics of the item, the layer depths in the containers, and the temperature in the sterilizer. Minimum times of exposure may vary considerably, from 6 minutes, unwrapped, at 400° F (204° C) to 6 hours at 250° F (121° C), depending on container amounts and manufacturers' recommendations (4, p. 268).

LOW-TEMPERATURE STERILIZATION

Low-temperature sterilization processes are useful for temperature- and moisture-sensitive critical medical devices and supplies that must be sterilized.

Ethylene Oxide

Ethylene oxide (EtO) has been the most widely used low-temperature sterilization process. EtO may be used for heat- and moisture-sensitive critical items.

- Healthcare facilities are now considering alternatives to EtO because: (1) some states (New York, California, and Michigan) require EtO emission reductions of 90% to 99.9%, (2) potential toxic hazards to staff and patients exist, and (3) flammability is a risk. Also, EPA regulations of 1995 ban production of chloro-fluorocarbons such as CFC-12 and freon, which were used as stabilizing agents in combination with EtO. Alternative technologies to EtO with CFCs include 100% EtO, and EtO with an alternative stabilizing agent such as hydrochlorofluorocarbons (HCFCs) or carbon dioxide (10, pp. 393-394).

- EtO concentrations and mixtures available are 100% EtO and the following mixtures: 12% EtO with 88% CFC, 8.6% EtO with 91.4% HCFC, 10% EtO with 90% HCFC, and 8.5% EtO with 91.5% CO_2 (12, p. 800).

The following information applies to the EtO standard sterilizer:

- EtO requires long exposure times: $\geq$2 hours of exposure time to EtO, at 129° F (54° C), followed by prolonged aeration (about 12 to 14 hours) at 131° F (55° C). Aeration times are variable. Some products, such as polyvinylchloride (PVC) tubing, are extremely difficult to aerate and may require up to 24 hours of aeration time (5, pp. 225-226).

- Gas concentration and relative humidity, as well as contact time and temperature, affect the rate of EtO sterilization. A relative humidity of at least 35% but no more than 85% is needed for effective sterilization. Items should be free of visible moisture droplets when placed in the sterilizer (5, p. 225).

- At the completion of each EtO cycle, the sterilizer door should be opened approximately 2 inches and the area cleared of all personnel for 15 minutes before unloading. EtO loading carts should be pulled, not pushed, from the sterilizer to the aerator because air currents flowing over the load may accumulate a residual gas that could be inhaled. NOTE: Some chambers are a combination sterilizer/aerator, in which the load is removed only after aeration (4, p. 270).

- EtO gas must be vented from the sterilizer to the outside atmosphere to avoid personnel exposure. Locking and sealing mechanisms on the sterilizer door should be checked regularly for any breaks in integrity. Automatic controls must function properly so that the door cannot be opened until the gas is evacuated from the chamber (4, p. 270).

- Items should *not* be removed from an EtO aerator before the appropriate aeration cycle (mechanical or passive) is completed. Complete aeration must precede safe use of the sterilized items. This should be a written hospital policy (5, pp. 225-226; 2, p. 350).

- EtO is soluble in some solids such as rubber, plastics, and skin; unreacted EtO is released slowly from these substances. If EtO gas cannot freely escape from the skin, burns or blisters may result; however, relatively long exposure is necessary to cause such damage. If liquid EtO contacts skin, damage is almost instantaneous; it may cause serious burns if not removed immediately by thorough washing. If the EtO is mixed with a diluent, contact with skin can result in frostbite and chemical burns (5, p. 225; 4, pp. 270-271).

• Inhaled EtO gas can be irritating to mucous membranes. Overexposure causes nasal and throat irritation. Prolonged exposure may result in nausea, vomiting, dizziness, difficulty in breathing, and peripheral paralysis. Long-term exposure to EtO is known to be a potential occupational carcinogen, causing illnesses such as leukemia. It is also a mutagen, causing spontaneous abortion, genetic defects, chromosomal damage, and neurologic dysfunction (4, pp. 270-271).

• Patients can also be affected by contact with items, such as polyethylene, rubber, or silicone, that have been sterilized by EtO but improperly aerated. Care should be taken to avoid exposure of both patients and staff to EtO (4, p. 270).

• Both the Occupational Safety and Health Administration (OSHA) and the U.S. Environmental Protection Agency (EPA) have classified EtO as a possible human mutagen and carcinogen. Both acute and chronic exposure to EtO may have short- and long-term effects. To prevent occupational exposure to EtO, OSHA recommends routinely monitoring the area and personnel, using a highly ventilated area (at least 10 air exchanges per hour), and having a medical surveillance and continuing education program for all involved personnel (5, p. 226).

• OSHA standards limit an employee's exposure to EtO to 1 part per million (ppm) of air averaged over an 8-hour period to an active level of 0.5 ppm, and to a short-term limit of 5 ppm averaged over a 15-minute period. Monitoring devices should be used (4, p. 270).

Gas-Plasma Systems

The Sterrad 100 and Sterrad 50 systems each consist of a single diffusion stage (hydrogen peroxide vapor) and a plasma stage.

• The advantages of these systems are that there are no toxic residues (the by-products are water and oxygen), they are environmentally safe, no aeration is necessary, they are simple to operate, and they have a relatively fast cycle time of approximately 75 minutes.

• The disadvantages of these systems are the limited ability to penetrate lumens—endoscopes or medical devices with lumens or channels of >40 cm in length or a diameter of <3 mm cannot be processed in the United States now—and the inability to process paper (cellulose), linens (especially wrappers), and liquids (9).

NOTE: Introduction of the Sterrad 50 system allows for a shorter exposure time of 45 minutes.

Peracetic Acid (Steris) Systems

These systems are liquid immersion sterilization processes that are fully automated. They are suitable for processing devices such as flexible and rigid endoscopes. Lumened scopes must be attached (by channel connectors) to the fluid ports in the Steris System 1 (low temperature method—122° to 131° F [50° to 55° C]) to affect an increased, directed flow of fluid. The sterilant, 35% peracetic acid, and an anticorrosive agent are supplied in a single-dose container. The container is punctured as the lid is closed and the process begins (10, p. 395).

• The advantages of this system are that the by-products—acetic acid, oxygen, and water—are environmentally safe, and the cycle time of 30 to 45 minutes is relatively short.

• The disadvantages of this system are that it is used for immersible instruments only, a small number of instruments are processed in a cycle, there is no long-term sterile storage (only just-in-time sterilization), it is costly, there is some material incompatibility, and the costly biological indicator may not be suitable for routine monitoring (10, p. 395). NOTE: Failures with this system have been associated with the incorrect use of adaptors and channel connectors. The importance of sterilant contact with the inner channel of an endoscope was demonstrated by Rutala and Weber (12, p. 804), who showed that rigid endoscopes without connectors that allow sterilant flow-through were not rendered sterile by the Steris System 1.

• Currently, only the Steris System 1 is FDA cleared for use with flexible endoscopes. This system allows the sterilant to flow continuously through the endoscope channels of flexible endoscopes when connected to channel irrigators (12, p. 804).

NOTE: The Steris system is referred to as a "just-in-time" or "point-of-use" process for immediate use as an endoscope sterilizer. In this context, the process can be labeled as a method of flash sterilization (sterilization for immediate use). (See the chapter "Flash Sterilization.")

OTHER STERILIZATION METHODS

Most of the sterilization methods in this section use low temperatures.

Gamma Ray Sterilization

Some commercially available products are sterilized by irradiation. Cobalt-60 is a radioactive isotope capable of disintegrating to produce gamma rays and is the source for irradiation sterilization most commonly used today. Irradiation sterilization with beta or gamma rays is limited to industrial use. Irradiation can be used to sterilize heat- and moisture-sensitive items but may alter the physical properties of some materials. Gamma rays can penetrate large bulky objects and cartons ready for shipping, making the process cost-effective for manufacturers (4, pp. 276-277).

Microwave Sterilization

Microwave sterilization is another form of radiation sterilization. This process uses low-pressure steam with the non-ionizing radiation to produce the localized heat that kills microorganisms. Small tabletop units may be useful for rapid sterilization of a single instrument or a small number of instruments. Current models have a small chamber size of 1 to 3 cubic feet (4, p. 276).

Ozone Gas Sterilization

This simple and inexpensive method sterilizes by oxidation, destroying organic and inorganic matter. The sterilizer generates its own agents using the hospital's oxygen, water, and electrical supply. Ozone gas sterilization provides an alternative to EtO gas sterilization of some heat- and moisture-sensitive items. Ozone can be corrosive to metals, however, and it also destroys natural rubber such as latex, natural fibers, and some plastics. FDA clearance for clinical use must be verified (4, p. 274).

New Technologies

Other sterilization methods that may become useful in the future include vapor-phase peracetic acid, vaporized hydrogen peroxide, gaseous chlorine dioxide, and pulsed light. These technologies are under development for use in healthcare facilities, and FDA clearance will be required before their widespread introduction into the marketplace (12, p. 799).

PACKAGING

- Items must be prepared and packaged so that their sterility can be achieved and maintained to the point of use (2, p. 347).

- Instruments should be held open and unlocked. Preparation and assembly procedures should consider the type of surgical instruments, total set weight, and density. These factors are more important than arbitrary weight limits (2, p. 347).
- The type of packaging selected should optimize the sterilization process, maintain the sterility of the product, and allow for aseptic delivery of the item. Packaging must allow the adequate removal of air, the adequate penetration of the sterilant, and direct contact with the item. The central processing manager must be aware of and compare all packaging options to ensure that the best selection is made (3, p. 85).
- Minimal operational requirements for packaging systems include the following:
  - They are appropriate to items and method of sterilization
  - They completely and securely enclose the items
  - They have a tamperproof closure or seal
  - They protect the package contents from physical damage
  - They allow for adequate air removal
  - They allow for penetration, release, and removal of the sterilizing agents
  - They are tear, puncture, and abrasion resistant
  - They are fluid resistant
  - They are free of holes
  - They are free of toxic ingredients
  - They are low-linting
  - They maintain barrier properties
  - There is aseptic presentation/delivery of product
  - They have a positive cost/benefit ratio
  - They are used according to manufacturers' written instructions (3, p. 85; 1, p. 299)

Textiles and Fabrics

Not all reusable textiles are the same. Reusable textiles have evolved from 144-thread-count, 100% cotton muslin to the current 100% polyester continuous filament material. Nonwoven fabrics include a range of paper wraps, from kraft paper, which is the oldest, to newer synthetic fabrics, such as spunbonded polyolefin. The effectiveness of each is dependent on adherence to packaging procedures recommended by the manufacturer (3, pp. 85, 87).

Reusable woven fabrics should be freshly laundered before use and should maintain a protective barrier through multiple laundering and sterilization processings. If repair of a woven fabric is needed, it should be done with double-vulcanized, heat-sealed patches according to manufacturers' written instructions. These patches should never be stitched to woven packaging materials as a way of repairing holes because stitching reduces barrier efficacy by creating permanent holes (1, p. 300).

SUPERHEATED STEAM

Steam at a temperature higher than the saturated temperature is called superheated steam (SHS). SHS can occur in prevacuum sterilizers when the jacket or steam supply pressure is set too high. It can also occur within fabric packs that have been stored in a hot, dry environment before placing in the sterilizer. SHS is similar in sterilization efficiency to dry heat sterilization (16, p. 125). NOTE: SHS can also occur when dehydrated materials (e.g., reusable woven wrappers that have not been prewashed) are used for packaging, leading to alteration of the bacteriocidal/sporicidal properties of steam. SHS should be avoided.

WRAPPING OF PACKAGES

- Packages should be wrapped to permit sterilization (and aeration, if needed) of the contents and to maintain sterility until packages are opened (1, p. 299).
- Sequential wrapping is a double-wrapping procedure that creates a package within a package, while simultaneous wrapping is wrapping with two sheets of wrap at the same time, using typical wrapping methods (1, p. 303).
- Double-thickness sequential wrapping, serving as a more tortuous path for contaminants after the sterilization process, and to assist in accommodating aseptic presentation, has been the traditional and accepted wrapping method. It is acceptable, however, to have double thickness without sequential wrapping, or double thickness that is bonded together, provided that aseptic technique is possible and packaging is used according to instructions by the manufacturer (1, p. 301). NOTE: The newer envelope-sleeve type of wrapping and packaging is also being used. No published information on this process was found.

WEIGHT OF INSTRUMENT SETS

- The usually cited maximum desirable weight for an instrument set is 16 to 17 pounds, and 7 pounds for a basin set. Sets weighing much less may have drying problems if they contain a concentrated metal mass. It is generally considered unwise to exceed 25 pounds when preparing a set of instruments for steam sterilization. Sets weighing more than 25 pounds are often difficult and unsafe for workers to handle and are more difficult to dry after sterilization. The more a set weighs, the greater the risk of back injury if it is not carried properly, even when using good body mechanics (6, p. 160; 14, pp. 152-153).

- Wrapped instrument sets should be of a weight specified by manufacturers of instruments, sterilizers, and container systems (excluding the weight of the wrapping materials). If instrument sterilization/container systems are used, the manufacturers' written instructions for maximum weight, set preparation, sterilizer loading procedures, exposure times, and drying cycles should be followed. Scientific supporting data should be provided by manufacturers (2, pp. 347-348).
- The bottom-line answer to, How much can an instrument set weigh? is dependent on many factors that are very specific to each hospital and each set of instruments (14, p. 153).

POUCH PACKAGING

- Pouch packaging is available as paper and/or plastic pouches that can be used for steam and EtO and Tyvek/plastic pouches that can be used for steam, EtO, and plasma sterilization. Some pouches have a self-seal; others require heat sealing. All allow for visibility of the contents (3, p. 90).
- Peel packages should have as much air removed as possible before sealing because expansion of air may cause rupturing of packages. They must also provide a seal of proven integrity. Peel packages should open without tearing, linting, shredding, or delaminating (1, p. 301).
- Double-pouch packaging should be used when an inner, or secondary, pouch is needed to ensure aseptic presentation (e.g., when several small items could fall out during opening, or to protect sharp points) and to protect an implant on the sterile field until time of use. An inside pouch should be sequentially placed, without folding, into the outer pouch. Plastic side to side allows for penetration of the sterilant (3, p. 90).
- Double-peel packages should be used in such a manner as to avoid folding the inner package to fit into the outer package. Folding edges of inner peel packages may allow for air entrapment, which could inhibit the sterilization process (1, p. 301).
- A peel-open seal, for sterile presentation, may be preformed on one end. The open end is either heat-sealed or closed with indicator tape after the item is inserted into the pouch or tube. All air is expressed from the package before sealing. Self-sealing pouches with adhesive flaps that do not require heat sealing are also available (4, p. 259).
- Peel packages made of plastic and paper combinations should be used according to the manufacturers' instructions. During

sterilization of double-peel packages, the paper portions should be placed together to ensure penetration and removal of sterilant, air, and moisture. The paper portions of the peel packages allow penetration of the sterilizing agents; the plastic portions of the package allow items to be seen (1, p. 301).

RIGID CONTAINERS

Rigid containers can be made of stainless steel, aluminum, polymers, and polymer/metal combinations and are available in a variety of sizes. Some containers use a filter system that includes filter paper and a retention frame, some use a filter incorporated in the seal, and some use a valve system. All have a locking mechanism and external handles. Rigid containers can be decontaminated after use in most automatic equipment (3, p. 88).

Before adoption and use, information should be obtained from each rigid container manufacturer on the following:

- Recommendations for cleaning agents
- Decontamination processes
- Inspection routines
- Preparation of instruments
- Securing and labeling
- Exposure times and sterilization instructions
- Test packs
- Barrier claims supported by scientific testing (3, pp. 88-89)

It is important to remember that the coolest areas and therefore the most difficult areas to sterilize in a rigid container system are under the lid and in each of the four corners (3, pp. 88-89). Also, see the section on rigid containers in the chapter "Opening and Setting Up Rooms."

STERILIZATION OF MISCELLANEOUS ITEMS AND MATERIALS

If sterilization of miscellaneous items is contemplated, the specific processes, compatibility of the material with the sterilizer and the process, and sterilization guidelines should be obtained in writing from the manufacturer of the sterilizer or the item.

Oils: Use only commercially available sterilizable oils, according to manufacturers' written instructions.

Powders: Prepackaged sterile talc is commercially available. If talc must be sterilized, however, refer to reference 4, p. 268.

Wood: Sterilization of wood is discouraged. One author comments (4, pp. 265-266):

> During sterilization, lignocellulose resin (lignin) is driven out of wood by heat. This resin may condense onto other items in the sterilizer and cause reactions if it gets into the tissues of a

patient. Therefore, wooden items must be individually wrapped and separated from other items in the sterilizer. Repeated sterilizing dries wood; steam may become superheated and lose some of its sterilizing power. The use of wood products that require steam sterilization should be minimized and their repeated sterilization avoided.

Batteries: A battery's lifetime is degraded by heat in the autoclave cycle. To preserve the life of the battery and ensure enough energy to safely run equipment, the manufacturers' written instructions should be followed (15, pp. 102-104).

EtO sterilization of miscellaneous items: In EtO sterilization, porous materials such as plastic, silicone, rubber, wood, and leather absorb a certain amount of EtO gas that must be removed. The thicker the walls of items, the longer the aeration time required (4, p. 272).

Since dry heat is the recommended process for sterilizing some miscellaneous items and materials, the reader should refer to the earlier section on dry-heat sterilization in this chapter.

References

1. AORN: Recommended practices for selection and use of packaging systems. In *Standards, recommended practices and guidelines,* Denver, 2000, Author, pp 299-304.
2. AORN: Recommended practices for sterilization in perioperative practice settings. In *Standards, recommended practices and guidelines,* Denver, 2000, Author, pp 347-358.
3. Eagleton AJ: Packaging: selection and use. In Reichert M, Young JH: *Sterilization technology for the health care facility,* ed 2, Gaithersburg, Md, 1997, Aspen, pp 85-98.
4. Fortunato N: *Berry & Kohn's operating room technique,* ed 9, St Louis, 2000, Mosby.
5. Gruendemann BJ, Fernsebner B: *Comprehensive perioperative nursing,* vol 1, *Principles,* Boston, 1995, Jones & Bartlett.
6. Lee SA: Steam sterilization: troubleshooting wet pack problems. In Reichert M, Young JH: *Sterilization technology for the health care facility,* ed 2, Gaithersburg, Md, 1997, Aspen, pp 155-166.
7. Rutala WA: Disinfection and sterilization of patient-care items, *Infect Control Hosp Epidemiol* 17(6):377-384, 1996.
8. Rutala WA: Disinfection, sterilization, and waste disposal. In Wenzel RP, editor: *Prevention and control of nosocomial infections,* ed 3, Baltimore, 1997, Williams & Wilkins, pp 539-593.
9. Rutala WA: Disinfection and sterilization. Lecture, Annual APIC Conference, Baltimore, June 21, 1999.
10. Rutala WA, Gergen MF, Weber DJ: Comparative evaluation of the sporicidal activity of new low-temperature sterilization technologies: ethylene oxide, 2 plasma sterilization systems, and liquid peracetic acid, *Am J Infect Control* 26(4):393-398, 1998.
11. Rutala WA, Shafer KM: General information on cleaning, disinfection, and sterilization. In Olmsted R, editor: *APIC infection control and applied epidemiology, principles and practice,* St Louis, 1996, Mosby, pp 15-1—15-17.

12. Rutala WA, Weber DJ: Clinical effectiveness of low-temperature sterilization technologies, *Infect Control Hosp Epidemiol* 19(10):798-804, 1998.

13. Rutala WA et al: Levels of microbial contamination on surgical instruments, *Am J Infect Control* 26(2):143-145, 1998.

14. Schultz JK: Steam sterilization: recommended practices. In Reichert M, Young JH: *Sterilization technology for the health care facility,* ed 2, Gaithersburg, Md, 1997, Aspen, pp 146-154.

15. Waldo R, Kamino A, Phippen ML: Providing instruments, equipment, and supplies. In Phippen ML, Wells MP: *Patient care during operative and invasive procedures,* Philadelphia, 2000, WB Saunders, pp 97-111.

16. Young JH: Steam sterilization: scientific principles. In Reichert M, Young JH: *Sterilization technology for the health care facility,* ed 2, Gaithersburg, Md, 1997, Aspen, pp 124-133.

Suggested Reading

1. Adler S, Scherrer M, Daschner FD: Costs of low-temperature plasma sterilization compared with other sterilization methods, *J Hosp Infect* 40(2):125-134, 1998.

2. Donaldson J: Auditing sterile processing practices, *Infection Control Today* 4(1):28, 30, 34, 2000.

3. Glaser ZR: Ozone as a sterilant, *Infection Control and Sterilization Technology* 5(3):36-37, 1999.

4. Reichert M, Schultz JK: Finding ways to avoid wet packs, *OR Manager* 15(12):22, 24, 1999.

5. Reichert M, Schultz JK: Is it sterile? How do you know? *OR Manager* 15(10):32-33, 1999.

6. Sheperd W: Safe ethylene oxide sterilizing, *Infection Control Today* 3(9):66-67, 1999.

E. Flash Sterilization

Flash sterilization (FS), the rapid sterilization of unwrapped items for immediate use, is a controversial procedure. FS has been and continues to be used for the purpose of convenience (e.g., when inventories are sparse, when fast turn-over times demand immediate sterilization between procedures, and when unsterile instruments and implants are brought in from the outside and need immediate sterilization). "Flashed" instruments are often carried in open trays through corridors from distant sterilizers, thus increasing the risk for contamination during transport.

Most flashing takes away the safeguards normally associated with routine sterilization: thorough cleaning, proper packaging and monitoring, avoidance of moisture issues, instruments that are cool to the touch, and safe modes of delivery to the sterile field. Because of the lack of safeguards, FS is now discouraged by some standard-setting organizations as a routine method of sterilization (see the definitions and descriptions section of this chapter). In some cases and in some states, FS is prohibited except in true emergency situations.

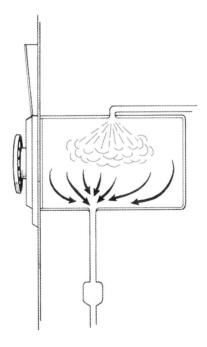

Not in question is whether devices can be sterilized as effectively in flash cycles as in conventional sterilization cycles because FS, in and of itself, is a safe and effective procedure. In question are the processes that take place before and after flashing (e.g., adequate cleaning, decontamination, and preparation, and a method of delivery to the sterile field that *ensures,* through biological indicator [BI] testing, the maintenance of sterility). FS is meant to be used not as a routine procedure but only when absolutely necessary.

DEFINITIONS AND DESCRIPTIONS

NOTE: Not all definitions and descriptions of FS are alike. The following, along with their sources, are presented here for the reader's consideration.

• *Association for the Advancement of Medical Instrumentation (AAMI):* FS is the process designated for steam sterilization of patient care items for immediate use. It is essential for healthcare personnel to properly carry out the complete multistep process, including decontamination and preparation, when FS is used. When performed correctly, FS is safe and effective for the sterilization of medical devices intended for use in contact with compromised tissue or the vascular system, as might occur during surgery or obstetrical delivery. The exposure times used in FS cycles are capable of producing appropriate lethality, as compared with the exposure times used to sterilize wrapped items (2).

• *The Centers for Disease Control and Prevention (CDC) Surgical Site Infection guideline* uses AAMI's definition of FS and goes on to explain that during any operation, the need for emergency sterilization of equipment may arise (e.g., to reprocess an inadvertently dropped instrument). However, FS is not intended to be used for reasons of convenience, nor as an alternative to purchasing additional instrument sets, nor to save time. Also, FS is not recommended for implantable devices because of the potential for serious infections. FS should be performed only on patient care items that will be used immediately (10, pp. 261, 268).

• *AORN:* FS should be used only in carefully selected clinical situations when certain parameters are met:

  • Work practices dictating proper cleaning and decontamination, inspection, and arrangement of instruments in the sterilizing tray or containers are followed.

  • The department of work area physical configuration provides for direct delivery of sterilized items to the point of use.

- Defined procedures for aseptic handling and personnel safety during the transfer of sterilized items to the point of use are followed and audited (1, pp. 348-349).
- *AORN (ambulatory surgery text):* FS should be used only in carefully selected clinical situations. The three previously mentioned AORN parameters must be met (3, pp. 55-56).
- *Association for Professionals in Infection Control and Epidemiology (APIC):* Although FS is as efficacious as longer, wrapped steam cycles, it does not have a drying cycle; therefore instruments are hot and wet. This compromises most forms of subsequent aseptic transport and storage of sterilized items. FS should be restricted to unplanned or emergency situations unless there are peer-reviewed, published references supporting expanded usage (4, pp. 95-3—95-4).
- *Joint Commission on Accreditation of Healthcare Organizations (JCAHO):* JCAHO has no written standard on FS; policies and procedures that are based on current literature should be left up to the facility (11).
- *Rutala:* FS should be restricted to emergency situations; it should not be used to compensate for inadequate inventories of instruments (13, p. 575).
- *Koch:* FS is any steam sterilization procedure that processes the items for immediate use, either with no packaging or with insufficient drying time to ensure continuing integrity of a wrapped package. The process can be carried out in any type of steam sterilizer—either gravity-displacement or dynamic air removal systems. In an emergency situation, with no alternative, FS is the only means of sterilization to provide the needed item. In this situation, a BI should always be used (8, pp. 168-170).
- *Fortunato:* FS should be used only in urgent, unplanned, or emergency situations, such as when individual items have been inadvertently dropped or forgotten and no alternative method exists. FS should not be used for routine sterilization of complete instrument sets. Specially designed surgical suites with in-room sterilizers may provide an acceptable form of FS. A flash/high-speed pressure sterilizer may have either a gravity-displacement or a prevacuum cycle; the gravity-displacement is the most common. Items to be permanently implanted in the body are not flash sterilized for immediate use unless the results of biological monitoring are immediately available. Sterility is not ensured without the results of BI testing (6, p. 264).
- *Gruendemann:* FS refers to the process of quickly sterilizing goods in an unwrapped fashion for immediate use (7, p. 218).

- *Lee:* FS is safe and efficacious when all of the recommended practices are followed. However, an important thing to remember when flash sterilizing is this: If there is not time to do it correctly the first time, when will there be time to do it over? (9, p. 47).

USE SPECIFICATIONS
Recommendations
NOTE: AAMI recommendations (also referenced by AORN and CDC) are presented in this section, followed by recommendations of other sources. Most of these recommendations are similar.
- AAMI recommendations for FS:
  I. For gravity-displacement sterilizers
     A. Metal, no lumens, nonporous items: 3 minutes at 270° F (132° C)
     B. Metal, with lumens, porous items such as rubber and plastic that are sterilized together: 10 minutes at 270° F (132° C)
  II. For prevacuum sterilizers
     A. Metal, no lumens, nonporous items: 3 minutes at 270° F (132° C)
     B. Metal, with lumens, porous items that are sterilized together: 4 minutes at 270° F (132° C) (2)
  Manufacturers' instructions must be followed for other types of sterilizers and other items to be flash steam sterilized.
- FS is sterilization of an unwrapped object at 270° F (132° C) for 3 minutes at 27 to 28 pounds of pressure in a gravity-displacement autoclave (13, p. 575).
- The minimum exposure time for FS is 3 minutes at 270° to 275° F (132° to 135° C) for unwrapped nonporous, uncomplicated stainless steel items without lumens. When porous items or instruments with instrument marking tape or lumens are included in the load, timing is increased to 4 minutes or longer in a prevacuum sterilizer and to 10 minutes or longer in a gravity-displacement sterilizer. With these cycles, the entire time for starting, sterilizing, and opening the sterilizer is a minimum of 6 to 7 minutes. Steam should be maintained in the jacket at all times (6, p. 264).
- FS can be accomplished in either a gravity-displacement or prevacuum sterilizer. A FS cycle is 3 or 10 minutes, depending on the item being sterilized (7, p. 220).
- FS is always performed at ≥270° F (132° C), with exposure times varying according to the type of item being sterilized. For example, the minimum exposure time for nonporous items requiring surface sterilization is 3 minutes, while the minimum exposure

time for porous items or items with spring hinges and/or channels is 10 minutes (8, p. 169).
• Exposure times for FS are shorter, but no less lethal, than those of
   longer cycles. There is still the same safety factor (usually at least
   50% more than the time needed to provide a sterility assurance
   level of 10^6) as in the standard sterilization cycles for wrapped
   goods (7, p. 220).

Special Considerations
Powered equipment
FS of powered equipment (e.g., drills, saws) is not generally recommended, but if FS is necessary, the prevacuum method should be
used. Some manufacturers may provide instructions for FS of powered equipment, using a 10-minute gravity cycle, but the equipment
may require special positioning (8, p. 169). NOTE: Written manufacturers' instructions should always be followed.

Use of single wrapper
• FS using a single wrapper is now available from at least one
   sterilizer manufacturer. This cycle consists of a 4-minute
   exposure time at 270° F (132° C) with a 3-minute dry time. There
   are, however, some conditions under which this method cannot
   be used (e.g., with paper/plastic peel pouches, or for complex
   medical devices such as powered instruments). Also, items flash
   sterilized using a single wrapper are intended for immediate
   use; the tray should be handled as though it had no wrapper
   (9, pp. 43-44).
• Some sterilizers have a flash cycle that allows the use of a single
   wrapper (e.g., an abbreviated prevacuum and pulsing gravity cycle). The exposure time is 4 minutes, and only simple all-metal or
   glass instrumentation can be sterilized. No complex devices,
   items with lumens, or nonporous materials other than the wrapper should be included (3, p. 56).

Flash sterilization containers
Container systems that protect items during transfer from the sterilizer to the sterile field are available for FS. The container manufacturers should provide scientific evidence of the suitability of the containers for the sterilizer in use (6, p. 264). NOTE: Containers should
be validated for the specific cycle being used for FS.

Implants
• Implantable medical devices should not be flash sterilized, but if
   this is done, the physical parameters of time, temperature, and

pressure should be monitored, recorded, and examined for each cycle (3, p. 56).

- Implantable medical devices should not be flash sterilized because of possible patient complications. Careful planning, appropriate packaging, and inventory management can eliminate the need to flash sterilize implantable medical devices. If an implantable device is flash sterilized, the device must be used immediately after a negative biological readout. If not used, the device must be reprocessed before future use (1, p. 350; 13, p. 575; 6, p. 264).

MONITORING

- A sterilization process monitoring device (SPMD) should be used with each load undergoing FS. BIs intended for flash sterilizers should be used daily according to manufacturers' written instructions (3, p. 56; 1, p. 350).
- The routine use of chemical process indicators and BIs is recommended (8, p. 171).
- Flash sterility is not ensured without results of BI testing (6, p. 264).
- Monitoring of flash cycles includes (1) *physical monitoring:* observing the real-time assessment of rounds charts, computer printouts, and gauges before a new cycle is initiated, during the cycle, and before each load is released for use; (2) *chemical monitoring:* a chemical indicator is used in each tray; (3) *prevacuum residual air testing:* known as the Bowie-Dick test, should be performed according to the manufacturers' instructions; (4) *biological monitoring:* a biological test product, appropriate for the type of flash cycle being employed (9, pp. 44, 46).
- Enzyme-based products entered the market in the early 1990s. The Rapid Readout product contains *Bacillus stearothermophilus,* just as other steam BIs do. This product tests for a naturally occurring enzyme that is present in a layer of the natural spore coat. A special dye is added to the growth medium through a test for fluorescence.

  Following a steam sterilization cycle, the indicator is placed in an incubator for 30 to 120 minutes and then read to determine whether the enzyme was inactivated. The lack of detectable enzyme is highly correlated with a successful sterilization cycle. Once the enzyme readout has been completed, the ampule *could* be placed in the incubator, then read in 7 days as a true BI. The Rapid Readout is registered with the U.S. Food and Drug Administration (FDA) as a BI because it contains spores. A second enzyme product, the RSI Rapid Indicator, contains only enzymes, not spores. The RSI is considered by the FDA to be a multiple interactive bacterial enzyme indicator. Responsible hospital personnel need to decide whether either the Rapid Readout or the RSI is appropriate for use in a sterility assurance program and under what circumstances (12, pp. 33-34).

See the section on rapid detection systems in the chapter "Monitoring of Sterilization Processes."

DOCUMENTATION

- Documentation should always include results of chemical and biological monitoring, as well as quality improvement data.
- FS records should be maintained for as long as is required by state and local statutes (9, p. 46).
- It is advisable to maintain a log of flash sterilizer use. Documentation provides a record of what transpired, especially if an infection control or legal inquiry occurs. It is not uncommon for the JCAHO surveyor to request the flash log for review. Documentation should include:
  - Patient identification
  - Operator identification
  - Sterilizer identification
  - Date and time of cycle
  - Load contents
  - Time and temperature of the exposure
  - Monitoring results

These records should be retained for the duration of the statute of limitations for the particular state in which the facility is located (5, pp. 274, 276).

PROBLEMS AND ISSUES

- It is erroneous to think that FS is somehow less effective than wrapped sterilization. However, there are some issues with FS that generally preclude its routine use: problems with the preparation of items (e.g., inadequate cleaning because of pressure to reprocess a device rapidly when large instrument sets are routinely flashed between procedures), the problem of post-sterilization handling of unwrapped items, and having the sterilizer positioned not immediately adjacent to the intended point of use (7, p. 218).
- FS has a smaller margin of safety than other methods of sterilization because the sterilization cycle parameters are the minimal requirements for sterilization. Deviations from exposure time, temperature, or pressure can result in failure of sterilization. In addition, the sterilized items will not be protected by packaging after sterilization, increasing the possibility of exogenous contamination (13, p. 575).

- Transferring instruments from the sterilizer to the sterile field always presents problems. Prevention of contamination during the transfer is the main concern. Two options are as follows:
  1. Use of a single wrapper to cover or wrap instruments. Some sterilizers provide such an option; specific instructions from the manufacturer must be followed (see previous discussion on single wrappers).
  2. Use of rigid containers designed for FS. These containers protect the sterility of the items during removal from and transport from the sterilizer. The manufacturers' recommendations should scientifically verify the safety of this process. For example, recommended temperature and exposure times for specific items should also be validated by the manufacturer (see previous discussion on container systems) (8, pp. 169-170).
- FS can result in clinical burns to patients after inadequate cooling of the instruments. A recent report cites burn injuries to two patients following the use of flashed instruments. One patient received a partial-thickness burn to the thigh from a hot shaver housing; the other patient suffered a full-thickness thigh burn from a retractor weight that had not been sufficiently cooled (14, p. 458).

References

1. AORN: Recommended practices for sterilization in perioperative practice settings. In *Standards, recommended practices and guidelines,* Denver, 2000, Author, pp 347-358.
2. Association for the Advancement of Medical Instrumentation: *Flash sterilization: steam sterilization of patient care items for immediate use, ANSI/AAMI ST 37-1996,* Arlington, Va, 1996, Author.
3. Association of Operating Room Nurses: *Ambulatory surgery principles and practices,* Denver, 1999, Author.
4. Earl A: Operating room. In Olmsted R, editor: *APIC infection control and applied epidemiology, principles and practice,* St Louis, 1996, Mosby, pp 95-1—95-7.
5. Fogg DM: Clinical issues, *AORN J* 69(1):272-274, 276, 1999.
6. Fortunato N: *Berry & Kohn's operating room technique,* ed 9, St Louis, 2000, Mosby.
7. Gruendemann BJ, Fernsebner B: *Comprehensive perioperative nursing,* vol 1, *Principles,* Boston, 1995, Jones & Bartlett.
8. Koch FA: Steam sterilization: recommended practices for flash sterilization. In Reichert M, Young JH: *Sterilization technology for the health care facility,* ed 2, Gaithersburg, Md, 1997, Aspen, pp 167-172.
9. Lee SA: Flash sterilization: practical insights for appropriate use, *Infection Control Today* 3(5):42-44, 46-47, 1999.
10. Mangram AJ, Hospital Infection Control Practices Advisory Committee (HICPAC), Centers for Disease Control and Prevention: Guideline for prevention of surgical site infection, 1999, *Infect Control Hosp Epidemiol* 20(4):247-278, 1999. (Reprinted, in part, in Appendix B.)

11. Personal communication, Joint Commission on Accreditation of Healthcare Organizations, June 1999.

12. Reichert M, Schultz JK: What's best for monitoring steam? *OR Manager* 15(7):33-34, 1999.

13. Rutala WA: Disinfection, sterilization, and waste disposal. In Wenzel RP, editor: *Prevention and control of nosocomial infections,* ed 3, Baltimore, 1997, Williams & Wilkins, pp 539-593.

14. Rutala WA, Weber DJ, Chappell KJ: Patient injury from flash-sterilized instruments, *Infect Control Hosp Epidemiol* 20(7):458, 1999 (letter to the editor).

Suggested Reading

1. Barrett T: Why not flash sterilization? ican News & Commentary, Editorial Commentary, icanPREVENT (www.icanPREVENT.com). Updated 9/8/00, accessed 9/8/00.

2. Joint Commission crackdown: are you doing flash sterilization properly? *Same Day Surg* 23(9):101-103, 1999.

3. Mayworm D: Sterilization problems: implants, *Infection Control and Sterilization Technology* 5(3):34-35, 1999.

4. Rhyne L, Ulmer BC, Revell L: Monitoring and controlling the environment. In Phippen ML, Wells MP: *Patient care during operative and invasive procedures,* Philadelphia, 2000, WB Saunders, pp 147-166.

F. Monitoring of Sterilization Processes

The importance of routinely monitoring the quality of sterilization procedures has been established (7, p. 261). Sterilizer efficacy should be monitored at regular intervals with a biological indicator (BI) (1, p. 354).

In order to ensure effectiveness of sterilization processes, several types of monitoring indicators and processes can be used. The types of monitoring indicators are physical or mechanical, chemical (including air-removal tests), and biological.

The indicators and processes that are appropriate for flash sterilization, including a section on rapid readout indicators, are discussed in the chapter "Flash Sterilization." Rapid readout indicators are also discussed in this chapter.

PHYSICAL OR MECHANICAL INDICATORS

Temperature and pressure gauges and recorders are the primary sources of information about proper mechanical, or physical, operation of sterilizers (5, p. 230).

Sterilizers have gauges, thermometers, timers, and/or other devices that monitor their functions. Records are reviewed and maintained for each cycle. Test packs or special diagnostics should be run at least once daily to monitor functions of each sterilizer, as appropriate. Such tests can identify process errors (3, p. 257).

It is not possible to measure steam temperature at every location in a steam sterilizer. Therefore reliance must be placed on secondary indications of conditions in the chamber. Appropriate information

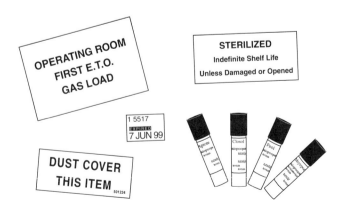

may be provided by mechanical indicators, such as chamber and jacket pressure and temperature gauges, and chart recorders. The information obtained from these mechanical indicators is then accompanied by additional data obtained from electronic sensors and displays, air leak tests, and process indicators (biological and chemical) (11, p. 116).

The sterilizer manufacturer should provide comprehensive routine and preventative care and maintenance instructions, as well as instructions for proper use and functioning (3, p. 257).

CHEMICAL INDICATORS AND AIR-REMOVAL TESTS

- A sterilization process monitoring device (SPMD) or chemical indicator such as chemically treated paper, pellets sealed in a glass tube, or pressure-sensitive tape should be used on (and/or in) each package to be sterilized, including items being flash sterilized. When the monitoring device is not visible from the outside of the package, a separate process indicator should be used on the exterior of the package (1, p. 354).

- The purpose of *external* process indicators is to differentiate between processed and nonprocessed items. Although SPMDs do not verify sterility, they help detect procedural errors and equipment malfunctions (1, p. 354).

- SPMDs ascertain whether items have been subjected to sterilization conditions. Sterility of the sterilizer load is evidenced by the killing of all spores on biological test indicators (1, p. 354).

- The following are six classes of chemical indicators:

  1. *Internal and external process indicators:* For example, autoclave tape, indicators on peel pouches, instrument protectors, and load record cards.

  2. *Bowie-Dick (air-removal) test for vacuum steam sterilizers:* Assesses the efficiency of the vacuum pump and the presence of air leaks and/or gases in the steam. Does *not* determine if sterilization parameters have been met.

  3. *Single-parameter indicators:* Assess minimum temperature, for example, by the melting of a chemical or changing of color.

  4. *Multiparameter indicators:* Contain ink that changes color when exposed to the correct combination of sterilization parameters; are sterilant specific.

  5. *Integrating indicators:* Respond to all sterilization parameters over a specified range of sterilization temperatures. The International Standards Organization (ISO) definition states that the performance of integrators can be compared to the inactivation of a test organism.

6. *Emulator:* Being developed; not currently available commercially. Its performance will be based on a specified sterilization cycle and is expected, when available, to be very cycle specific (8, pp. 105-107).

- An air-removal test for prevacuum steam sterilizer cycles (e.g., any sterilizer that has assisted air removal as part of the cycle) should be performed daily in an empty chamber. This air-removal test detects residual air in the sterilizer chamber, which would prevent steam contact with items in a load and interfere with the sterilization process (1, p. 355).

BIOLOGICAL INDICATORS

- One component of a sterilization assurance program is biological monitoring. Biological monitoring evaluates the ability of a sterilization process to operate effectively regardless of the equipment, medical device sterilized, or sterilizing agent used (9, pp. 37-38).
- Biological monitoring involves the use of a device impregnated with a known number and type of microorganism and is used to verify that all of the conditions necessary for sterilization have been met. The use of a BI does not guarantee sterility but rather provides an additional mechanism for monitoring the sterilizer cycle beyond the graphic temperature-pressure recording and the physical chemical indicators (6, p. 101).
- BIs that are used to monitor sterilization processes represent a worst-case microbial challenge to the sterilization process. Inactivation of the BI organisms provides a very high level of assurance that naturally occurring organisms are also inactivated. Standard BI preparations are available only for sterilization processes and cannot be applied to disinfection or sanitization (4, p. 8).
- Spore strip BIs are the only process indicators that directly measure sterilization. A disadvantage is the delay in getting results due to incubation times (10, p. 15-13).
- Sterilizer efficacy should be monitored at regular intervals with a BI. Additional monitoring of several consecutive cycles should be done after sterilizer installation, major repair, major redesign, or relocation (1, p. 354).
- The following is a list of sterilizers and the BIs that are used to monitor them:
  - Steam: *Bacillus stearothermophilus* spore testing should be done at least weekly and preferably daily (and with each load of implantables).
  - EtO: *Bacillus subtilis* spore testing should be done with each load.

- Low-temperature hydrogen peroxide gas plasma: *B. subtilis* spore testing should be done at the same interval as other sterilizer testing in the facility.
- Low-temperature liquid peracetic acid: *B. stearothermophilus* spore testing should be done at least weekly and preferably daily with products designed for this specific process.
- Dry heat: *B. subtilis* var. *niger* indicators should be used on installation and after any major testing. For tabletop gravity convection units, sterilizer loads should be monitored with a BI at least once a week (1, p. 354; 3, p. 257).
- Positive BI results must be reported immediately to appropriate personnel so that corrective action can be taken. All BI test results, including control results, must be interpreted by qualified personnel and included in the sterilization records (1, p. 354).
- BIs ascertain whether products have been subjected to sterilization conditions. Sterility of the load is evidenced by the killing of all spores on biological test indicators (1, p. 354).
- BIs are used to monitor sterilization processes involving steam, dry heat, gaseous sterilants, and radiation. Commercially available BIs are made with spores of organisms that are stable, reproducible, and highly resistant to the mode of sterilization that they monitor; several types are available (2, p. 111).
- BIs may be supplied in a self-contained system, on dry spore strips or disks in envelopes, or in sealed vials or ampules of spores in suspension. Each of these units contains the spores to be sterilized and a control BI that is not sterilized. Some also incorporate a chemical indicator (3, p. 257).
- An "every-load" biological monitoring system may be chosen after a sterilizer process fails, for example, when a patient has been potentially harmed or a physician notified about a potentially negative patient outcome. In most cases, quarantine and every-load biological monitoring are the most practical and least expensive operational processes that also meet the ethical responsibilities to the patient (9, pp. 40-41).
- BIs need to conform to the testing standards of the U.S. Pharmacopeia (USP). A control test is performed at least once weekly in each sterilizer. Every load of implantables is monitored, and implants should not be used until negative test results are known. All test results are filed in permanent records for each sterilizer (3, p. 257).

Interpretation of Biological Indicator Results

- BIs are used to show only that sterilizing conditions were attained at the sites monitored by them. As long as a device can be sterilized in the generic recommended time; it is properly cleaned, prepared, packaged, and placed on the sterilizer cart; and the BIs are placed in the most difficult-to-sterilize locations, it is reasonable to accept that the device is sterile if the activated BIs demonstrate no growth (i.e., negative results) (2, p. 114).

- Before any conclusions about sterility are made, the control BIs must be evaluated. A *positive control BI* is a BI that is activated and incubated without being subjected to the sterilization process. This control should be positive, indicating that there are viable spores on the spore strip. If the control is negative, a potential sterilization failure may not be detected (2, p. 114).

- When a BI (not a control) is positive, it is indicative of a possible sterilization process failure. All products processed since the last negative BI should be recalled (2, p. 114).

Rapid Detection Systems

- An advance in biological monitoring has been the development of rapid readout monitors. These monitors use the fluorimetric detection of a spore-bound enzyme at 60 minutes rather than the observation of spore growth, which normally requires a minimum of 24 hours for assessment of sterilizer effectiveness. More rapid results would allow recall of potentially inadequately sterilized devices either before patient use or before the end of surgery (10, p. 15-13).

- One type of a self-contained BI contains a rapid detection system, based on the interaction of an enzyme in the bacterial spore with a substrate in the growth medium. Fluorescence occurs when the viable BI is exposed to ultraviolet light. This BI is particularly valuable in the operating room or ambulatory setting where products may be sterilized unwrapped in a gravity displacement ("flash") sterilizer. This type of BI can be read within 3 hours when used in specified steam sterilizers, in certain cycles (2, p. 111).

- A rapid readout BI, developed specifically for monitoring a high-speed pressure steam sterilizer with a gravity displacement cycle, is based on the fluorimetric detection of a *B. stearothermopilus*–bound enzyme, rather than on spore growth. The enzyme becomes fluorescent yellow within 60 minutes as the spores are killed (3, p. 257).

  NOTE: Additional rapid detection devices have become available—some claiming very short readout times (e.g., 20 seconds). Manufacturers' instructions should be carefully followed. (See the section on enzyme-based products in the chapter "Flash Sterilization.")

QUALITY CONTROL

Quality control parameters for the sterilization process should include the following:

- Sterilizer maintenance history
- Sterilization process monitoring by biological, chemical, or mechanical devices
- Air removal testing, such as the Bowie-Dick type, of prevacuum steam sterilizers (i.e., sterilizers that have assisted air removal as part of the sterilization cycle; this is *not* a test for sterility)
- Visual inspection of packaging
- Lot control and traceability of load contents (1, p. 353)

Documentation, including routine biological monitoring results, is necessary for every cycle, wrapped or unwrapped, of every sterilizer within a healthcare facility. Documentation of sterilization produces a record of cycle performance and establishes accountability in the practice setting (1, p. 353).

References

1. AORN: Recommended practices for sterilization in perioperative practice settings. In *Standards, recommended practices and guidelines,* Denver, 2000, Author, pp 347-358.
2. Berube R, Oxborrow GS: Sterilization process monitoring: biological indicators. In Reichert M, Young JH: *Sterilization technology for the health care facility,* ed 2, Gaithersburg, Md, 1997, Aspen, pp 110-115.
3. Fortunato N: *Berry & Kohn's operating room technique,* ed 9, St Louis, 2000, Mosby.
4. Graham GS: Decontamination: scientific principles. In Reichert M, Young JH: *Sterilization technology for the health care facility,* ed 2, Gaithersburg, Md, 1997, Aspen, pp 1-8.
5. Gruendemann BJ, Fernsebner B: *Comprehensive perioperative nursing,* vol 1, *Principles,* Boston, 1995, Jones & Bartlett.
6. Japp NF: Packaging: shelf life. In Reichert M, Young JH: *Sterilization technology for the health care facility,* ed 2, Gaithersburg, Md, 1997, Aspen, pp 99-103.
7. Mangram AJ, Hospital Infection Control Practices Advisory Committee (HICPAC), Centers for Disease Control and Prevention: Guideline for prevention of surgical site infection, 1999, *Infect Control Hosp Epidemiol* 20(4):247-278, 1999. (Reprinted, in part, in Appendix B.)
8. Proietti RM: Sterilization process monitoring: chemical indicators. In Reichert M, Young JH, editors: *Sterilization technology for the health care facility,* ed 2, Gaithersburg, Md, 1997, Aspen, pp 104-109.
9. Ross ES: Using biological monitoring to reduce infection, risk, and cost, *Surgical Services Management* 4(7):37-38, 40-41, 1998.
10. Rutala WA, Shafer KM: General information on cleaning, disinfection, and sterilization. In Olmsted R, editor: *APIC infection control and applied epidemiology, principles and practice,* St Louis, 1996, Mosby, pp 15-1—15-17.
11. Schneier ML: Sterilization process monitoring: mechanical indicators. In Reichert M, Young JH: *Sterilization technology for the health care facility,* ed 2, Gaithersburg, Md, 1997, Aspen, pp 116-123.

G. Event-Related Sterility, Expiration Dating, and Storage of Sterile Items

Many questions remain regarding how long a sterile package can stay sterile and if outdating can be completely eliminated. Today, both time-related and event-related sterility processes are in place in healthcare facilities in the United States. The standard in most facilities, however, is event-related sterility (ERS). The issue of time-related versus event-related sterility is not a simple one and requires that facilities and processing departments carefully evaluate and justify their practices (6, p. 99).

Policies and procedures that designate either time-related or event-related sterility for hospital sterilized items, and also for commercially prepared sterile items that do not have an expiration date, are required by the Joint Commission on Accreditation of Healthcare Organizations (JCAHO). In addition, the JCAHO requires that the established policies be consistent in intent and application throughout the facility (2).

This chapter includes a discussion on both the recommended ERS, including protocols for use, and the occasionally used time-related expiration dating. Packaging, storage, and sterility maintenance are also discussed.

EVENT-RELATED STERILITY

Since the early 1990s ERS has become a well-accepted standard in the processing of sterile healthcare devices and supplies. This trend was brought about not only by the advent of new packaging materials, but also by the desire of healthcare managers to reduce the costs of reprocessing and resterilizing many devices and supplies that, al-

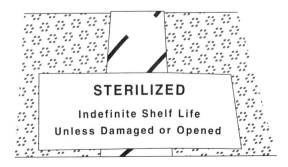

though their packages were intact, had expired sterility dates. Quality improvement methods were used to assess the appropriateness of protocols that did not seem cost effective in terms of time, labor, and productivity.

The idea behind ERS is that if a sterile item (packaged according to acceptable protocols) and its packaging have not been compromised, the item is considered to be sterile and safe for use. With ERS, sterile items packaged are assumed to be sterile as long as the package is intact; length of time since sterilization is irrelevant.

Manufacturers have used ERS for many years. The techniques used during processing produce a totally sealed package made of materials that are impervious. Typical ERS package labels read, "Contents sterile unless package is open or damaged. Inspect before use."

In any situation, each package of sterile items must always be carefully inspected by the end user for any break in integrity—regardless of expiration date or event-related processes. Breaks in integrity can include evidence of holes and tears, water marks that may indicate that the item was wet after sterilization, and defects in peel-pouch seals. Inspection for these breaks is a priority when handling any packaged sterile item or device.

STERILITY EXPIRATION DATING

With time-related sterility expiration dating, sterilized items are packaged and labeled with expiration dates. An expiration date is based on the method of packaging used and the length of time since sterilization. An item is considered sterile until the package has reached its expiration date, at which time the item is repackaged, resterilized, and assigned a new expiration date.

Expiration dates are still used in certain situations. Some products, such as pharmaceuticals, latex products, and specialized catheters, may degrade or change over time and therefore have designated shelf lives of their own that take precedence over ERS considerations.

- Expiration dates can be used to ensure proper inventory turnover and to conserve storage space. The appropriate use of expiration dates serves as a reminder that packages are susceptible to contamination and helps to facilitate the rotation of supplies to ensure that older items are used first. Expiration dates do not guarantee either sterility or lack of sterility (9, p. 15-15).
- Deterioration of a packaged product after a specified period and general rotation of items are the only plausible reasons for shelf-life dating (1, p. 66).

EVENT-RELATED STERILITY AND SHELF LIFE

- The shelf life of a packaged sterile item is event related. An event must occur to compromise package content sterility. Events that may compromise package sterility include multiple handling that can lead to seal breakage or loss of package integrity, moisture penetration, and airborne contamination (3, p. 353).
- The shelf life of a packaged sterile item is event related and depends on the quality of the wrapper material, conditions during storage and transport, and the amount of handling prior to use (6, p. 101).
- Event-related shelf life practice recognizes that the product should remain sterile until some event causes the item to become contaminated. Examples of events are tears in packaging, the packaging becoming wet, the package being dropped on a contaminated surface such as a floor, and any compromise that destroys the barrier effectiveness of the packaged material (9, p. 15-15).
- Sterility is lost when an event takes place that is capable of introducing microorganisms into a package. Such an event can occur at any time. Examples of events are touching warm and damp packs or instrument trays just removed from the sterilizer (microorganisms on hands may penetrate wrappers); finding tears or pinholes in wrappers; and sneezing or coughing on a package that is not totally sealed, such as a wrapped instrument set (8, pp. 20-21).
- Most contaminating events probably happen as a direct result of frequent or improper handling. Dust or particulate matter on packages can be carried into the package during handling. Lack of cleanliness of storage shelves is a contributing factor, and conditions outside of the surgical suite where sterile supplies are stored should also be assessed (8, pp. 20-21).
- The optimum number of times an item should be handled is three: (1) when removing an item from the sterilizer cart and placing it on a storage shelf, (2) when placing the item on a case cart or supply exchange cart, and (3) when picking up the item to open for use (8, p. 20).
- In ERS, a protocol should also ensure that oldest items are used first. Sterilized items should be marked with the date of sterilization. At regular intervals stock should be rotated so that items with the oldest sterilization dates are in the front of the shelf or bin. These items should be used first to avoid prolonged opportunities for contaminating events to occur (2).
- The sterility of a package can be assured in one of two ways: (1) prevention—ensuring that events that would compromise

the integrity of a package are eliminated, or (2) protection—protecting sterile products with a plastic sterility maintenance cover (dust cover) or a sealed Tyvek pouch package (8, p. 21).

• An effective event-related policy is an example of the practice of sound infection control techniques (7, p. 38).

ESTABLISHING ERS PROTOCOLS

• Too often the transition from expiration dating to an ERS maintenance program merely involves removal of the expiration dates. There is much more to the process than that. The following steps should be taken to ensure an effective ERS program:
  • Investigating and assessing the environment
  • Minimizing events that could compromise the sterility of a package
  • Controlling inventory to minimize the time between sterilization and use
  • Selecting and using appropriate packaging materials and techniques
  • Reinforcing the need to inspect packages prior to use (8, pp. 20-21)
• Issues to consider include:
  • Barrier characteristics of materials
  • Methods of microbial contamination
  • Size of particles that can penetrate barriers
  • Packaging materials suitable for the method of sterilization
  • Whole-package challenge testing of barrier materials (e.g., testing of peel-pouch seals)
  • Proper sealing of peel pouches (e.g., two pouches applied plastic to plastic to allow for sterilant penetration and removal)
  • Vulnerability of packaging materials to contamination while still hot, with water vapor inside (such as after steam sterilization)
  • Number of times the package will be handled between sterilization and actual use
  • Consistency of workers in the selection and application of wrappers
  • Environmental conditions (e.g., relative humidity and ventilation)
  • Methods of transport
  • Cleanliness of storage areas inside and outside of the surgical suite
  • Care and handling at point of use (6, p. 99; 8, pp. 20-21)
• It is the responsibility of each processing manager to assess the environment and develop a system that ensures that products will be sterile at the point of use (6, p. 102).

- Hospitals and other healthcare facilities have two strong incentives for changing to an ERS policy: (1) the cost of reprocessing due to expiration dates can be significantly reduced, and (2) by taking all the steps needed to implement the policy, hospitals can identify several areas where they can improve internal processes, thus reducing cost, expediting work flow, and enhancing productivity (7, p. 31).

PACKAGING

- Effective packaging materials should provide adequate barriers to microorganisms or their vehicles. The FDA classifies sterilization wrap as a Class II medical device intended to allow sterilization of the enclosed device and maintenance of sterility of the device until used (7, pp. 32-33).
- Healthcare facilities need to carefully review the technical documentation of barrier performance supplied by wrap manufacturers (7, p. 32).
- Factors that compromise the bacterial barrier efficiency and integrity of a package material include the following:
  - *Airborne bacteria:* may be forced into the package by incorrect or excessive handling
  - *Dust, soil, gross contamination:* may be forced into the package by incorrect or excessive handling, poor storage facilities, or improper techniques
  - *Moisture:* may be absorbed into the package
  - *Holes, tears, breaks, rupture of seals:* allow direct entry of microbes
  - *Improper opening of the package:* may lead to the introduction of microbes (9, p. 15-15)
- A double-wrapped package will reduce the possibility of contamination during unwrapping. Sterilized items (except those in rigid containers or peel pouches) should be wrapped in two thicknesses of paper or nonwoven fabrics (6, p. 101).
- Double-thickness sequential wrapping has been the traditional and accepted wrapping method; however, it is acceptable to have double thickness without sequential wrapping or double thickness that is bonded together, provided aseptic presentation can be maintained and packaging is used according to manufacturers' written instructions (2).
- A dust cover (sealed, airtight plastic bag) protects a sterile package from dust, dirt, lint, moisture, and vermin during storage. After sterilization and immediately following aerating or cooling to room temperature, infrequently used items may be sealed in plastic 2 to 3 mm thick. A dust cover will protect the integrity of a package (5, p. 278).

• Protective packaging, commonly referred to as sterility maintenance covers (SMCs), or dust covers, is used to maintain the
sterility of items. The sterilized product is sealed within the
SMC immediately after cool-down. As long as the impervious
SMC is sealed and intact, the item is protected from the contaminating effect of various events. This protective cover is usually 3 mm thick and is available in a variety of preformed, perforated tear sizes. Some have a self-seal; others require heat
sealing (4, p. 91).

  The reader should also refer to the section on packaging in the
chapter "Sterilization."

STORAGE

• Appropriate storage conditions for sterile packs include the
following:
  • Limited access to the storage area or closed cabinets
  • Separate storage of clean and sterile supplies
  • Clean, dry, dust-free, lint-free area
  • Area with a temperature between 65° and 72° F and a humidity
    level between 35% and 50%
  • Materials storage 8 to 10 inches from the floor, 18 to
    20 inches from the ceiling (to allow for functioning of sprinkler
    systems), and 6 to 8 inches from an outside wall (to avoid
    condensation and subsequent contamination) (9, p. 15-15)
• Sterile packages should not be crushed, bent, or compressed.
Supplies must not be stored under or next to sinks, water or
sewer pipes, or in any area where they might become wet. Only
designated shelves, counters, or carts should be used. Storage is
generally on carts or designated shelving, either fixed or portable.
Both open and closed shelves are used, but closed shelving is
preferred (6, p. 102).

STERILITY MAINTENANCE

• Sterility maintenance is dependent on having measures in place
to eliminate events that could compromise packaging and to
protect the integrity of the package (6, p. 101).
• Two practices that facilitate rapid use of sterile supplies and can
contribute to sterility maintenance, are inventory control to prevent overstocking and rotation of supplies to ensure that older
stock is used before newer stock (9, p. 15-15).
• Sterile items remaining on shelves and unused for a period of
over 1 year should be evaluated with regard to the continued
need for considering the item sterile. Items remaining on shelves
for extended periods represent poorly managed inventory. Slow

inventory turnover should be carefully evaluated to determine the necessity of stocking such items (2).

• By closely examining exactly what happens as a sterile item moves through the system, hospitals not only reinforce the principles of sterility maintenance but also can find ways to improve their processes, even if they do not adopt an event-related policy (7, p. 33).

• Developing a process-oriented system to eliminate possibilities of compromise to sterility is one of the prime objectives of an ERS maintenance policy (7, p. 32).

DROPPED STERILE ITEMS

• If a sterile package is dropped, the item may be considered safe for immediate use only if it is enclosed in an impervious material and the integrity of the package is maintained. Dropping items wrapped in woven materials could force air and contaminants through the wrapper; therefore such dropped items should not be used (5, p. 172).

• It was once recommended that if a sterile package is dropped on the floor, it should be discarded or reprocessed. However, with the switch to ERS, this practice has changed. Contamination occurs because an event has allowed penetration of the packaging. Nevertheless, if a package is dropped on the floor, it is always considered contaminated. Whether a package was sterilized in the hospital or commercially should not be a factor (2). (See the chapter "Opening and Setting Up Rooms.")

• The following questions should be answered before deciding whether an item wrapped in a sterile package is contaminated after the package has been dropped:
  • Is the package material impervious?
  • Is the package material woven or nonwoven?
  • Is the surface on which the package was dropped clean? dry? unknown?
  • Does the wrapper surface have tears, holes, or questionable areas (2)?

References

1. Alexander D: Packaging: pouches. In Reichert M, Young JH: *Sterilization technology for the health care facility,* ed 2, Gaithersburg, Md, 1997, Aspen, pp 62-69.
2. AORN Online Clinical Practice FAQ Database, 1999, www.aorn.org/_results/clinical.asp (accessed 2000).
3. AORN: Recommended practices for sterilization in perioperative practice settings. In *Standards, recommended practices and guidelines,* Denver, 2000, Author, pp 347-358.

4. Eagleton AJ: Packaging: selection and use. In Reichert M, Young JH: *Sterilization technology for the health care facility,* ed 2, Gaithersburg, Md, 1997, Aspen, pp 85-98.

5. Fortunato N: *Berry & Kohn's operating room technique,* ed 9, St Louis, 2000, Mosby.

6. Japp NF: Packaging: shelf life. In Reichert M, Young JH: *Sterilization technology for the health care facility,* ed 2, Gaithersburg, Md, 1997, Aspen, pp 99-103.

7. Kovach SM, Taylor JR: Implementing an event-related sterility maintenance policy, *Infection Control and Sterilization Technology* 1(3):31-33, 38, 1995.

8. Reichert M, Schultz JK: The dating game 25 years later, *OR Manager* 16(4):20-21, 2000.

9. Rutala WA, Shafer KM: General information on cleaning, disinfection, and sterilization. In Olmsted R, editor: *APIC infection control and applied epidemiology, principles and practice,* St Louis, 1996, Mosby, pp 15-1—15-17.

Suggested Reading

1. American Society for Healthcare Central Service Professionals of the American Hospital Association: *Training manual for central service technicians,* Chicago, 1997, Author.

2. AORN: Recommended practices for selection and use of packaging systems. In *Standards, recommended practices and guidelines,* Denver, 2000, Author, pp 299-304.

3. Association for the Advancement of Medical Instrumentation: *Good hospital practice: steam sterilization and sterility assurance, ANSI/AAMI ST 46-331, 1994,* Arlington, Va, 1994, Author.

4. Jenich D: Keeping patients safe: disposable wraps offer numerous benefits, *Infection Control Today* 4(1):58-60, 2000.

5. Key P, Wehmer MA: Microbial transference in dropped sterile items, *Infection Control Today* 3(6):36, 38, 40, 42, 1999.

6. Mayworm D: Probably sterile, *Infection Control and Sterilization Technology* 1(3):7, 1995.

H. Parametric Release

Validation of the entire sterilization process may be done through a process called parametric release (PR). This process is used by medical device manufacturers in the United States and by hospitals for steam sterilization in Europe.

With PR, predetermined conditions in the sterilizer and the load must be met. This is in contrast to the use in most U.S. healthcare facilities of a single biological indicator (BI) to determine conditions inside a steam sterilizer.

Sophisticated monitoring systems are a prerequisite for PR, as are strong quality systems, whether in industry or healthcare facilities. PR uses process control parameters.

PR is a relatively new term to central service personnel in the United States, but it is becoming better known.

DESCRIPTION AND USE

- PR uses BIs for sterilization cycle development and validation, but *not* for routine monitoring of sterilization processes. Rather,

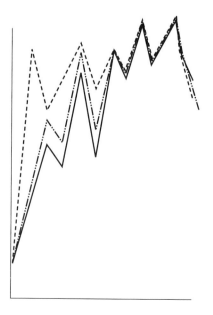

the critical parameters of the process are constantly monitored during the cycle (1, p. 128).

- Medical device manufacturers who employ PR use process controls and validation procedures that are at the heart of good manufacturing practices (GMPs) to verify the sterilization process. These GMPs include environmental monitoring, equipment qualification, cycle development and validation using BIs, packaging evaluations, and strict process control and documentation to ensure the reliability of sterilization. Biological and chemical indicators are considered part of process controls (1, p. 121).

- Since all critical parameters needed for steam sterilization (e.g., temperature, pressure, and time) can be routinely monitored during a cycle, the load may be released for use based on the attainment of predetermined physical parameters at various parts in the chamber and load during the cycle. This PR process is widely used in industry for moist heat sterilization processes (4, pp. 174-175).

- PR is possible only if all of the components of the sterilization process (e.g., cleaning, preparation, packaging, and drying) conform to predetermined limits and are under strict and continuous control and validation (4, pp. 174-175).

- The advantages of PR include the immediate use of items without concern for the outcome of BIs. At best, BIs detect only catastrophic failure of sterilization processes. Information obtained during PR validation, routine cycle monitoring, and ongoing use of process controls is more reliable in predicting sterility than a single BI (4, pp. 174-175).

- The validation of a sterilization process in industry (PR) includes:
  - Correct installation and functioning of equipment
  - Verification of process specifications (cleaning, inspection, loading, and exposure to the proper physical conditions)
  - Performance qualifications based on attainment of physical parameters (time, pressure, and temperature) and microbial lethality using well-established, scientific criteria (5, p. 12)

- The use of PR, in particular the exclusion of routine use of BIs, would establish a single standard of care for the sterilization of all patient care devices and would lead to considerable cost savings associated with the reprocessing of sterile supplies (5, p. 12).

- It is impossible to measure the sterility of items by simple inspection or observation. Therefore either (1) the system must be validated as having met the specifications known to sterilize devices (PR), or (2) BIs must be used to validate that sterilizing conditions were met. A validation process based on BIs is slow (3, p. 32).

- PR is the release for use of items processed within a system capable of providing and validating predetermined physical specifications. The method used to obtain the documented evidence that the system has met specifications is called process validation. Process validation is the obtaining of proof that the process performs as it was intended. Under PR, a healthcare facility would use mechanical monitors and chemical integrators as documented evidence of successful completion of the cycle under controlled conditions. A quality system must be used in the facility (3, p. 32).

FUTURE USE

- In U.S. industry, PR is practiced routinely for radiation sterilization and steam sterilization and increasingly with ethylene oxide. PR is being proposed for use in U.S. hospitals, but it is too early to gauge whether PR will be accepted as standard procedure by the hospital central sterilization community (1, p. 121).
- In Europe, standards for steam sterilization of medical devices apply equally to industry and healthcare facilities; no longer are there two different sets of standards. In many developed countries of the world, this single approach is being used effectively. PR (the industrial model) is known to be the most rigorous in terms of ensuring sterility. Adoption of PR, however, requires much forethought and planning and the implementation of some new practices, especially for hospitals. The concepts of PR, along with international standards for steam sterilization, are gaining acceptance in healthcare facilities throughout the world (4, pp. 173, 177).
- PR involves monitoring of the critical parameters of sterilization procedures without the routine use of BIs and is used in both industry and hospitals in Europe. The possibility of using this approach in U.S. hospitals is being considered by standard-setting organizations (1, p. 131).
- In the United States the document, American National Standards Institute (ANSI) and Association for the Advancement of Medical Instrumentation (AAMI) ST 46, *Good Hospital Practice: Steam Sterilization and Sterility Assurance (1996)* is under review for potential updating. Also, the International Standards Organization (ISO) Standard 13683, relating to the validation and control of steam sterilization in healthcare facilities, is being considered as an alternative, providing optional election of a system employing

PR. An AAMI Technical Information Report helps to explain PR (2, p. 23).

- Currently PR is not required in the United States, but U.S. surgical services managers should prepare for its introduction (2, p. 23).

References

1. Favero MS: Developing indicators for monitoring sterilization. In Rutala WA, editor: *Disinfection, sterilization and antisepsis in health care,* Washington, DC, Association for Professionals in Infection Control and Epidemiology; Champlain, NY, Polyscience, 1998, pp 119-132.

2. Hancock CO: Parametric release, a new standard for steam sterilization? *Surgical Services Management* 4(7):19-20, 22-23, 1998.

3. Hancock CO: Parametric release: what is it? *Infection Control and Sterilization Technology* 5(4):32, 38, 42, 1999.

4. Schultz JK: Steam sterilization: ISO standards and the future of parametric release. In Reichert M, Young JH: *Sterilization technology for the health care facility,* ed 2, Gaithersburg, Md, 1997, Aspen, pp 173-177.

5. Sharbaugh R: Sterilization in health care facilities: towards parametric release, *APIC News* p 12, Sept/Oct 1998.

I. Reuse and Reprocessing of Single-Use Devices

Healthcare is under considerable pressure to reduce costs. Many institutions are examining practices to determine better and more cost-efficient approaches to patient care. One avenue that hospitals may consider for cost reduction is the reprocessing of single-use devices (SUDs). However, reuse of SUDs is a very controversial issue. At the center of the controversy is the question, Is it a safe practice?

A *SUD,* also referred to as a disposable device, is defined by the U.S. Food and Drug Administration (FDA) as a device that is intended to be used on one patient during a single procedure. It is not intended to be reprocessed (cleaned, disinfected, or sterilized) and used on another patient. The labeling may or may not identify the device as single use or disposable and does not include instructions for reprocessing. *Reuse,* again defined by the FDA, is the repeated use (multiple use) of any medical device, including devices intended for both reuse and single use, with reprocessing (cleaning, disinfection, or sterilization) between uses. *Reprocessing* includes all of the steps performed to make a contaminated device—whether reusable or single use—safe for use on another patient. The steps may include cleaning, functional testing, repackaging, relabeling, disinfection, or sterilization. *Resterilization* is the application of a terminal process designed to remove or destroy all viable forms of microbial life, including bacterial spores, to an acceptable sterility assurance level, to a device that has previously undergone a sterilization process (6, p. 40).

There is very little scientific literature to support or discourage the practice of reusing SUDs. In an effort to scientifically evaluate this issue, the Centers for Disease Control and Prevention (CDC) examined all outbreaks of infection associated with reprocessed medical devices from January 1986 to April 1996. A total of 115 on-site investigations of outbreaks were performed, and of these, 13 (11.3%) of the outbreaks were associated with reprocessed medical devices. All of the outbreaks involved the dialysis setting. Of the 13 outbreaks, 11 were associated with reprocessed dialyzers used during hemodialysis and included both bloodstream infections and pyrogenic reactions. The remaining two involved the reprocessing of a needle device used for intravenous access for hemodialysis or a transducer. The majority of these outbreaks were associated with the use of water of inadequate quality, a hose or spray device (water pick), or an overdiluted disinfectant (10, p. 17).

In this CDC study it is stated that in the United States, hemodialyzers are the most common FDA-approved SUDs to be reprocessed and reused. The majority of dialysis centers reprocess and reuse hemodialyzers (for use on the same patient) and do so with no evidence of adverse effects and with considerable cost savings. Safety with such processes is dependent on solid infection control facility infrastructures that include surveillance systems, policies, procedures, and education on appropriate methods of reprocessing and reuse (10, p. 22).

In the United States, reprocessing of medical equipment designed for single or multiple uses is an *infrequent yet important cause of nosocomial outbreaks.* Any reprocessing or reuse must be supported by standardized systems, plus adherence to manufacturers' instructions and both the CDC and industry recommendations (10, p. 18).

Central to this issue was the issuance by the FDA in late 1999 and early 2000 of draft guidelines relating to reprocessing and reuse of SUDs. These guidelines set forth factors that the agency would consider in categorizing the risk associated with SUDs that are reprocessed. The risk categories would then be used to set the FDA's enforcement priorities and schemes.

The FDA revised the draft reuse strategy based on comments received and on August 2, 2000, issued the document, *Enforcement Priorities for Single-Use Devices Reprocessed by Third Parties and Hospitals* (6). This guidance document receives considerable attention in this chapter.

In this chapter we will explore the issues surrounding reprocessing from a financial, ethical, legal, safety, clinical and operational standpoint and examine two approaches to implementing a reuse program: (1) developing an internal reprocessing program and (2) outsourcing the reprocessing to a third-party reprocessor.

CONTROVERSIAL ISSUE

- The Health Industry Manufacturing Association (HIMA) has chastised the FDA for previous lack of regulation of the practice of reprocessing single-use devices and states that its concerns are product quality, safety, and liability (21, pp. 44-45).
- The Association for Professionals in Infection Control and Epidemiology (APIC) maintains a neutral position on the issue of reuse, per se. APIC, as an organization, has been supportive of stricter regulation for the reprocessing of critical devices only and has engaged in dialogue with the FDA and other stakeholders on this issue. APIC will continue to work with the FDA to ensure that reprocessing remains a viable option for users, while also being safe and effective for patients (1).

- On the other side of the controversy is the Association of Medical Device Reprocessors (AMDR), stating that healthcare providers need to provide quality care at the lowest possible cost. The AMDR states that third-party reprocessing offers hospitals a way to realize significant cost savings without compromising patient safety (9).
- The American Hospital Association's (AHA's) position is that proper reprocessing for certain medical devices is a safe, effective means of providing quality patient care (4).
- The Joint Commission on Accreditation of Healthcare Organizations (JCAHO) recommends the following:
  - Reprocessing should not be done unless the institution can justify the position.
  - A decision should be made whether or not the patient should be charged for the reused item; the decision must have supporting data.
  - Patients should be provided with the choice between a SUD and a reused device (11).
- AORN does not take an official position on the practice of reprocessing and refers to the deficit of scientific literature to explain their stance. However, AORN does state that reuse of SUDs should be considered on an item-by-item basis after careful validation of the safety and efficacy of each device after reprocessing. A SUD that cannot be cleaned and resterilized or disinfected without damage to its integrity or function should not be reprocessed. Patient safety should be the major concern (5, pp. 1014, 1017).

So, practically speaking, what does all of this mean to the clinician? How should this controversial issue of reuse and reprocessing of SUDs be addressed? Should an institution consider reprocessing? Before making a decision, an institution should explore ethical, legal, financial, safety, clinical, and operational considerations. Once the decision to reprocess is made, an institution should develop an implementation approach: either outsource to a third-party vendor or maintain the process internally. The FDA's new regulatory document will now be an influencing factor in decision-making by hospitals.

ISSUES AND TRENDS
Financial Issues
Before 1970 reusable equipment was commonly used. Several circumstances are credited with the later advent and proliferation of SUDs:

1. The HIV crisis and fear of transmission
2. The reduced liability for device manufacturers

3. Payers' willingness to absorb the cost of SUDs
4. The development of new plastics and sterilization techniques (12, p. 62)

Rising healthcare costs in the 1980s and 1990s encouraged healthcare institutions to look for ways to reduce costs. SUDs are believed to increase the cost of care and create disposal problems. Hospitals produce tons of waste per year, with considerable cost going toward hazardous waste disposal. Some institutions consider reprocessing SUDs a means for reducing this cost (12, p. 62).

When considering whether to reprocess SUDs, an institution should perform a cost/benefit analysis, taking into account the following:

- Original cost of the product
- Estimated number of reuses
- Estimated cost of reprocessing
- Total number of devices used annually (13, p. 15)

Ethical and Legal Issues

The following three ethical considerations should be taken into account before implementing a reuse program for SUDs:

1. Billing practices for SUDs: Will the institution bill the same amount for reprocessed SUDs that it bills for the new devices?
2. Patient notification and informed consent: Many institutions that reprocess SUDs do not notify the patient and obtain prior consent.
3. Distribution of care: Is the cost of SUDs preventing certain patient populations from access to certain medical procedures or therapies? This is particularly relevant in third-world countries that cannot afford the expense of SUDs (20, pp. 11-13).

Legal implications prevent many institutions from considering reuse programs. When an institution maintains an in-house reprocessing program, the institution is subject to the same regulations as the manufacturing industry. The institution, in essence, becomes a manufacturer (16, p. 236).

The FDA's position is this: when a hospital or third-party reprocessing company reprocesses a device designed for single use, the device has been altered and is considered a new device. HIMA has been critical of the FDA for not enforcing these regulations (21, p. 44; 18). NOTE: The FDA will now be enforcing these regulations.

According to the previous FDA draft guidelines, the reprocessor (hospital or third party) is subject to applicable FDA requirements, including premarket notification or approval, good manufacturing practice compliance, device labeling, and medical device reporting (21, p. 44).

Regulatory Issues

Before 2000, the FDA had not heavily regulated the reuse of SUDs. Although the third-party reprocessors fell under FDA regulations and were considered manufacturers by the FDA, standards to this effect did not receive much emphasis. In late 1999 the FDA released several documents soliciting input from the industry on this controversial issue. The FDA's change of position was driven by pressure from the device manufacturers, as well as legislative provisions to fund better regulation of the reuse of SUDs. In addition, the FDA indicated that the following issues called for increased regulation:
- The increase in the practice of reusing SUDs
- The industry expansion of third-party reprocessors
- The types of SUDs being reprocessed (e.g., the examination of safety issues and informed consent are needed) (4, pp. 156-157)

Safety Issues

In a thoughtful analysis of medical device reprocessing, Alfa questions the variability in precleaning processes, especially with regard to the precleaning of critical devices such as long and narrow-lumened cardiac catheters, and cautions that reuse of critical SUDs is highly controversial. Because cardiac catheters are often inserted into blood vessels, process validation is crucial when reprocessing them on a routine basis. Ensuring consistent compliance with reprocessing protocols and determining margins of safety are substantial challenges for the quality assurance program personnel of most reprocessing centers (either hospitals or third-party reprocessors) (2, p. 497).

Steam sterilization is the most preferred and cost-effective method for sterilization of medical devices, but it cannot be used for heat-sensitive devices. Alternative low-temperature sterilization methods currently in use in many hospital settings include ethylene oxide (long turnaround times because of lengthy aeration processes), plasma (poor penetration ability in long or narrow lumens), and liquid chemical sterilization (designed for "point-of-use" sterilization with no feasible method of long-term sterile storage). All of the low-temperature sterilization methods have poorer penetration of organic and inorganic materials (debris) than steam sterilization (2, pp. 496-497).

Reprocessed medical devices must be guaranteed sterile and suitable for use on other patients. The issues surrounding the reprocessing of single-use critical medical devices are highly complex and need additional study (2, pp. 496-497).

THE FDA REGULATORY DOCUMENT

The FDA document, *Enforcement Priorities for Single-Use Devices Reprocessed by Third Parties and Hospitals,* issued August 2, 2000, provides guidance to third-party and hospital reprocessors regarding their responsibility as manufacturers engaged in reprocessing devices labeled for single use (6). Third-party and hospital reprocessors of SUDs are subject to all regulatory requirements currently applicable to original equipment manufacturers (OEMs), including premarket submission requirements. The following excerpts are from this FDA document. (All FDA excerpts are in reduced text.)

Definition of Terms

For the purpose of this guidance, FDA has defined the following terms:

Hospital: A hospital is an acute health care facility.

Single-use device: A single-use device, also referred to as a disposable device, is intended to be used on one patient during a single procedure. It is not intended to be reprocessed (cleaned, disinfected/sterilized) and used on another patient. The labeling may or may not identify the device as single-use or disposable and does not include instructions for reprocessing.

Opened-but-unused: Opened-but-unused devices are single-use, disposable devices whose sterility has been breached or compromised, or whose sterile package was opened but has not been used on a patient, that is, they have not been in contact with blood or bodily fluids.

Reuse: The repeated use or multiple use of any medical device including devices intended for reuse or single-use, with reprocessing (cleaning, disinfection or sterilization) between uses.

Reprocessing: Reprocessing includes all the steps performed to make a contaminated reusable or single-use device patient ready. The steps may include cleaning, functional testing, repackaging, relabeling, disinfection or sterilization.

Resterilization: Resterilization is the application of a terminal process designed to remove or destroy all viable forms of microbial life, including bacterial spores, to an acceptable sterility assurance level, to a device that has previously undergone a sterilization process.

Background

On November 3, 1999, FDA released a proposed strategy on the reuse of single-use devices (SUDs). This proposal identified the steps under consideration in the development of the agency's SUD reprocessing policy. These steps were:

1. Develop a list of commonly reprocessed SUDs;
2. Develop a list of factors to determine the degree of risk associated with reprocessing devices;

3. Apply those factors to the list of commonly reprocessed SUDs and categorize them into three categories—high, moderate, and low; and

4. Develop priorities for the enforcement of premarket submission requirements for third party and hospital reprocessors based on the category of risk.

In addition to publishing the proposed strategy document for public comment, FDA also sponsored a teleconference . . . and convened an open public meeting . . . to obtain comments on the proposed strategy. As a result of the comments we received, FDA published on February 11, 2000, two companion draft guidances entitled "Reprocessing and Reuse of Single-Use Devices: Review Prioritization Scheme" ("RPS guidance") and "Enforcement Priorities for Single-Use Devices Reprocessed by Third Parties and Hospitals" ("SUD Enforcement guidance"). These draft guidelines set forth factors that would be considered in categorizing risks and enforcing premarket submission requirements.

The following is a summary of the major comments received:

- Strong support for the agency's decision to actively regulate third party and hospital reprocessors.
- Concern that the Risk Prioritization Scheme lacked clarity and was too subjective.
- Concern that FDA was imposing burdensome regulations on hospitals.
- Concern that many hospitals are not prepared to comply with the agency's premarket requirements due to their lack of experience in this area or to their limited financial resources.
- Support for FDA's decision to exclude "opened-but-unused" SUDs from this enforcement strategy. . . . [The] current policy for "opened-but-unused" products remains unchanged.
- Several stakeholders identified additional SUDs that they were currently reprocessing or were considering reprocessing in the future that were not on FDA's current list of frequently reprocessed SUDs.

Revision of Final Document

As a result of the comments the agency received [on the draft guidelines], FDA has revised the final SUD regulatory strategy as follows:

1. The proposed Risk Prioritization Scheme will not be used to determine the timing of FDA's enforcement priorities for the premarket requirements. Rather, FDA will use the device classification listed in the Code of Federal Regulations (CFR) (i.e., class I, class II, or class III) to set its enforcement priorities for the premarket submission requirements.

2. FDA intends to enforce premarket submission requirements within six (6) months of issuance of this final SUD Enforcement guidance document for all class III devices; within twelve (12) months for class II devices; and eighteen (18) months for class I devices. At a later date, FDA intends to examine on a case-by-case

basis, the need to revoke exemptions from premarket requirements for class I and II exempt products based upon the risks that
may exist due to reprocessing.
3. For hospital reprocessors, FDA intends to establish a one (1)
   year phase in for active enforcement of the Act's non-premarket
   requirements (e.g., registration, listing, medical device reporting, tracking, corrections and removals, quality system, labeling). The agency will use the one-year period following the issuance of this final guidance document to educate hospitals
   about their regulatory obligations. FDA does not anticipate that
   the one-year extension of enforcement discretion following the
   issuance of this guidance document will pose any significant
   public health risks because the agency has no evidence at this
   time to demonstrate that reprocessing and reuse of SUDs is pos-
   ing any imminent danger to public health.
4. The "List of Frequently Reprocessed SUDs" [Appendix A of the
   document] has been expanded to include additional SUDs that
   are currently being reprocessed.

Box 4-1 contains a list of samples of SUDs in each of the risk
categories.

| BOX 4-1 | Classification and Examples of Devices |

Class I—Low Risk
Blood pressure cuffs
Tourniquets (pneumatic and nonpneumatic)
Gas masks and breathing circuits
Surgical scalpels, forceps, and clamps
Stomach- and intestinal-suturing devices
Surgical drills
Orthopedic saw blades
Laparoscopic scissors
Staplers
Suction catheters
Inflatable external extremity splints

Class II—Moderate Risk
Surgical gowns
Angiography catheters
Cardiovascular guide wires
Cardiovascular oximeters
Vascular clamps
Compressible limb sleeves
Laparoscopes
Biopsy forceps
Cytology brushes
Urological catheters

Continued

BOX 4-1   **Classification and Examples of Devices—cont'd**

Class II—Moderate Risk—cont'd
Endoscopic blades
Hypodermic needles
Laparoscopic insufflators
Electrosurgery units

Class III—High Risk
Intra-aortic balloon catheters
Percutaneous transluminal coronary angioplasty (PTCA) catheters
Percutaneous tissue-ablation electrodes
Implantable infusion pumps
Endotracheal tube changers
Needle-destruction devices

Our primary goal is to ensure a reprocessing and reuse regulatory program based on good science that protects public health, while ensuring that our regulatory requirements are equitable to all parties. FDA does not believe that the changes to its final SUD regulatory strategy pose any significant public health risks. Rather, we believe that these changes may facilitate the implementation of the reuse policy. For example, FDA believes that using the existing CFR device classification system may reduce the chance for delaying implementation of the final SUD policy by eliminating confusion or misunderstanding regarding a device's risk category and the timing of premarket submissions.

The major change in FDA's plan is the use of the traditional device classification scheme rather than the draft Risk Prioritization Scheme to establish enforcement priorities for the premarket submission requirements. FDA was concerned about significant differences between the risk category assigned to a SUD by FDA and by stakeholders. The existing CFR device classification system is an established categorization system that is familiar to all device manufacturers and many device users.

This SUD enforcement guidance document sets forth FDA's priorities for enforcing premarket submission requirements, based on the device's Code of Federal Regulations (CFR) classification (i.e., class I, class II, and class III). Upon issuance of this guidance document, the agency intends to enforce premarket submission requirements within six (6) months for all class III devices; within twelve (12) months for all class II non-exempt devices; and within 18 months for all class I non-exempt devices. At a later date, the agency will evaluate, on a case-by-case basis, the need to revoke exemptions from premarket submission requirements for class I and class II exempt products. Revocation of exemptions will be based on the agency's determination that premarket submissions for reprocessed devices in those classifications are necessary to ensure that these devices are safe and effective for reuse after reprocessing. The issuance of this guidance document does not preclude FDA from taking immediate action against any particular product that is causing significant harm.

Requirements

NOTE: The following information is summarized from the FDA document, *Enforcement Priorities for Single-Use Devices by Third Parties and Hospitals.*

The requirements that apply to third-party and hospital reprocessors are:

1. *Registration and listing:* Owners and operators of establishments that process devices must register their establishment with the FDA and provide a list of their devices.

2. *Medical device reporting:* Manufacturers' reporting requirements and other requirements under this regulation are more extensive than device user facility requirements. Hospitals that engage in manufacturing activities such as reprocessing are subject to manufacturer reporting requirements for the SUDs that they reprocess as well as user facility reporting requirements. In addition, they must adhere to user facility reporting requirements for all other medical devices that they use. Hospitals that reprocess SUDs may need additional guidance on how to submit manufacturer adverse-event reports.

3. *Medical device tracking:* The purpose of medical device tracking is to ensure that manufacturers of certain devices establish tracking systems that will enable them to promptly locate devices in commercial distribution in the event that corrective actions or notifications about the device are necessary. Manufacturers are not subject to this requirement unless and until the FDA issues a direct order to the manufacturer. Accordingly, reprocessors will not be subject to this requirement unless the FDA issues an order for the specific device(s) being reprocessed.

4. *Medical device corrections and removals:* All device manufacturers must report to the FDA within a specified time certain types of device corrections and removals. In addition, each manufacturer must maintain records of all corrections and removals. Each device manufacturer also must submit a written report to the FDA of any correction or removal of a device initiated by the manufacturer if the correction or removal was undertaken to reduce a risk to health posed by the device or to remedy certain violations of the Act. The term *correction* is defined as "the repair, modification, adjustment, relabeling, destruction, or inspection (including patient monitoring) of a device without its physical removal from its point of use to some other location." The term *removal* is defined as the "removal of a device from its point of use to

some other location for repair, modification, adjustment, re-labeling, destruction, or inspection."

5. *Quality system regulation:* Current good manufacturing practice requirements that govern the methods used in and the facilities and controls used for the design, manufacture, packaging, labeling, storage, installation, and servicing of all finished devices are set forth in this regulation. These requirements include design controls, corrective and preventive action requirements, and process validation requirements.

6. *Labeling:* The FDA has general labeling requirements regarding the name and place of manufacture and the inclusion of adequate directions for use.

7. *Premarket requirements:* There are two types of premarket submissions (1) a premarket notification (or 510[k]) and (2) a premarket approval application (PMA). The type of submission used depends on the CFR classification of the device.

Unless the classification regulation specifically exempts a device, a premarket notification (510[k]) submission is required for class I and class II devices. Class III devices may require either a 510(k) or a PMA, depending on the particular type of class III device. The classification regulation for each type of class III device indicates whether a premarket approval application is required. Appendix A of the FDA document is a listing of known reprocessed SUDs and the type of marketing application that is required for each type of device.

A 510(k) submission must contain enough information for the FDA to determine whether the device is as safe and effective as (substantially equivalent to) a legally marketed predicate device. The information submitted must compare the unique characteristics of the device with the predicate device, establishing that the devices are equivalent with respect to safety and effectiveness factors.

The FDA's basis for approval of a PMA is a finding that the device has a reasonable assurance of safety and effectiveness for its intended use based on valid scientific evidence. Submission of clinical data may be necessary in order to establish the safety and effectiveness of a device. A PMA application should evaluate the unique characteristics of the device. The FDA requires a satisfactory inspection of the manufacturing facilities, including identification of all appropriate manufacturing controls, before a PMA application can be approved.

Premarket (510[k]) submissions and PMA applications are device specific; the FDA requires a 510(k) or a PMA for each device. Only closely related variations of the same type of device should be grouped in one submission or application. The FDA advises reprocessors to examine device groupings that original equipment manufacturers (OEMs) have developed in previous submissions as models that may be useful in considering the groupings of reprocessed SUDs.

Purpose

The purpose of this SUD Enforcement guidance document is to describe FDA's enforcement priorities to third parties and hospitals that reprocess SUDs. The enforcement priorities for premarket submission requirements are based on the device's CFR classification. Appendix A [of the document] contains a list of SUDs known by FDA to be currently reprocessed for reuse in humans. This list is not comprehensive; it represents the agency's current knowledge of the types of SUDs that are being reprocessed. This list also contains information such as device classification, CFR regulation number and product codes (i.e., procodes) that the reader may find useful.

Scope

This guidance document is applicable to third party and hospital SUD reprocessors. The enforcement priorities set forth in this guidance do not apply to:

1. Permanently implantable pacemakers. The reuse of permanent pacemakers is addressed in Compliance Policy Guide 7124.12 (issued on October 1, 1980 and revised in March 1995);
2. "Opened-but-unused" SUDs;
3. Health care facilities that are not hospitals; or
4. Hemodialyzers. The reuse of hemodialyzers is addressed in "Guidance for Hemodialyzer Reuse Labeling" (final draft issued on Oct. 6, 1995). A copy of this guidance is available on FDA's web site at www.fda.gov/cdrh/ode/dilreuse.pdf.

FDA is aware that hospitals are not the only health care facilities that reprocess devices labeled for single use. At this time, the agency is limiting its focus to SUDs reprocessed by third party and hospital reprocessors. In the future and following experience with implementation of this guidance document, FDA intends to examine whether other establishments that reprocess SUDs should be included.

FDA believes that a phased-in approach for enforcement of regulatory requirements for third party and hospital reprocessors is appropriate for several reasons, including:

1. The agency believes that the health risk associated with reprocessing SUDs varies with each device and the agency's regulatory activities should be implemented in accordance with the device's CFR classification.

2. A phased-in implementation period may avoid any unintended and unpredictable consequences, such as potential shortages in certain hospitals, of an agency decision to immediately enforce all the requirements.
3. Establishments, such as hospitals, may be unfamiliar with FDA regulations, and a phased-in implementation approach will allow those facilities time to learn about the requirements and to develop programs to comply with them.
4. The agency's limited resources do not permit immediate enforcement of all regulatory requirements on third party and hospital reprocessors.

However, FDA emphasizes that nothing in this guidance document, including the phased-in enforcement approach that the agency intends to implement, precludes the agency from taking immediate action against any particular product that is causing harm.

The entire FDA regulatory document, along with the Appendix A listing of more than 200 frequently reprocessed SUDs, can be accessed online at www.fda.gov/cdrh/comp/guidance/1168.pdf. The FDA's press release on the Final Guidance Document (7) and the FDA's reuse web page (8) are also available online (see references for web addresses).

Predictions

The effects of the new 2000 FDA regulatory policy are difficult to foresee. However, it is predicted that many hospitals now reprocessing SUDs will begin sending them to third-party reprocessors because of the difficulty in meeting the FDAs new premarket requirements for demonstrating that the devices are safe (19).

Moving from in-house to third-party reprocessing will increase costs for hospitals because third-party reprocessors often charge half the cost of a new device for their service. Hospitals usually can reprocess items for substantially less cost. Also, the outsourcing of reprocessing increases the wait time for the return of the devices compared with doing the reprocessing in house (19).

The FDA and hospitals have no experience working together, and this could complicate the process. Furthermore, the FDA has no existing mechanism for inspecting hospitals; however, the FDA may partner with an agency such as the JCAHO to accomplish this task (19).

At the same time there are predictions that device manufacturers, who have generally opposed reprocessing, may begin reprocessing their own products. Device manufacturers are already well versed in preparing 510(k) submissions and premarket approval documents and therefore could open their own reprocessing plants (19).

Representatives of the major reprocessing companies think that the FDA regulations will both increase their business and make reprocessing more acceptable. Quality control processes are already in place in most of these companies (19).

The FDA regulatory policy will have far-reaching effects on hospitals, device manufacturers, and the industry of third-party reprocessing.

HOSPITAL REUSE AND REPROCESSING PROGRAMS

An organization's decision to reprocess SUDs should be a multidisciplinary decision. Suggested involvement includes medical staff, senior management, a product evaluation committee, biomedical engineering, infection control, sterile processing, finance, risk management, and the quality departments (13, pp. 14-15).

The multidisciplinary committee should:

I. Examine the ethical, legal, regulatory, financial, and clinical implications before moving forward with a reprocessing program.

   A. The financial implications should include a cost/benefit analysis, evaluating costs associated with outsourcing versus maintaining an internal program. Reference 16 provides an excellent discussion and design for a cost model.

   B. The legal implications should include a risk analysis that addresses:

      1. The probability that the device will be dirty or nonsterile and that its use will result in an infection.

      2. The probability that the device will be damaged during processing and result in a patient injury.

      3. The probability that toxic levels of chemicals may remain on the device after processing and cause injury to a patient (16, p. 237).

II. Generate a list of SUDs and consider devices independently, evaluating each as high, moderate, or low risk using the FDA's scheme. A suggested approach is to create a table of devices similar to the FDA list (Appendix A of the FDA regulation).

III. Provide clinicians with a list of devices and their risk assignments according to the FDA. Interviews or surveys should be conducted to determine the number of clinicians willing to reuse the different SUDs listed. NOTE: If clinicians simply opt to use the SUD on the shelf rather than the reprocessed item, the program may result in additional expense.

IV. Reach a decision. If the multidisciplinary team decides to proceed with a reuse program, the next major step is the consideration of outsourcing versus maintaining an internal reprocessing program.

There are two basic approaches for hospitals in developing a reuse program: develop an internal program or outsource the program to a third-party reprocessor. Before implementing a program, both avenues may be considered.

Internal Reprocessing

Development of an internal program requires that an institution be prepared to demonstrate:

- Proper cleaning and sterilization techniques
- That the device integrity has not been compromised by reprocessing
- That the device is safe and effective for use

Historically, internal hospital reprocessing programs have not followed good manufacturing practices (GMPs). A recommendation is that hospital internal programs follow GMPs, having in place the following:

- An organizational structure and staff to sufficiently support an internal program
- A quality assurance program, including all documentation, policies, and procedures
- A process developed that maintains a sterility assurance level of 10^{-6}
- A quality review of all aspects of the program, including:
  - Production records
  - Manufacturing materials
  - In-process materials
  - Packaging materials
  - Labeling
  - Finished devices
- A verification process that ensures that problems are identified, documented, and corrected
- Scheduled audits of the quality process, with reports reviewed by management
- Recordkeeping of written and oral complaints about device performance, quality, safety, durability, and effectiveness; and documentation of each complaint (16, pp. 236-237)

The processing procedure is critical to the success of an internal reprocessing program. Before developing a processing procedure, a device should be "destroyed and examined" (17). The purpose of this procedure is to examine the channels, lumens, and internal works of the device. If any of the construction involves areas that appear to be difficult or impossible to clean, the device should not be considered for reprocessing (17, pp. 108-109).

The processing program must demonstrate measurable outcomes, pass/fail inspection criteria, and process control. Process control should include either tag spore or a protein assay test. The following is the device processing procedure:

1. The device arrives in central processing within an established timeframe from the original point of use
2. The device is consistently transported to central processing with minimal variation in process
3. The device is effectively decontaminated
4. The device is tested and demonstrates functionality that is measurable and well documented
5. The device is removed from service at the predetermined point of discard (e.g., "after three uses, the device is discarded")
6. The device is properly prepared, packaged, and labeled
7. The device is appropriately sterilized and aerated
8. The device is sterile at time of use (16, pp. 236-237)

The specifications for each of these steps must be clearly and operationally defined. Each step of the process should be outlined and documented with policies and procedures. It is recommended that the institution request information from the manufacturer on proper processes used to produce, test, and sterilize the device (16, p. 237).

Information on acquiring or selecting the appropriate sterilizer, certifying the sterilizer, validating the efficacy of the sterilization process, and checking appropriate levels of ethylene oxide and by-product residues may be found in:

1. American National Standards Institute: *Medical devices: validation and routine control of ethylene oxide sterilization,* Arlington, Va, 1994, AAMI, ANSI/AAMI/ISO 11135.
2. American National Standards Institute: *Biological evaluation of medical devices,* Arlington, Va, AAMI, 1995, ANSI/AAMI/ISO 10993.

Outsourcing of Reprocessing

Any institution considering reprocessing should consider the possibility of outsourcing to a third-party reprocessing company, from which there are several to choose. An institution should evaluate reprocessing vendors and determine which company best meets its needs. Suggested standards for a third-party reprocessing company are as follows:

1. The company should meet all FDA requirements and be prepared to provide documented evidence.
2. The company's functionality testing and sterilization should meet the same specifications as the original manufacturer of the device.
3. The company should be prepared to provide documentation that product testing verifies the effectiveness of the device after processing.
4. The company should have product indemnification and liability insurance up to $25 million aggregate coverage.
5. The company should demonstrate superior quality and be certified with ISO 9000 standards. (ISO is an international standards organization that requires a company to have well-defined procedures for quality monitoring) (22, pp. 43-44).

Additional information on evaluating a third-party reprocessor can be obtained from references 15, 14, and 3. Reference 15 provides an excellent flowchart decision-making tool to assist the reader with evaluating and selecting a third-party reprocessor.

CONCLUSION

The reprocessing of SUDs may be a viable avenue for cost savings. The scientific literature to support or discredit this practice is virtually nonexistent, with the exception of the previously discussed study. The lack of scientific literature calls out to investigators to evaluate the safety and efficacy of this practice.

The FDA's regulatory document outlines reprocessing requirements that may force the officials of hospitals that already have internal programs to discontinue these programs and begin outsourcing reprocessing services to a third-party reprocessor. Although meeting the FDA requirements may result in safer practices, the implementation of programs that meet these requirements is costly.

References

1. Agencies issue policy notices, Association for Professionals in Infection Control and Epidemiology, February 2000 (press release).
2. Alfa MJ: Medical-device reprocessing, *Infect Control Hosp Epidemiol* 21(8):496-498, 2000 (editorial).
3. Examining liability risks in disposable reuse, *OR Manager* 12(6):10, 16, 1996.
4. FDA issues strategy for reuse of single-use medical devices, *ICP Report* 4(12):156-161, 1999.
5. Fogg DM: Clinical issues, *AORN J* 69(5):1014, 1017-1018, 1999.
6. Food and Drug Administration (FDA): *Guidance for industry and for FDA staff: enforcement priorities for single-use devices reprocessed by third parties and hospitals,* www.fda.gov/cdrh/comp/guidance/1168.pdf (August 2, 2000).

7. Food and Drug Administration (FDA): Press release on final guidance, www.fda.gov/bbs/topics/ANSWERS/ANS01027.html (August 2000).

8. Food and Drug Administration (FDA): Reuse web page, www.fda.gov/cdrh/reuse/index.shtml (August 2000).

9. Furman P: Health policy: Association of Medical Device Reprocessors' position on reprocessing single-use medical devices, *Surgical Services Management* 4(7):42-43, 1998.

10. Jarvis WR: Outbreaks associated with reprocessed medical devices: The Hospital Infections Program, Centers for Disease Control and Prevention experience, January 1986—April 1996. In Rutala WA, editor: *Disinfection, sterilization and antisepsis in health care,* Washington, DC, Association for Professionals in Infection Control and Epidemiology; Champlain, NY, Polyscience, 1998, pp 17-23.

11. JCAHO and FDA comment on reuse of single-use items (report of the month), *North Carolina Statewide Program for Infection Control and Epidemiology* III(6):1-2, 1999.

12. Krowech K, Lester BR: Reuse of medical devices: issues and trends, *Infection Control Today* 4(1):62-63, 78, 2000.

13. Pedley A: Reusing single-use medical devices: one organization's strategy for evaluating proposed reuse programs, *Surgical Services Management* 4(7):14-16, 1998.

14. Reichert M: Choice to reuse disposables requires factual assessment, *OR Manager* 12(6):8-9, 1996.

15. Reichert M: Investigate outsourcing companies with care, *OR Manager* 12(6):10-11, 1996.

16. Reichert M: Reuse of single-use devices. In Reichert M, Young JH: *Sterilization technology for the health care facility,* ed 2, Gaithersburg, Md, 1997, Aspen, pp 236-250.

17. Reichert MF: Single use versus reusable devices. In Rutala WA, editor: *Disinfection, sterilization and antisepsis in health care,* Washington, DC, Association for Professionals in Infection Control and Epidemiology; Champlain, NY, Polyscience, 1998, pp 107-117.

18. Reprocessing issues taking users down "slippery slope," *OR Manager* 12(6):1, 7, 1996.

19. Roos R: New regulatory wave may drive hospitals out of reprocessing, ican News and Features, Commentary, icanPREVENT (www.icanPREVENT.com). Updated 9/5/00, accessed 9/5/00.

20. Schultz JK: Ethical considerations for reusing single-use medical devices, *Surgical Services Management* 4(7):11-13, 1998.

21. Singer N: Health policy: the Health Industry Manufacturers Association's position on reprocessing single-use medical devices, *Surgical Services Management* 4(7):44-45, 1998.

22. Speer J: Reprocessing single-use medical devices, *Infection Control Today* 3(9):42-44, 46, 1999.

Suggested Reading

1. Becker C: To reprocess or not to reprocess, *Modern Healthcare,* p 34, July 24, 2000.

2. FDA issues reuse requirements, *OR Manager* 16(9):7, 2000.

3. FDA moving on reuse regulation, *OR Manager* 16(2):7, 2000.

4. FDA warns reprocessing company, *OR Manager* 16(2):5, 2000.

5. Greene VW: Reuse of disposable medical devices: historical and current aspects, *Infect Control* 7(10):508-513, 1986.

J. Cleaning of Rooms

"Confine and contain" has always been the mantra for environmental cleaning in surgical settings. To confine and contain is to follow the directive that all things contaminated should be contained within as small a space as possible and immediately cleaned and decontaminated.

Perioperative personnel bear the prime responsibility for this cleaning, but all surgical staff members, including environmental cleaning personnel, share accountability for ensuring that the surgical environment is sanitary, hygienically clean, and conducive to safe patient care.

Sanitation protocols for cleaning and disinfection are required before, during, and after each procedure. Environmental cleaning is the framework and basis for all aseptic practices. It is a preparatory phase that must never be omitted.

In this chapter, several topics are discussed around three central themes: *before procedure cleaning, during procedure cleaning,* and *after procedure cleaning.* Other topics related to environmental cleaning, such as airborne contamination, contaminated procedures, and construction and renovation, are discussed in various other chapters of this book.

- Cleaning should be performed on a scheduled basis and should provide a safe, visibly clean environment for patients. The same cleaning protocols should be implemented for all surgical procedures, for protection of both patients and staff, because all surgical procedures are considered contaminated (1, p. 255).
- Although some patients are infected with known pathogenic organisms, others are infected with unknown organisms. Therefore every patient should be considered a potential contaminant in the surgical environment. Clean-up procedures should be rigidly followed to confine and contain contamination of known and unknown organisms (2, p. 549).
- Protocols for proper environmental cleaning that are implemented on a consistent basis decrease the risk of cross-infection from patient to patient and patient to healthcare worker (HCW). The use of Standard and Universal Precautions should be followed during all environmental cleaning (7, p. 12). (See the chapters "Standard Precautions" and "Bloodborne Pathogens and Safety Issues.")
- The role of housekeeping (environmental services) personnel in breaking the chain of infection is to clean the environment

in which infectious agents may reside, thus eliminating the reservoirs, portals of exit, and vectors of transmission (14, p. 68).

CLEANING BEFORE PROCEDURES

- Proper cleaning reduces the amount of exogenous microorganisms, dust, and debris in surgical environments, and it helps to reduce airborne contaminants that may travel on dust and lint and settle on surfaces. Rooms should be visually inspected before any supplies or case carts are brought in (1, p. 255).
- All horizontal surfaces within the operating room (OR) (e.g., furniture, surgical lights, and equipment) should be damp-dusted before the first scheduled surgical procedure of the day. Damp-dusting is done with a clean, lint-free cloth moistened with an Environmental Protection Agency (EPA)-approved hospital disinfectant (1, p. 255).
- Lights and overhead tracks become contaminated quickly with dust, debris, and microorganisms, which can fall onto sterile surfaces or into wounds during surgical procedures. Therefore lights and overhead tracks should be cleaned on a daily basis before the first procedure of the day (6, p. 174).

CLEANING DURING PROCEDURES

- During a procedure, contamination should be confined and contained to as small an area as possible. Appropriate protective devices (e.g., gloves, instruments, eyewear, and gowns) are used when handling contaminated articles (13, p. 160). (See the chapter "Standard Precautions.")
- Accidental spills of contaminated debris (e.g., blood, tissue, or body fluids) in areas outside the surgical field should be cleaned as promptly as possible with an EPA-approved hospital disinfectant (1, p. 256).
- Blood and body fluid spills should be contained and cleaned by a person wearing gloves and using absorbent materials such as paper towels. After the initial cleaning, a spill should be appropriately disinfected with an EPA-approved disinfectant. Various dilutions of bleach are often recommended, especially for blood spills, but bleach solutions are generally corrosive and can easily be replaced by EPA-approved disinfectants available in the facility (8, p. 249).
- Contaminated items should be handled using personal protective equipment (PPE). Use of PPE protects HCWs from direct exposure to potentially infectious pathogenic microorganisms (1, p. 256).

- Soiled sponges are placed in a plastic-lined bucket, not on a draped table or spread out on an impervious barrier on the floor. Sponges are counted and then sealed in an impervious bag (13, p. 160).
- All disposable sharps (e.g., needles, scalpels, electrosurgical tips, and pins) are considered infectious waste and should be placed in puncture-resistant containers that are labeled as containing biohazardous material (1, p. 257).
- Contaminated disposable items used in patient care should be discarded in leak-proof, tear-resistant containers (1, p. 256).
- Gloves are worn when handling contaminated linens or trash. According to the Occupational Safety and Health Administration (OSHA), disposable items that are so grossly contaminated with blood and tissue that they would produce dripping on compression are confined in leak-proof containers or bags that are color-coded, labeled, or tagged for easy identification as infectious or regulated medical waste. Other disposable items that do not pose a hazard because of compression dripping are placed in separate containers and handled as nonregulated hospital waste (11, p. 64175; 13, p. 160).

CLEANING BETWEEN AND AFTER PROCEDURES

- All trash is collected in sturdy plastic or impervious bags. Double bagging of laundry and trash is not necessary unless the outside of a bag has been contaminated or a bag is punctured. Disposition of potentially infectious waste must comply with local, state, and/or federal regulations. Appropriately labeled and color-coded leak-proof bags for infectious waste and puncture-resistant containers for sharps should be used (2, p. 552). Any recycling of items is done at this time, according to facility policies.
- Plaster of Paris clogs regular plumbing; therefore it is discarded in a sink or hopper with a plaster trap. All plaster drip and bucket contents should be washed down this sink. If no plaster trap is available, the plastic-lined bucket should be stored until the plaster in the bucket hardens, after which time the water is emptied and the plastic liner bag containing the hardened plaster is discarded. Reusable buckets are cleaned thoroughly (2, p. 680).
- All horizontal surfaces and surfaces that have come in immediate contact with a patient or body fluids, or with electrosurgical or laser plume, are cleaned with an EPA-approved disinfectant solution. Protective eyewear, a mask or face shield, an apron or gown, and gloves should be worn when disposing of suction

container fluids if this procedure is part of the protocol (13, p. 160). (See the chapter "Waste Management" for a discussion of liquid waste disposal.)

- All horizontal surfaces of tables and equipment should be cleaned with an EPA-approved disinfectant solution. The disinfectant can be applied from a squeeze-bottle dispenser and wiped with a disposable wipe or a clean cloth that is changed frequently. The use of spray bottles can cause the disinfectant solution to become aerosolized and therefore should be avoided for routine use (6, p. 174).

- The OR bed is cleaned, and all surfaces and mattress pads are wiped with a disinfectant-soaked, lint-free cloth. Particular attention is given to all surfaces of the OR bed, mattress, and positioning aids where contamination with blood or other fluids may have taken place (13, p. 160).

- After being cleaned, the OR bed is moved to the periphery of the room so that access is gained to the center of the room, the bed area. Cleaning of this area is done if the area is visibly soiled. When moving the OR bed, the casters should be moved through the cleaning solution (13, p. 160).

- After removal of trash, linen, and instruments, the floor area within a 3- to 4-foot (1- to 1.3-m) perimeter around the operative field is cleaned if visibly soiled. The area cleaned is extended as necessary to adjacent contaminated areas. A wet-vacuum and disinfectant/detergent or a clean mop and mophead soaked in a fresh disinfectant/detergent solution are used. When a reusable mophead is used, it is discarded into a laundry hamper (13, p. 160; 4, pp. 872-873).

- There are no data to support cleaning the entire floor after each procedure, or cleaning or mopping the floor between procedures if there is no visible floor soil (4, pp. 872-873).

- Overhead lights should be spot-cleaned as necessary. After cleaning, the operative light reflector shields should be wiped with 70% isopropyl alcohol to remove cleaning detergent film (13, p. 160).

- After the room is cleaned, gloves are removed, hands are washed, and the room is prepared for the next patient. New liner bags are placed in the appropriate trash and linen receptacles. The OR bed is prepared with fresh linen and a clean safety belt. Clean suction canisters and tubing are set up according to facility policy (13, p. 161).

- Walls are not considered contaminated and need not be washed between surgical procedures unless soiled with blood, organic debris, or other contaminants during the procedure. In that case, the soiled areas should be cleaned with an EPA-approved hospital disinfectant (6, p. 175).

- Fogging has been used to fill the air in a room with aerosolized disinfectant solution in an attempt to control microbial contamination. Action on airborne contaminants is temporary because the agent dispersed through the air settles on surfaces or is exhausted through the ventilating system. Fogging is not recommended because it is potentially toxic to personnel and patients, and it is too impractical and ineffective to be an acceptable method of disinfection in OR suites (6, p. 285).

TERMINAL CLEANING

- All ORs should be terminally cleaned, regardless of whether they are used during the 24-hour surgery period (5, p. 1018).
- The OR floor should be wet-vacuumed after the last operation of the day or night with an EPA-approved hospital disinfectant (10, p. 268).
- Many facilities do not have access to wet-vacuum equipment or have found the practice to be too time consuming and costly. As an alternative to wet-vacuuming, a floor can be "flooded" with a disinfectant/detergent solution, with one clean mop used to apply the solution and a second used to take up the solution. Each mophead is placed in a laundry hamper after a single use (3, p. 295).
- Overhead lights, doors, handles on cabinets, and remaining furniture or room equipment are wiped with a disinfectant. The floor is flooded with a disinfectant/detergent for 5 minutes and thoroughly scrubbed with a floor scrubber; the solution is removed with a wet-vacuum, or a freshly laundered or single-use mophead. Last, the housekeeping equipment is cleaned (13, p. 161).
- At the end of each day, all procedure rooms, substerile areas, scrub sinks, scrub or utility areas, hallways, furniture, and equipment are terminally cleaned. All portable equipment in the room, such as kick buckets and suction canisters, are removed from the room and cleaned with a disinfectant/detergent. Reusable soap dispensers are disassembled and cleaned before filling as needed (13, p. 161).
- Cabinets and doors should be cleaned, especially around handles or push plates, where contamination is common (6, p. 176).

SCHEDULING CLEANING

Schedules should be established for routine cleaning of cabinets and shelves; walls; ceilings and recessed ceiling tracks, such as overhead lighting tracks and lighting fixtures; air conditioning and heating grills, vents, ducts, and filters; sterilizers; warming cabinets; refrigerators and ice machines; offices; lounges; locker rooms; workrooms; and corridors (13, p. 161; 1, p. 258).

DISINFECTANT USE IN CLEANING

- An appropriate EPA-approved hospital disinfectant cleaner should be used for environmental cleaning. Most disinfectants used for cleaning the environment perform both the cleaning and disinfection steps. The choice of agent depends on the nature of the item or surface to be cleaned, the level of microbial kill required, cost, safety, and ease of use. Instructions on labels should always be followed (14, p. 69).
- The environmental surfaces category for cleaning and disinfection carries the least risk of disease transmission but may potentially contribute to secondary cross-contamination by contact with the hands of HCWs or by contact with equipment that subsequently comes into contact with the patient (14, p. 69).
- Antibiotic-resistant organisms are a major infection-control concern. At the present time, however, there are no data suggesting that antibiotic-resistant strains of bacteria are more resistant than ordinary strains of bacteria to chemical disinfectants. This is because disinfectants work by a chemical mechanism that destroys the cell wall of the organism, but antibiotics work by a metabolic mechanism. Therefore no special cleaning agents or disinfectants are required (14, p. 69).
- Cleaning and disinfecting environmental surfaces (e.g., bedside tables, door knobs, and faucet handles) with an appropriate quaternary ammonium compound or a phenolic is acceptable practice (14, p. 69).

Revised OSHA Policy

- The OSHA policy on the use of disinfectants with an EPA approval against human immunodeficiency virus (HIV) and hepatitis B virus (HBV) was revised in 1997. Regarding this policy, the memorandum from OSHA's Directorate of Compliance Programs (12, p. 10) states:

> The policy requiring the use of EPA-registered tuberculocidal disinfectants and/or a diluted bleach solution to decontaminate contaminated work surfaces should be expanded to include EPA-registered disinfectants that are effective against both HIV and HBV.
>
> OSHA's [newly revised] policy is that EPA-registered disinfectants for HIV and HBV meet the requirement in the Bloodborne Pathogen Standard and are "appropriate" disinfectants to clean contaminated surfaces,

provided such surfaces have not become contaminated with agent(s) for which higher level disinfection is recommended.

NOTE: This revised policy can be simplified and interpreted as follows: Disinfectants for routine use on contaminated surfaces in ORs now need not be EPA-registered *tuberculocidal* agents, as previously required in the OSHA Bloodborne Pathogen Rule, unless there is evidence that the tubercle bacillus is present on the surface to be cleaned. EPA-registered disinfectants that are effective against HIV and HBV (and not the tubercle bacillus) are now acceptable for use on contaminated environmental surfaces. For further discussion of this OSHA directive, see the chapter "Disinfection."

- The OSHA Bloodborne Pathogen Standard requires that employers ensure clean and sanitary worksites that prevent worker exposure to blood or other potentially infectious materials. OSHA's "appropriate disinfectants" previously included an EPA-registered tuberculocidal disinfectant or a 5.25% sodium hypochlorite (bleach) solution diluted between 1:10 and 1:100 with water. An intermediate-level disinfectant was required in order to satisfy this directive. The 1997 directive, previously discussed, added another type of agent that would satisfy the requirement: EPA-registered disinfectants for HIV and HBV. If bloodborne agents other than HIV or HBV are of concern, only the first two disinfectants mentioned are considered acceptable. When selecting a quaternary ammonium product, for example, assurance must be present that the product has been approved for HIV and HBV disinfection (9, pp. 40, 42).

References

1. AORN: Recommended practices for environmental cleaning in the surgical practice setting. In *Standards, recommended practices and guidelines,* Denver, 2000, Author, pp 255-260.
2. Atkinson LJ, Fortunato NH: *Berry & Kohn's operating room technique,* ed 8, St Louis, 1996, Mosby.
3. Conner R: Clinical issues, *AORN J* 70(2):295-297, 1999.
4. Fogg DM: Clinical issues, *AORN J* 67(4):870, 872-874, 1998.
5. Fogg DM: Clinical issues, *AORN J* 69(5):1014, 1017-1018, 1999.
6. Fortunato N: *Berry & Kohn's operating room technique,* ed 9, St Louis, 2000, Mosby.
7. Grahs PJ: Environmental cleaning in the operating room, *Infection Control Today* 3(3):12, 16, 18, 1999.
8. Gruendemann BJ, Fernsebner B: *Comprehensive perioperative nursing,* vol 1, *Principles,* Boston, 1995, Jones & Bartlett.
9. Krystofiak S: Selection of surface disinfectants, *Infection Control Today* 3(10):38, 40, 42, 44, 1999.

10. Mangram AJ, Hospital Infection Control Practices Advisory Committee (HICPAC), Centers for Disease Control and Prevention: Guideline for prevention of surgical site infection, 1999, *Infect Control Hosp Epidemiol* 20(4):247-278, 1999. (Reprinted, in part, in Appendix B.)

11. Occupational Safety and Health Administration: Occupational exposure to blood-borne pathogens: final rule, *Federal Register* 56(235):64175-64182, 1991.

12. OSHA update: news and letters, *Infection Control Today* 3(9):10, 1999.

13. Rhyne L, Ulmer BC, Revell L: Monitoring and controlling the environment. In Phippen ML, Wells MP: *Patient care during operative and invasive procedures,* Philadelphia, 2000, WB Saunders, pp 147-166.

14. Young M: Housekeeping's role in infection control, *Infection Control Today* 3(9): 68-70, 1999.

Suggested Reading

1. Jacobs PT et al: Cleaning: principles, methods and benefits. In Rutala WA, editor: *Disinfection, sterilization and antisepsis in health care,* Washington, DC, Association for Professionals in Infection Control and Epidemiology; Champlain, NY, Polyscience, 1998, pp 165-181.

2. Peers JG: Cleanup techniques in the operating room, *AORN J* 19(1):53-60, 1974. (Classic article.)

3. Rutala WA et al: Stability and bactericidal activity of chlorine solutions, *Infect Control Hosp Epidemiol* 19(5):323-327, 1998.

4. Rutala WA et al: Susceptibility of antibiotic-susceptible and antibiotic-resistant hospital bacteria to disinfectants, *Infect Control Hosp Epidemiol* 18(6), 417-421. 1998.

5. Wells P: Confine and contain approach to OR cleanup, *AORN J* 25(1):61-62, 1977. (Classic article.)

K. Opening and Setting Up Rooms

Personnel who work in surgical settings should have a sound working knowledge of aseptic principles and techniques. These must be internalized and made an integral part of conscientious practice. However, there are many gray areas and questions that occur even during "simple tasks" such as creating a sterile field or opening sterile supplies.

SETTING UP ROOMS

Following cleaning of the operating room (OR), all furniture and supplies should be organized in preparation for the procedure (5, p. 170). Sterile equipment and solutions should be assembled immediately prior to use (7, p. 268).

- Tables, Mayo stands, and ring stands should be grouped and organized, side by side, in an area that is away from traffic patterns and at least 18 inches away from walls, cabinets, and other nonsterile furniture (e.g., the linen hamper and trash or biohazard waste container). Unneeded supplies and equipment should be removed. Suction should be set up and checked for proper functioning (5, pp. 170-171).

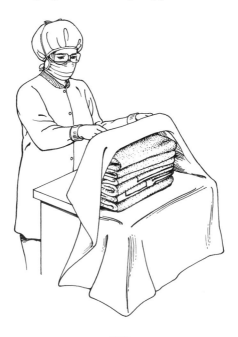

- A clean sheet, lift sheet, armboard covers, and safety strap should be placed on the OR bed. Clean pressure and warming devices should be available for use (5, p. 171).
- A waterproof hamper for soiled linen and properly marked containers for biohazardous waste and sharps should be placed away from sterile items (5, p. 171).
- An impervious plastic liner should be placed in each kick bucket, with the cuff folded over the edge (5, p. 171).
- Supplies that are checked and ready to open are placed on appropriate tables (5, p. 171).

ESTABLISHING A STERILE FIELD

Rigorous adherence to the principles of asepsis by all scrubbed personnel is the foundation of surgical site infection prevention. Others who work in close proximity to the sterile field also must abide by these principles (7, p. 263). Nonsterile equipment or furniture, such as the Mayo stand, should be covered appropriately with sterile barrier materials if it is to be used during the procedure. Only sterile items should touch or extend over sterile surfaces (3, p, 344).

Opening Packs

Sterile drapes establish an aseptic barrier that minimizes the passage of microorganisms between nonsterile and sterile areas (3, p. 342). The drape pack should be placed on a clean, dry surface and unfolded by touching only the outside of the wrapper. The inside of the outer wrapper becomes the table drape and base of the sterile field. Care must be taken so that the inside or sterile portion of the wrapper does not touch any part of the nonsterile surface. Inspection for tears, holes, or areas of strike-through should be performed immediately, before additional items are placed on the sterile field (5, p. 171). When opened, the edges of the drape are considered nonsterile below the level of the table or other flat surface.

- If the pack has sequential double wrappers, the outer wrapper is considered the dust cover, and the inner wrapper the microbial barrier (5, p. 171).
- Large items (e.g., instrument sets and basins) are usually four-corner wrapped and should be opened on a table or other flat surface. It is important not to reach over the sterile field when opening packs (11, p. 98).
- An early reference based on a limited research study states that if insects, hair, or other foreign materials are found in a pack, the hair is sterile and can be handed off on a hemostat, and the setup used (8, pp. 679-680). NOTE: This statement and practice bears scrutiny. Customary practice has been to discard the

contents and pack if insects or other foreign materials are found in them. Technically hair could be sterilized, but being a foreign material, it should not be considered an acceptable component of a sterile pack. In some instances it would not be possible to determine whether the item in question was in the pack before opening or had inadvertently found its way there later. (See the section on draping guidelines in the chapter "Draping.")

Use of Custom Packs

A custom pack is a preassembled collection of items sterilized as a single unit. Contents of a pack may be standardized for general use in many facilities or specified by the purchaser for an individual OR with input from the surgeon or group of surgeons according to the needs for specific procedures (e.g., laparotomy, lumbar discectomy with fusion). Packs are sterilized by ethylene oxide or gamma radiation according to government regulations for testing that ensures sterility (5, p. 178).

- Some consider the use of standardized procedure packs a means of reducing personnel time spent on handling supplies, consolidating storage space needs, facilitating inventory control, encouraging standardization, reducing waste, and increasing cost effectiveness (2, p. 262).
- Because fewer individual sterile packs will need to be opened, the risk of contamination from physical activity around the sterile field, which disperses lint and dust, will be decreased. Thus, infection rates will possibly be decreased (5, p. 179). NOTE: Personnel should be aware of the specific contents of each custom pack to avoid mistakenly opening supplies already contained in the packs, which increases cost, waste, and the potential for contamination.
- The use of custom packs may increase costs if surgeons' preferences change. Some supplies within the custom packs may not be used, and additional supplies may need to be opened. Many custom pack processors have addressed the problem of changing surgeon preferences by offering to supply the packs in small quantities (5, p. 179).

OPENING STERILE ITEMS

Before presentation to the sterile field, all sterile items should be inspected for proper packaging, processing, seal, package integrity, and the inclusion of a sterilization indicator and expiration date, if indicated (3, p. 343).

- Surgical supplies should be opened only when there is reasonable certainty that they will be used during the procedure (2, p. 261).

- Items that are introduced to the sterile field must be sterile and remain sterile until they are used. Secure packaging, sterilization, delivery to the field, and handling during use should provide that assurance (5, p. 230).
- Items introduced onto a sterile field should be opened, dispensed, and transferred by methods that maintain sterility and integrity (3, p. 343).
- Some sterile items (e.g., suture packages) are designed to be "flipped" onto the sterile field. The inner edge of the seal of the peel package is considered the sterile boundary. With instruction and practice, items can be safely flipped onto the sterile field without contaminating the field by reaching over it (1).

Wrapped Supplies

Wrapped supplies should be opened by a nonscrubbed person, unfolding the wrapper flap farthest away from the body first, and the flap nearest to the body last, while being careful not to reach over the sterile contents. Wrapper edges on hand-held packages should be secured in the hands so that they do not flip back and touch the item as it is introduced (3, p. 343).

A nonscrubbed person should open items that are heavy or difficult to open without contaminating them. The nonscrubbed person should present the items to the scrubbed person, who places them on the sterile field. These items can also be placed on a separate flat surface and opened so that the wrapper becomes a sterile field and the scrubbed person can remove the items without contaminating them (3, p. 343).

Heat-Sealed Peel Pack Items

Heat-sealed peel pack items should be opened by peeling the edges apart (while controlling the edges) and uncovering the contents. The scrubbed person removes the contents without touching the edges of the pack cover or the hands of the nonscrubbed person (11, p. 98). If the nonscrubbed person introduces the item to the sterile field, the outside wrapper should be folded back so that one edge covers the hand and inner forearm. This allows the arm to be covered with the inside of the wrapper. If the arm is adequately covered, the sterile item can be held a short distance over the sterile field where it can be released safely. Care must be taken to keep the contents from touching the edges of the packaging material as it is presented to the sterile field. The edges of the pack cover are considered contaminated (11, p. 98).

Rigid Containers

Rigid containers should be inspected to make sure the operational filters and/or valve systems are intact. If damaged, the contents should be considered contaminated (11, p. 98). The seal on the outside and the chemical indicator on the inside of the container should be checked for integrity and indication of proper processing. The inner basket of instruments should be lifted straight out of the container because the edges and outside of the container are not considered sterile (5, p. 172).

Dropped Items

If a sterile package is dropped, the item may be considered safe for immediate use only if it is enclosed in impervious packaging that was not punctured or torn on impact. If the wrapper is impervious and the area of contact is dry, the item may be transferred to the sterile field. Dropped items wrapped in reusable woven fabric materials should not be transferred to the sterile field because these materials allow air to implode into the package. A dropped package should not be put back into sterile storage (5, pp. 172, 230).

POURING SOLUTIONS AND MEDICATIONS

When delivering solutions to the sterile field, the scrubbed person should hold the receiving container or place it near the table edge.

- Solutions should be poured slowly to avoid splashing. Liquids should not run down the sides of the container. The spout or lip of the container is considered contaminated after the cap has been removed. The remainder of the solution is discarded (11, p. 98).
- Medications should be delivered to the sterile field using strict aseptic technique. The scrubbed person should place the receiving container close to the edge of the table so that the nonscrubbed person does not reach over the sterile field (11, p. 98). NOTE: Depending on the dispensing container, medications may either be poured into a sterile container on the sterile field or withdrawn from the dispensing container by the nonscrubbed person using a syringe and needle, then delivered to the sterile field. All medications on the sterile field should be labeled, and labels must be checked by both the scrubbed and nonscrubbed persons for correctness, expiration date, and dosage.

MOVEMENT AROUND A STERILE FIELD

- Movement within and around the sterile field is kept to a minimum to avoid contamination of sterile items or persons (3, p. 344).
- Conversation in the presence of a sterile field should be kept to a minimum (3, p. 344).

• The number of personnel entering the operating room should be limited to those necessary to perform the procedure (7, p. 267).
• Reducing the number of personnel in the room decreases the amount of shedding and the possibility of accidental contamination of sterile items. Reducing individual room traffic also keeps air turbulence at a minimum. This requires planning ahead for supplies and equipment that will be needed during the procedure (6, p. 287).

CONTROVERSIAL PRACTICES
Covering a Sterile Field

• Currently there are no scientific data to support the practice of either covering or not covering sterile fields. Removing a table cover without contaminating the sterile area of the table cannot be done because the drape below the level of the tabletop is considered contaminated, and the cover would touch the sterile tabletop during removal. Agencies or departments that choose to cover sterile fields should meet preapproved criteria established by the infection control committee in the practice setting (3, pp. 343-344).
• Another reference states that sterile supplies should not be opened until they are ready to be used. Tables should not be prepared and covered for use at a later time. Uncovering the table is difficult and the process may compromise sterility. Also, unless the table is under constant surveillance, sterility of any setup cannot be adequately defended (5, p. 172).

Leaving Setups Unattended

It is important to continuously monitor all sterile areas for possible contamination. Event-related sources of possible contamination can occur at any time. These include personnel, airborne contaminants, liquids, and insects (3, p, 344).

• Sterile fields should be prepared as close as possible to the time of use because the potential for contamination increases over time (3, p, 343).
• Direct observation increases the likelihood of detecting breaches of sterility (3, p. 344).
• An unguarded sterile field should be considered contaminated (5, p. 233).

Use of a Setup from a Canceled Procedure

If a patient is taken into the OR and the surgical procedure is canceled, the sterile field, drapes, and supplies on the tables should be torn down and the room cleaned as if the surgical procedure had taken place. The setup is considered contaminated and may not be used for another patient. Disposable items may be saved and used for employee orientation or in-service education (5, p. 172).

Leaving a Sterile Field Open for Later Use

- When prepared, the opened sterile field should be constantly guarded to protect against inadvertent contamination. Considerations to be included in the decision to use an already open sterile field are the expected length of the surgical procedure, engineering practices (e.g., OR air exchange rates), and infection control practices (e.g., traffic control). When the length of the delay is unknown, it may be possible to use all or part of the sterile setup for another procedure if the patient has not entered the room, rather than discarding the entire sterile setup. If the setup is used for another procedure, that procedure must be performed in the room where the sterile supplies were opened. Moving to another room could result in contamination (4, p. 104; 10, p. 1064).
- AORN recommended practices for maintaining a sterile field state that a sterile field should be maintained and monitored constantly. Bacterial growth increases with the passage of time. Several things should be considered when determining the appropriate amount of time to keep a sterile setup open: (1) the type of procedure, (2) the duration of the procedure, (3) the availability of staff members to monitor the setup, and (4) infection control practices (10, p. 1063).
- Healthcare facilities can establish internal policies that limit the amount of time the sterile field remains open before the start of the surgical procedure. The policy will serve as a guideline for staff members and provide the same level of care to all surgical patients. The policy should include constant monitoring of the open setup. Monitoring does not have to be done by a registered nurse but can be done by anyone who has been properly trained to monitor a sterile field. It is not appropriate to tape the doors of the OR closed as an alternative to monitoring (10, pp. 1063-1064).

Moving Sterile Setups

If a sterile setup is prepared for one procedure and it is canceled, it may be used for another procedure if that procedure is performed in the same room where the sterile supplies have been opened. Moving the opened sterile setup from one room to another may result in contamination (4, p. 104).

Whether setting up the room, scrubbing, or circulating, the nurse and OR team members must have an automatic response to any break in aseptic technique. All team members must maintain both an individual and a collective surgical conscience. The goal of this collective surgical conscience is not to excuse error but to readily admit breaks in technique and to take steps to rectify the mistake (9, p. 61).

References

1. AORN: *Flipping sterile supplies onto the sterile field,* AORN Online FAQ Database (www.aorn.org/_results/clinical.asp), 2000.
2. AORN: Recommended practices for environmental responsibility. In *Standards, recommended practices and guidelines,* Denver, 2000, Author, pp 261-265.
3. AORN: Recommended practices for maintaining a sterile field. In *Standards, recommended practices and guidelines,* Denver, 2000, Author, pp 341-346.
4. Fogg DM: Clinical issues, *AORN J* 62(1):104, 1995.
5. Fortunato N: *Berry & Kohn's operating room technique,* ed 9, St Louis, 2000, Mosby.
6. Gruendemann BJ, Fernsebner B: *Comprehensive perioperative nursing,* vol 1, *Principles,* Boston, 1995, Jones & Bartlett.
7. Mangram AJ, Hospital Infection Control Practices Advisory Committee (HICPAC), Centers for Disease Control and Prevention: Guideline for prevention of surgical site infection, 1999, *Infect Control Hosp Epidemiol* 20(4):247-278, 1999. (Reprinted, in part, in Appendix B.)
8. McWilliams RM: The experts research Q & A, *AORN J* 20(4):679-680, 1979.
9. Mews PA: Establishing and maintaining a sterile field. In Phippen ML, Wells MP: *Patient care during operative and invasive procedures,* Philadelphia, 2000, WB Saunders, pp 61-93.
10. Petersen C: Clinical issues, *AORN J* 70(6):1063-1064, 1999.
11. Waldo R, Kamino A, Phippen ML: Providing instruments, equipment, and supplies. In Phippen ML, Wells MP: *Patient care during operative and invasive procedures,* Philadelphia, 2000, WB Saunders, pp 97-111.

L. Preparing the Patient's Skin

The goals of patient skin preparation ("prepping") are to cleanse the skin and bring both the resident and transient bacterial counts to an irreducible minimum, thus reducing the risk of wound contamination and subsequent surgical site infection (SSI). Skin preparation is comparable to the surgical scrub routine performed by the surgical team.

Because most wound infections are associated with endogenous microbes (e.g., the patient's own microbial flora), prepping the patient's skin prior to surgery is an extremely important procedure. Care and attention must be given to ensure optimal preparation of the surgical site by maximal reduction of microorganisms.

The purpose of skin preparation is to:
- Remove soil and debris from the patient's skin (7, p. 203)
- Reduce the microbial count to a minimum (7, p. 203; 2, p. 329)
- Inhibit regrowth of microorganisms with the least possible skin irritation (7, p. 203; 2, p. 329)
- Reduce the number of microorganisms entering the wound (5, p. 503)

PREOPERATIVE SKIN CLEANSING AND HAIR REMOVAL
- Showering or bathing with an antiseptic agent no earlier than the night before surgery but preferably the morning of surgery is recommended for patients. Chlorohexidine gluconate (CHG) reduces the colony count 9-fold, which is a significantly greater reduction than either povidone-iodine (1.3-fold) or triclocarban-

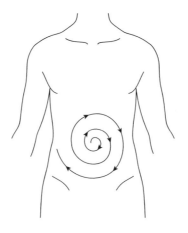

medicated soaps (1.9-fold). With CHG-containing products, repeated antiseptic showers are usually indicated. Although preoperative showers reduce the microbial colony counts on skin, they have not been shown to definitively reduce SSI rates (12, pp. 257, 267). (See the chapter "Preoperative Patient Preparation.")

- Skin should be assessed for abrasions, open sores, cuts, and scars before preoperative hair removal or cleansing (7, p. 204; 2, p. 329).
- The chart should be checked and the patient interviewed regarding allergies to antimicrobial products. If indicated, the plan of care should be changed and the change documented (7, p. 204).
- Hair should not be removed unless it will interfere with access to the operative area or fall into the wound (7, p. 204; 12, pp. 257, 266).
- If hair removal is necessary, it should be done as close to the time of the surgical procedure as possible. With increased time between hair removal and surgery comes increased incidence of SSI. This increased incidence of SSI has been attributed to microscopic cuts in skin serving as foci for microbial growth (7, p. 204; 2, p. 329; 12, p. 257).
- If hair is to be removed, it should be removed in an area outside the room where the surgical procedure is to be performed (2, p. 330).
- Hair should be removed by a method that preserves skin integrity. The use of either clippers (either battery powered or electric with disposable or reusable heads) or a depilatory cream is preferred over a hand razor. However, depilatory creams may cause skin irritation. If clippers and reusable blade assemblies are used, they should be disassembled and disinfected. Single-use heads should be replaced after each use (2, p. 330; 12, p. 257).
- If shaving needs to be done, wet shaving is recommended because wet hair is softer and easier to remove than dry hair, thus there is less risk for skin abrasion (2, p. 330).

Body Jewelry
All body jewelry that pierces the skin should be removed and the pierced area cleaned thoroughly prior to the surgical skin preparation (4, p. 120). For more details, refer to the section on body jewelry in the chapter "Preoperative Patient Preparation."

SKIN PREPARATION
Use of Antimicrobial Agents
Antimicrobial skin preparation agents should:
- Reduce number of microorganisms on intact skin (7, p. 203)
- Be broad spectrum, fast acting, and persistent (7, p. 204; 10, p. 254)

- Be virucidal and active against protozoa and yeasts (5, p. 505)
- Contain a nonirritating antimicrobial agent (5, p. 505)
- Be noninflammable for use with laser, electrosurgical, or other high-energy devices (5, p. 505)

The iodophors, alcohol-containing products, and CHG are the most commonly used agents (12, pp. 257-258). However, several other agents are available. The most popular prepping agents are iodophors, CHG with alcohol 70%, parachlorometaxylenol (PCMX), and triclosan. It is important to follow manufacturers' directions for application and, if recommended, removal after the procedure (13, p. 79).

General Guidelines

- The skin should be cleansed until it is free of gross contamination. This should be done prior to the sterile skin preparation procedure (12, p. 267; 10, p. 262).
- The patient should be assessed for any allergy or previous reaction to prepping agents (10, p. 262).
- Sterile gloves should be worn for the prepping procedure, and the procedure should be carried out using sterile technique (7, p. 205).
- The area prepared should be wide enough to include the surgical site and a substantial surrounding area to allow for manipulation of the skin, extension of the incision, and placement of drains. The size of the fenestration in the drape and possible movement of the drape should also be considered (7, p. 204; 2, p. 331; 12, p. 258).
- Sterile towels should be used to isolate the prep area from nonsterile areas. This practice prevents pooling of the prep solutions and thus reduces the risk of chemical burns (7, p. 205; 5, p. 506).
- Skin preparation begins at the proposed incision site with application of the antiseptic solution in concentric circles. It is very important not to return to the incision site with the used applicator (7, p. 204; 5, p. 507; 12, p. 258).
- The procedure should continue with new applicators for both cleansing and final solutions (7, p. 204; 5, p. 507).
- Electro-dispersive pads, tourniquets, and electrocardiogram (ECG) leads should be covered by a liquid-proof barrier if they are close to the area to be prepped. This practice reduces the risk of chemical burns (13, p. 79; 2, p. 331).
- The final application of solution should be accomplished with prep sticks using a no-touch technique so that there is no possible contamination from gloves used in previous preparation steps (5, p. 507).
- Modification of the standard skin preparation procedure may include removing or wiping off the antiseptic agent after

application, using an antiseptic-impregnated adhesive drape, or painting the skin with an antiseptic in lieu of a complete skin preparation procedure. None of these modifications have proven to have an advantage (12, p. 258).

- Using a *sterile* versus *clean* skin preparation kit also has not been shown to represent an advantage in infection reduction (6, p. 494; 12, p. 258). NOTE: The use of sterile versus clean prep kits continues to be controversial.

- During skin preparation the most bioburdened areas, such as the perineum, anus, vagina, and axilla, should be prepared last. Each sponge should be discarded and not reused. The exception to this rule is the umbilicus. It should be prepared first by soaking the area with the prep solution or using cotton-tipped applicators and prep solution that are contained in most prep kits (7, pp. 204-205).

- Multiple incision sites should be prepared separately, using different prep kits (5, p. 507).

- Special areas of the body such as the eyes or ears may require that special solutions be used or that regular solutions be diluted. Chlorhexidine is contraindicated for facial preps, and iodophors are used with caution around the eyes. Both can cause corneal damage if accidentally introduced into the eyes. They can also cause sensorineural deafness if the agents enter the inner ear (5, p. 508).

- When preparing the patient for skin grafting, separate setups and skin preparation procedures are needed for donor and graft sites 5, p. 507).

- Most povidone-iodine skin prep solution products contain labels warning against solution warming. Warming of prep solutions should not be done unless manufacturers' instructions are consulted and the practice is found to be safe. Manufacturers' written recommendations for storage, heating, and proper use of all skin prep solution products should be followed. If a manufacturer has not provided specific instructions on heating, the manufacturer should be contacted for clarification before any prep solution is warmed (3, p. 1244).

- If flammable solutions are used, adequate time must be allowed for drying before the drapes are applied (13, p. 79).

- Preparing the skin before cancer surgery may be done by using the paint solution only. Vigorous rubbing that may loosen cancer cells should be avoided (5, p. 506).

- Prepping after cast or dressing removal may require soaking the skin or wound with sterile solutions to remove skin squames or adherent dressings (13, p. 79).

PREPPING CONTAMINATED AREAS

Surgical procedures such as abdominal-perineal and abdominal-vaginal need to be prepped as two separate procedures using different prep trays, solutions, and gloves. In the former, the perineal prep should be performed first, with the perineal area covered with sterile towels during the abdominal prep. The rationale for performing the abdominal prep last is to avoid contamination of the already prepared abdominal area by the splashing or aerosolization of solutions while the perineum is being prepped and the Foley catheter inserted (15; 4, pp. 120-121).

- If povidone-iodine solution is used, only the paint should be used on mucous membranes of the vagina (14).
- Other contaminated areas of the body need special consideration and modification of the standard skin preparation procedure. Stomas from a colostomy, ileostomy, or other ostomy can first be sealed off with a sterile adhesive drape. If the stoma is within the area to be prepped, sterile gauze can be placed over it. The remainder of the surgical area should be prepared, the gauze removed, and the stoma cleaned last, following the clean-to-dirty guideline. Care should be taken not to spread contaminated solution over the remainder of the prepared area (5, p. 507; 13, p. 79).
- The vagina, anus, skin ulcers, and draining sinuses are considered contaminated and should be prepared last (5, p. 507).
- Traumatic wounds may require a copious amount of wound irrigation as part of the skin preparation. The wound may be packed with sterile gauze while the remainder of the skin is thoroughly and vigorously prepared. The wound is prepared last, when there is less risk of contamination from the rest of the skin (5, p. 507; 13, p. 79).

Procedure

Surgeon preference for the size of the skin area to be prepped should be verified and complied with. Agency policy or perioperative references for instructions on specific surgical incision sites should be consulted (5, pp. 508-510; 13, pp. 79-85). Individual supplies or a kit should be opened and assembled on a small table (7, p. 205). Sterile prep kits have not been found to be preferable to clean ones (6, pp. 486-495). NOTE: If solutions are not supplied in the kit, they can be added or poured before sterile gloves are donned.

The patient's privacy is maintained by exposing only the area to be prepared. However, the area must be wide enough to comply with accepted skin preparation guidelines and surgeon preference (7, p. 205). The skin is cleansed of gross contamination prior to beginning the sterile prep (12, p. 258). Sterile gloves are donned. Sterile towels are placed below, above, and at the side of the patient at table level to absorb excess fluid and prevent pooling of solution under the patient. This step reduces the risk of burns or chemical irritation from the prep solution (5, p. 506; 10, p. 262).

The most important rule of skin preparation is this: prepping always proceeds from clean to dirty (most bioburdened) areas. Mechanical friction is used in a circular pattern, moving outward from the proposed incision site. To do otherwise would risk microorganisms being brought from the periphery back to the proposed incision site; thus the incision area should always be prepared first. The prep solution applicator is discarded when the outer boundary is reached. The procedure is repeated with new applicators until the skin is thoroughly cleansed (13, p. 79; 7, p. 204).

The area is blotted with the sterile absorbent towels supplied in the kit. When placing or removing towels, it is important that the nonsterile edges of the towels are not dragged across the prepped area (13, p. 79). Also, care should be taken to not touch nonsterile areas such as blankets or bed linen with sterile gloves or prep sponges (5, p. 506).

A final antimicrobial solution is applied with sponge sticks. Care is taken not to touch the final prepped area with gloves that have touched nonprepped skin at the beginning of the procedure. Last, the border towels are removed and the contents of the tray and gloves discarded (13, p. 79; 5, p. 506).

New Products

Topical gels are being used for skin preparation. Most contain a povidone-iodine agent combined with alcohol in a thick gel (7, p. 204). Manufacturers state that the higher viscosity of the solution, usually a povidone-iodine agent combined with alcohol in a gel, reduces the risk that the solution will run down the operative site and pool under the patient, causing skin irritation or burns (1, p. 2).

- In vitro testing showed that the 30-second application of one alcohol-gel product delivered an efficacy equivalent to a 5-minute application of povidone-iodine. The gel has a long-lasting effect of up to 24 hours if not washed off (9, p. 488).
- Manufacturers' instructions for application should be consulted and followed. These will vary among products (11, p. 2).
- All alcohol-gel product application procedures differ significantly from the traditional skin preparation procedure. The most important difference is that alcohol-gel products are applied only once. The application is thorough and uniform,

starting at the incision site and moving outward in concentric circles until the periphery is reached (11, p. 2). NOTE: Manufacturers' instructions or agency policies regarding the use of sterile gloves for the prepping procedure should be followed.

- One brand of topical gel is not water-soluble and resists cleansing with water. The sticking quality of this gel enhances drape adhesion, which helps to maintain a sterile surface through surgery (11, p. 3).

- The high concentration of alcohol in alcohol-gel products presents safety concerns. These products should not be used on the mucous membranes of the mouth, eyes, nose, ears, or vagina. The solution is flammable when wet and therefore must dry completely before the patient is draped, the incision is made, or laser or electrosurgery is used (1, p. 2; 11, pp. 1-5).

- Manufacturers' instructions should be consulted before cleaning the skin after a procedure. Some alcohol-gel products can be removed with soap and water; others require special solutions for removal. Also, some alcohol-gel products should remain on the skin for up to 24 hours to provide continuous antimicrobial activity (1, p. 2; 11, p. 2).

- A new skin preparation product combines alcohol with emollients and preservatives that prolong antimicrobial persistence for up to 24 hours. These components also blend together for ease of application and a nonrunny consistency, along with a rapid, broad-spectrum antimicrobial action. The product has a fast drying time after a one-time application. As with alcohol-gel products, the solution should dry completely before incision, the use of electrosurgery, or laser procedures (8, p. 14).

Documentation

The area prepared, solutions used, condition of the skin, and the person performing the prep should be documented on the operative record (5, p. 511; 2, p. 331).

References

1. Allegiance Healthcare Corporation: *Prevail product insert instructions,* McGaw Park, Ill, 1998, Author.
2. AORN: Recommended practices for skin preparation of patients. In *Standards, recommended practices and guidelines,* Denver, 2000, Author, pp 329-333.
3. Conner R: Clinical issues, *AORN J* 69(6):1244-1248, 1999.
4. Fogg DM: Clinical issues, *AORN J* 70(1):120-121, 1999.
5. Fortunato N: *Berry & Kohn's operating room technique,* ed 9, St Louis, 2000, Mosby.
6. Gauthier DK, O'Fallon PT, Coppage D: Clean vs. sterile surgical skin preparation kits, *AORN J* 58(3):486-495, 1993.

7. Gruendemann BJ, Fernsebner B: *Comprehensive perioperative nursing,* vol 1, *Principles,* Boston, 1995, Jones & Bartlett.

8. Healthpoint: *Actiprep product monograph,* Fort Worth, Tex, 2000, Author.

9. Jeng DK, Severin JE: Povidone iodine gel alcohol: a 30-second, onetime application preoperative skin preparation, *Am J Infect Control* 26(5):488-494, 1998.

10. Larson E: Guideline for use of topical antimicrobial agents, *Am J Infect Control* 16(6):253-266, 1988.

11. 3M Health Care: *#8630 Duraprep surgical solution product insert instructions,* St Paul, Minn, 1999, Author.

12. Mangram AJ, Hospital Infection Control Practices Advisory Committee (HICPAC), Centers for Disease Control and Prevention: Guideline for prevention of surgical site infection, 1999, *Infect Control Hosp Epidemiol* 20(4):247-278, 1999. (Reprinted, in part, in Appendix B.)

13. Mews PA: Establishing and maintaining a sterile field. In Phippen ML, Wells, MP: *Patient cure during operative and invasive procedures,* Philadelphia, 2000, WB Saunders, pp 61-93.

14. Perdue Frederick Company: The use of microbicides on mucous membranes, December 7, 1999 (personal communication).

15. Questions and Answers: Abdominal/vaginal preoperative preparation, *Minim Invasive Surg Nurs* 10(1):7, 1996.

Suggested Reading

1. Michels M: Wound cleaning versus skin antisepsis, *Infection Control Today* 2(4):54-58, 1998.

2. Wong ES: Surgical site infections. In Mayhall CG, editor: *Hospital epidemiology,* Baltimore, 1996, William & Wilkins, pp 154-175.

M. Draping

Surgical draping is an art based on aseptic principles. Draping is the process of covering with sterile barrier materials the nonsterile area immediate to and surrounding the operative site. Draping is one of several procedures that creates a barrier or an isolated surgical site as free from outside contamination as possible. Setting up tables, gowning, and gloving are other barrier procedures.

Many questions are asked about drapes and draping. How extensive an area around the incisional site needs to be draped? Is "abbreviated" draping acceptable in outpatient surgical settings (e.g., four sterile towels as the drape for a dilatation and curettage [D & C])? How much draping is really necessary? Are several layers of drapes necessary? Are adhesive ("sticky") drapes effective in preventing surgical site infections (SSIs)? Which is better—reusable or single-use drapes?

The answer to many of these questions is, *It depends.* In other words, there are very few if any scientific studies that give one or two definitive answers to questions about draping. Wong, an expert on draping, explains the dilemma (23, p. 163): "The use of gowns and drapes to prevent surgical site contamination and infection is logical, and their value is implied, but not proven in clinical studies."

Prudent judgment and facility policy help to steer draping decisions. But factors such as condition of patient, risk of infection (patient diagnosis and comorbidities; the procedure itself and the extent of its "invasiveness," length of procedure, and amount of fluid contamination anticipated), and the nature of the surgical setting are also significant determinants. The prime emphasis, however, should be on the risk for infection that a patient or procedure poses, not on the clinical setting alone. The higher the risk, the more protection that is needed, and therefore the more extensive the drapes and draping should be.

In spite of the questions, draping is still considered a standard of patient care in the operating room (OR). This chapter has references that directly and indirectly address the comments and questions mentioned. The information necessary for rational decision-making regarding draping is also included.

NOTE: Since similar materials (both disposable and reusable) are used for both drapes and gowns, some of the information in this chapter (e.g., materials, materials testing, and desired characteristics) applies to both drapes and gowns. The discussion on a closely related issue—the criteria for choosing between disposable versus reusable drapes and gowns—is found in the chapter "Gowning."

PURPOSE

Draping occurs after the patient has been positioned and the area on and around the operative site has been prepared ("prepped") with appropriate antimicrobial agents. (See the chapter "Preparing the Patient's Skin.") Prepping reduces the number of microorganisms at the surgical site but does not render the skin sterile. Drapes serve as an additional barrier that helps prevent microbial contamination of the surgical incision both from *exogenous sources* (e.g., the OR team, environment, and contaminated instruments) and, more important, from *endogenous sources* (e.g., the patient's own skin flora). As mentioned elsewhere in this book and again in this chapter, endogenous microbes rather than exogenous contaminants are seen as the major sources of SSIs.

- Draping is done primarily for the protection of the patient, the surgical site, and the sterile field. Sterile surgical gowns and drapes are used to create a barrier between the surgical field and potential sources of bacteria. Gowns are worn by all scrubbed surgical team members and drapes are placed over the patient. The Centers for Disease Control and Prevention (CDC) states that there are limited data that can be used to understand the relationship of gown and drape characteristics to SSI risk (13, p. 262).

- Drapes and draping create a sterile field around or close to a surgical site. The sterile field helps to maintain sterility of instruments, sponges, and other devices and equipment used during the procedure. Drapes provide a margin of safety, allowing adequate room for instrumentation, sterile supplies, and movement of the surgical team around the surgical incision and the sterile field. In a laparotomy, for example, a full-body drape with fenestration is usually used because of the large margin of safety needed for the multiple staff members, extensive instrumentation and supplies, and relatively large incisional area. On the other hand, a patient having a cataract extraction probably would not need a full-body drape because of the need for less extensive instrumentation and fewer supplies, a smaller operative area, and fewer scrubbed staff at the sterile field.

- The patient, tables, and equipment are draped, isolating nonsterile from sterile surfaces and leaving only the incisional area within the sterile field exposed. Only sterile items placed within the sterile field and handled by gowned and gloved personnel can be used in the incisional area (9, p. 206).

- The main purpose of draping is to create an aseptic barrier between the surgical incision and the patient's nonprepared skin, guarding the wound from bacteria. Drapes may also help to keep the patient warm. Most draping practices have not been formally studied, but it is probable that draping plays a secondary role in infection control. This statement is made despite the fact that the main source of SSIs is endogenous (e.g., the patient's own microbes and skin). The secondary source of SSIs is exogenous, coming from the OR environment and the surgical team, and playing a more important role in clean than in contaminated procedures (16, p. 1).

- The primary routes of microbial transfer are air and touch. Through aseptic practice surgical personnel aim to cut these routes of transfer by using sterile instruments and supplies, gowns, masks, caps and gloves, and ventilation. Rising costs and an emphasis on outcomes are fueling closer scrutiny of secondary measures such as draping (16, pp. 1, 15).

DRAPE AND GOWN FABRICS

- Drapes and gowns are single use (disposable) or multiple use (reusable). The composition and porosity of the fabric affect the characteristics of drapes, gowns, and also towels as barriers to bacteria and body fluids. Cotton muslin with thread counts of 140 is easily penetrated by bacteria. An early study (5) showed that when drapes and gowns become wet, microbial penetration is enhanced by a wicking effect known as *strike-through*. Drapes and gowns made of a nonwoven or more tightly woven fabric (280-thread-count cotton) are more resistant to bacterial penetration than loosely woven fabrics, but whether this translates to lower SSI rates is unclear (23, p. 163).
- Regardless of what materials their fabrics are made from, drapes and gowns should be impermeable to liquids and viruses. Surgical drapes and gowns must be effective barriers—able to resist liquid penetration—when wet (13, pp. 262, 268).
- The protective barrier ability of surgical drapes and gowns is a primary concern when evaluating materials. The ability to withstand punctures, tears, fiber strains, and abrasions is necessary in order to prevent passage of microorganisms, particulates, and fluids from nonsterile to sterile areas. *Microbial passage is dual-directional.* If liquids are wicked or transferred through pressure between sterile and nonsterile surfaces, one or both sides may become contaminated (3, p. 268).
- There are two general categories of protective fabrics used in surgical drapes and gowns: (1) those that rely on repellent finishes and/or construction, and (2) those that rely on reinforcement by films. Even with the same product, one area or "zone" may be more resistant to liquid penetration than another.

For example, the area around the fenestration of surgical drapes is typically reinforced in some way to provide more resistance to liquid penetration than other portions of the drape (4, p. 7).

Single-Use Nonwoven (Disposable) Fabrics

- Most nonwoven single-use fabrics are composed of compressed layers of synthetic fibers (rayon, nylon, or polyester) combined with cellulose (wood pulp) and bonded together chemically or mechanically without knitting, tufting, or weaving. Nonwoven fabrics can be either nonabsorbent or absorbent and may contain other materials, films, or reinforcements such as polypropylene and foil. Nonwoven fabrics that establish an effective barrier are moisture repellent, retarding blood and aqueous fluid moisture strike-through to prevent contamination. They are also lightweight yet strong, lint free unless cellulose fibers are torn or cut, antistatic, flame retardant, and can be combined with contaminants for disposal. Nonwoven disposable fabrics are prepackaged and sterilized by the manufacturer, ready for use, eliminating the washing, mending, folding, and sterilizing processes for the end user (8, p. 512).
- Some nonwoven drapes are made with special reinforcement around the fenestrations to reduce instrument slippage. They also offer antimicrobial, absorbent reinforcements and attached plastic pouches in the critical areas to contain and control body fluids (15, pp. 86-87).
- Disposable nonwoven fabrics for drapes are composed of both natural and synthetic fibers of various types. The most widely used are a spunlace, wet-laid wood pulp and polyester fiber blend and a spun-bonded meltblown polyethylene. Both of these fabrics have polyethylene film laminated beneath the nonwoven fabric in the critical areas of drapes; this provides an effective fluid-proof sterile barrier. Areas that are not laminated with polyethylene provide an effective fluid-resistant sterile barrier (15, p. 86).
- Nonwoven fabrics are designed for single use. They are composed of processed cellulose and synthetic fibers randomly oriented in sheets and held together with binders, or they are fabrics produced by bonding fibers (3, p. 269).

Multiple-Use Woven (Reusable) Fabrics

- Thread counts and finishes of natural woven fibers determine the integrity and porosity of reusable fabrics. Tightly woven fabrics may inhibit the migration of microorganisms. For example, tightly woven 100% hydrophobic polyester reusable fabrics can repel water droplets but still allow vapor permeation, and when wet, cotton fibers swell and thus can inhibit liquid diffusion through woven fabrics (8, p. 512).

- Reusable drapes may be made of 270- or 280-thread-count pima cotton with a fluorochemical finish. This finish, in combination with a phenazopyridine or a melanin hydrophobe, produces a durable water-resistant fabric. Treated fabrics, however, may have the same heat-retaining qualities as plastic lamination and therefore should not be used for complete patient draping but rather for reinforcement around fenestrations in otherwise untreated drapes. Newer types of materials for reusable fabrics are polyester and composite sheeting, fabric reinforcements, and impervious films (8, pp. 512-513).

- Tightly woven polyester-cotton blends treated with chemicals were developed to improve barrier properties. Treatment renders these fabrics nonwicking and liquid resistant. Fabrics of polyester microfibers are durable, cool, and breathable, and have a water-repellent finish. In most cases, however, the barrier effectiveness achieved by waterproofing reusable fabrics deteriorates with multiple processings. The repeated processes of laundering and sterilization gradually disrupt the integrity of the fabric. Therefore a system should be established to monitor, control, and determine useful life when reprocessing fabrics made from woven materials (15, p. 86; 3, p. 267).

- Many reusable products are provided with a grid, bar code, or other device that can record each time the product is inspected before reuse (4, p. 27).

- Densely woven, treated cotton will become moisture-permeable after about 75 washings, untreated cotton after as few as 30 washings. Repeated drying, ironing, and steam sterilizing also changes the fabric structure. The number of uses, washings, and sterilizing cycles should be recorded, and drapes that are no longer effective as barriers should be taken out of use (8, pp. 512-513).

- A more recent development in reusable materials is a barrier fabric laminate bonded between two layers of lightweight polyester. The fabric is liquid-proof, durable, breathable, and prevents strike-through (15, p. 86). Most of the newer-generation reusable fabrics are chemically treated to enhance barrier performance.

MATERIALS TESTING OF DRAPE AND GOWN FABRICS
Barrier Testing

The American Society for Testing and Materials (ASTM) has developed two quantitative tests, F1670 and F1671, to assess fluid and viral penetration for surgical textiles (1; 2). The first test, F1670, measures synthetic blood penetration through surgical barrier fabrics and can be used to screen the liquid barrier properties of apparel materials. F1670 successfully discriminates between liquid-resistant and liquid barrier materials—in other words, those that inhibit visible penetration rather than prevent it (20, pp. 13, 15).

The second test, F1671, is a more sophisticated technique that detects viral penetration and measures how well fabric materials that have passed the first test will prevent the passage of viruses based on a surrogate virus test system. Materials that fail F1670 will also fail F1671. Materials that pass F1670 but fail F1671 may be classified as liquid barrier materials but not microbial barrier or liquid-proof materials because small amounts of liquid-carrying viruses may penetrate the fabric (20, pp. 13, 15).

Many groups, including Association for the Advancement of Medical Instrumentation (AAMI) and the U.S. Food and Drug Administration (FDA), have referenced the ASTM test methods as effective means for gauging medical fabric barrier performance. Only materials that consistently pass both tests can be considered liquid-proof, microbial barrier materials (e.g., preventing transmission of both liquids and microorganisms) (20, p. 15).

For both F1670 and F1671 a synthetic blood is applied to the fabric in a special test cell under fixed applied pressure. After exposure, the fabric is examined for evidence of visual penetration or microbiologically tested for evidence of viral penetration. The pressure recommended for these test methods is 2 psi (pounds per square inch) (17, p. 31).

Researchers tested four commonly used medical textiles for fluid penetration at various pressures:

1. Calendered treated polyester: failed at 1 psi
2. Spunlace nonwovens: failed at 0.5 psi
3. Spunlace-meltblown-spunlace (SMS) nonwovens: failed at 1.25 psi
4. Monolithic films (solid films that are relatively free of pores or defects): passed at up to 40 psi hydrostatic pressure (17, pp. 31-32)

In a surgical barrier material a nonwoven film laminate may provide the strength of a nonwoven with the barrier properties of the monolithic film. Because there is no universally accepted definition of *barrier* at this time, studies related to exerted pressures may help to shed light on efforts to produce such a standard (17, pp. 31-32).

AAMI's Technical Information Report outlines four categories of barrier materials:

1. Liquid resistant (inhibits the penetration of liquids)
2. Liquid barrier (prevents the visible penetration of liquids)

3. Microbial barrier (prevents the penetration of microorganisms)
4. Liquid proof (prevents the penetration of liquids and microorganisms)

These distinctions can be used to differentiate types of protective apparel available and to form a hierarchy of barrier protection (4; 20, p. 15).

One suggested hierarchy for predicting barrier effectiveness is:

Level 1: liquid-resistant materials (passing hydrostatic head and mason jar/spray impact testing)

Level 2: liquid barrier materials (passing ASTM 1670 testing)

Level 3: liquid-proof materials (passing ASTM 1671 testing); if fabrics pass Level 3, they pass all other listed tests

Applying these concepts to the clinical environment requires that surgical personnel know how much blood and body fluid penetration is acceptable, considering that the Occupational Safety and Health Administration's (OSHA's) Bloodborne Pathogen Final Rule mandates the reduction of exposure risk through the use of protective apparel that does not allow blood or fluids to penetrate under normal conditions (20, p. 19).

For readers who are in the process of choosing drape and gown materials, obtaining AAMI Technical Report No. 11-1994 (4) is a *must.*

Flammability Standards

The introduction of more high-energy ignition devices (e.g., lasers, fiberoptic illumination systems, and electrosurgery units) has created increasing numbers of potential fire hazards in surgical settings. Lasers and other advanced electrical equipment are now used in 60% to 80% of all surgical procedures (19, p. 41).

Although there are requirements for minimum performance of gowns, there are no federal, state, or local regulations that require a minimum performance for surgical drapes. Most surgical drape manufacturers, however, have adopted the same minimum performance levels for drapes as those required for surgical gowns (19, p. 42).

The National Fire Protection Agency (NFPA) *Standard (No. 702-1980) for Classification of the Flammability of Wearing Apparel* has four classes for rating wearing apparel (and drapes) by ignition and flame spread characteristics:

Class 1 (relatively slow burning): 20 seconds or more

Class 2 (moderately flammable): 8 to 19 seconds

Class 3 (relatively flammable): 3 to 7 seconds

Class 4 (relatively fast burning): less than 3 seconds (19, p. 43)

Even though the officially inactivated NFPA Standard is still referenced, surgical gowns (and drapes) are regulated by Consumer Product Safety Commission (CPSC) 16 CFR Part 1610, *Standard for the Flammability of Clothing Textiles,* and must exhibit a minimum flame spread rate of 3.5 seconds for a Class 1 rating. This test is less stringent than NFPA 702-1980 (19, p. 43).

The NFPA 702-1980 is listed by the FDA as the flammability reference test for surgical drapes and gowns. AAMI references both the NFPA and the CPSC as standard test methods for evaluating safety and performance characteristics for both surgical drapes and gowns (21; 4, p. 43). Although the NFPA 702-1980 was removed from the NFPA's list of "active" standards in 1987, the test is still referenced (4, p. 18).

OR personnel should look for statements regarding flammability on gowns, such as *The Base Fabric Meets the Class 1 Flammability Requirements for CPSR 16 CFR Part 1610* (19, p. 41).

Testing for Comfort

New thermophysiological models for clothing and methods of laboratory analysis help healthcare personnel to make intelligent purchasing decisions. Barrier qualities and comfort measurements are inherent criteria used (11).

CHOOSING DRAPES

Barrier material characteristics; requirements of the procedure itself and the extent to which the patient needs to be covered; and the amount of blood, body fluids, and irrigating fluid anticipated should all be considered when choosing drapes and draping materials.

- Barrier materials should be safe, comfortable, and appropriate for the intended use in the practice setting. Surgical drapes should be flexible in order to conform to patients' contours, to allow placement and manipulation of surgical instruments, and to appropriately drape specified equipment (3, pp. 268-269).
- Selection and use of barrier materials should be consistent with their intended purpose and should demonstrate a positive cost/benefit ratio. Barrier materials prevent the penetration of microorganisms, particulates, and fluids (3 p. 269).
- Used to create a sterile field and a sterile barrier, the barrier effectiveness of drapes and sheets varies depending on the material used. Some single-use, nonwoven drapes contain a

layer of plastic throughout the drape or in zoned areas to create a liquid-proof barrier to fluids. Woven or nonwoven fabrics alone are liquid resistant but not necessarily liquid proof (14, p. 45).

- The size of the sterile field, the location and size of the incision, the number of sterile persons at the operative field, and the sterile instrumentation and equipment on the field should all be considered (14, p. 45).

DESIRED DRAPE AND GOWN CHARACTERISTICS

Regardless of the materials they are composed of, drapes and gowns should have the following characteristics:

- As a barrier, resistant to the passage of blood and fluids (resistant to strike-through)
- Impermeable to moist microbial penetration, including viruses
- Resistant to tearing, puncture, or abrasion
- Lint free, to reduce airborne contaminants and shedding into the surgical site
- Flame resistant/flame retardant and antistatic (of special concern with the use of lasers, electrosurgical units, and other high-energy devices that provide an ignition source at the sterile field)
- Free of toxic ingredients (e.g., laundry residues and nonfast dyes)
- Porous enough to maintain an isothermic environment appropriate to body temperature, thus eliminating heat build-up
- Conformable and drapable for ease in use by surgical staff and for ease in draping patients, equipment, and furniture (9, p. 206; 8, p. 511)

NOTE: Since drape and gown materials are very similar, the reader is referred to the discussion on desired gown characteristics in the chapter "Gowning." Criteria for choosing single-use (nonwoven) versus reusable (woven) gowns and drapes are also included in that chapter.

TYPES OF DRAPES
General Drapes

- Numerous configurations, sizes, and types of drapes exist. Many drapes are designed for particular procedures or specialty areas and are named accordingly: laparotomy, laparoscopy, thyroid, breast, eye, kidney, hip, cesarean section, and perineal. Other types are fenestrated, aperture, split, major, minor, medium, single sheets, leggings, and towels. Sterile towels are commonly used to outline or "picture frame" a surgical site. The folded edge of each towel is placed toward the line of incision (8, pp. 511-514; 9, p. 206). Towel drapes, made either of disposable or clear plastic material, may have a band of adhesive along one end of the towel (15, p. 87).

- Drapes may be reinforced, especially around fenestrations, or treated to be totally impervious. Other draping materials may be impregnated with carbon to make them nonstatic (8, pp. 512-514).
- Aluminum-coated drapes may be safest for use with lasers, especially around the oxygen-enriched environment of the head and neck area. Since no drapes currently withstand thermal laser beam impact, as a safety precaution wet towels should be placed around the area where a laser will be used. Fluid-proof drapes should be applied under the wet towels to prevent strike-through and microbial migration. Research is being conducted to develop laser-resistant drapes (8, pp. 512-514; 15, p. 87).
- Some drapes are equipped with pouches or troughs along the sides to collect fluids such as amniotic fluid. Others have pockets, devices for holding suction tubing or electrosurgical cords, or other attachments. Other drapes are classified as table covers (8, pp. 512-514).
- An isolation drape is a plastic transparent hanging drape used to isolate the C-arm, x-ray equipment, and other nonsterile equipment from the sterile operative field (15, p. 87).
- Miscellaneous drapes are available for draping microscopes, endoscopes, cameras, and other surgical instrumentation and equipment. Sterile covers for light handles are also available. Care must be taken in attaching these covers to avoid contaminating sterile gloves by touching the nonsterile parts of the light or light handles.
- The procedure for pneumatic tourniquet draping is as follows: First, a nonsterile tourniquet cuff is placed around the extremity, wrapped with soft cast padding, before prepping the patient's skin. A nonsterile plastic drape placed over the tourniquet cuff can be used to isolate the cuff from the sterile field and protect it from prep solutions before the prep. A stockinette, which is a sterile seamless tubing of stretchable woven material, sometimes with an impervious covering, is used to drape and cover the prepped extremity within the sterile field. A sterile barrier drape that delineates the upper limit of the surgical area is carefully placed around the extremity immediately at or below the tourniquet cuff.

Adhesive Incise Drapes

Also known as adhesive plastic, plastic incise, incision, or sticky drapes, these drapes are applied to the patient's prepped skin at the operative site and the incision is made through the plastic. They are used in addition to drapes that simply cover the patient. Incise drapes protect against contamination of the wound by surrounding skin.

- An incise drape can define the surgical site and hold other drapes down, thus possibly eliminating the "squaring off" of the surgical site with sterile towels (14, p. 45).
- An incise drape, which is a self-adhering plastic film applied directly to the prepared dry skin, helps stabilize other drapes and isolates potential sources of infection such as stomas, colostomies, and fistulas (15, p. 87).
- The use of incise drapes is based on the belief that adherent coverage of skin up to the margin of the incision effectively prevents surgical site contamination from contiguous (surrounding skin and tissues) sites (23, p. 163).
- The most important feature of an incise drape is reliable adhesion. Drapes that lift fail to provide a sterile surface. An incise drape must adhere to wound edges even during heavy retraction or irrigation (14, p. 45).
- Researchers Cruse and Foord (6), in a study of 62,939 wounds, documented a higher infection rate when plastic adhesive drapes were used than when they were not used. Lilly, et al. (12), also studied the effect of adhesive drapes on contamination of operative wounds, and Jackson, Pollock, and Tindal (10) examined the value of plastic adhesive drapes in the prevention of SSIs. The results of these latter two studies demonstrated no difference in SSI rates when the use of plastic adhesive drapes was compared with the use of conventional drapes (23, p. 174).
- Another investigator studied the role of incision drapes on the bacterial contamination of wounds and concluded that incision drapes do little to reduce the bacterial count on wounds and that they do not reduce the frequency of wound sepsis (18, p. 528).
- Whyte, et al. (22), advocated draping the wound edge with wound edge drapes, thinking that the main source of wound contamination is at or near the wound edge with many bacteria residing either on the surface of the skin, in the lower layers of skin, or in the skin ducts themselves.
- Adhesive plastic drapes have not been shown to reduce infection rates, but many surgeons use them, particularly in contaminated and hard-to-drape areas (16, p. 16).

Antimicrobial Incise Drapes

These drapes contain impregnated antimicrobial agents. A film coated with an iodophor-containing adhesive, for example, slowly releases active iodine during the surgical procedure to effectively inhibit proliferation of organisms from the patient's skin (contraindicated when the patient is allergic to iodophors). Manufacturers' instructions should be followed. An alcohol skin wipe may be done and must be allowed to dry before such an antimicrobial incise drape is applied. Other antimicrobials such as triclosan may also be used (8, p. 511).

DRAPING GUIDELINES

• Sufficient time should be allowed to carefully establish a draping plan, have all items available, and use impeccable aseptic technique.
• Drapes are handled as little as possible.
• Care is exercised in picking up drapes so that they do not unfold prior to placement. Drapes should not be fanned or waved in the air.
• The scrub person stands away from the nonsterile OR bed to avoid contamination of sterile gown and gloves from the nonsterile areas; folded drapes are carried to the OR bed; the area closest to the scrub person is draped first.
• Drapes are held high enough to avoid touching nonsterile areas until they are over the proper area, at which time they are placed.
• Reaching across either a patient or an OR bed that has not been draped to place a drape is not acceptable.
• Sterile gloved hands are protected from contact with the patient by placing them under the drape (cuffing) as each drape is being placed.
• Once placed, drapes are not moved or rearranged.
• If towel clips are used to secure or stabilize towels or drapes, the nonperforating type should be used.
• If a wet drape is found, it should be discarded immediately; contaminated gloves should be changed and a new sterile drape applied.
• If a hole or defect is found in a drape after its placement, either the defect must be covered with a secondary sterile drape material or the entire drape must be discarded.
• If doubt exists regarding the sterility of a drape, or if a drape becomes contaminated, it should not be handled further but should be considered contaminated and must be discarded.
• Soiled drapes are carefully contained in the room and placed in appropriate containers.

- Any drape manufacturer or vendor of drape services should provide written instructions regarding the use and care of their drapes, as well as draping procedures. These instructions should be carefully followed (9, p. 206; 8, pp. 514-515).
- Procedure manuals and appropriate texts should be consulted for specific draping instructions and procedures. Facility policies, surgeons' preferences, and the guidelines and principles discussed in this chapter should all be used to determine and carry out meticulous, aseptically correct, safe draping procedures.

OTHER DRAPING TOPICS
Drapes Extending Over Edges

How far should a drape extend over the edge of a draped table or item? This questions arises occasionally when the issue is how extensive a drape is needed to adequately cover a table, ring stand, or the patient on an OR bed. There is no one definitive answer to this question, nor is there a rule for calculating the length of a drape as it extends over an edge of a table.

AORN has no official recommendation on this issue, stating that the question requires application of basic aseptic principles (e.g., draped tables are sterile only at table level). The edges and sides of the drape extending below table level are considered nonsterile. If this is used as a guiding principle, how far the drape extends over the edge of a draped surface becomes irrelevant because any portion of the drape beyond the flat surface is considered contaminated; only the top surface is considered sterile (7, p. 274).

NOTE: Another consideration in this issue is the *margin of safety* principle of asepsis. A margin of safety, that small extra distance or space, serves as a safety net, making it difficult to accidentally contaminate oneself when creating a sterile field or draping a patient. A drape that hangs at least 12 inches below table level, or 12 inches or more below the level of the operative site, provides that margin of safety that allows for necessary movement and activity around the sterile field while still keeping the sterile field and surrounding area intact throughout the procedure.

Layering of Drapes

Layering of drapes was commonly done when all drapes were made of reusable woven materials. Layers of drapes were added to counteract and prevent strike-through. Conventional wisdom at that time was that additional drapes and more layers equated with better and safer draping. With the advent of better technology, new materials, and single-use drapes, layering is seldom required and in addition usually only adds to the time required for and the cost of draping.

Many of the drapes used today, including impervious and reinforced-back table covers, require only a single layer for barrier protection.

In minor procedures and some ophthalmic surgery, for example, half drape sheets may be adequate. Also, incise drapes may be used in place of squaring off the incisional site with towels. A fluid-collection pouch incorporated into a drape can eliminate the need for extra drapes, and towels can also reduce the clean-up process in the OR (14, p. 45).

Manufacturers and providers of drapes should be contacted for recommendations related to efficacious draping, particularly the proper application of numbers and types of drapes and the reasons for changes in the need for layering.

Contaminated Areas on Drapes

Can a contaminated drape area be covered with a sterile towel or an incise drape? This topic is seldom discussed in the literature. However, it seems reasonable that a small contaminated area of a drape could be covered with a sterile drape of adequate size to maintain the sterile field. If the contaminated area is also wet, care must be taken that the reinforced sterile covering is liquid proof so that no strike-through is possible. Good judgment must always prevail when deciding whether a contaminated area can be satisfactorily covered to maintain and not compromise the sterile field, or whether re-draping is necessary.

Hair or Other Foreign Objects

If a hair is found on a drape, the hair can be removed with a hemostat and handed off the sterile field. The area is then immediately covered with a sterile towel or another piece of sterile draping material. Although hair can be sterilized, the source of a hair is usually unknown when it is found on a sterile drape (e.g. it could have fallen from a staff member's head). A foreign body reaction would result if the hair got into the wound.

NOTE: Although this information can be found in reference 8, page 515, it is considered a controversial recommendation. Some clinicians would consider any foreign object (e.g., hair, insects, or dirt) found in a sterile pack or instrument set to automatically render the setup contaminated and would tear it down and proceed with a new setup. Other clinicians would do as discussed above: rid the field of the foreign object, immediately consider any area or glove that was in contact with the object to be contaminated, and take steps to make those areas or attire as sterile as possible. (See the section on opening packs in the chapter "Opening and Setting Up Rooms.") Most important is that each surgical setting is prepared for thorny issues like this that could arise and has in writing the policies and procedures so that all staff members respond in the same way.

Reuse of Open, Unused Single-Use Drapes

Unused single-use surgical gowns and drapes should not be resterilized unless manufacturers provide written instructions for reprocessing. Single-use gowns and drapes may not be amenable to adequate resterilization and could be damaged in the process or may retain toxic residues. In addition, facilities that choose to reprocess single-use items may be subject to the FDA regulations that consider the responsibilities of facilities who reprocess to be similar to the responsibilities of manufacturers (3, p. 268; 15, p. 86). NOTE: The new August 2000 FDA guidance document does not apply to "open-but-unused" SUDs (single-use devices). For more information on the FDA regulations, the reader is referred to the chapter "Reuse and Reprocessing of Single-Use Devices."

References

1. American Society of Testing Materials (ASTM): *Standard test method for resistance of materials used in protective clothing to penetration by synthetic blood, F1670-98,* West Conshohocken, Penn, 1998, Author.
2. American Society of Testing Materials (ASTM): *Standard test method for resistance of materials used in protective clothing to penetration by bloodborne pathogens using Phi-X174 bacteriophage penetration as a test system, F1671-976,* West Conshohocken, Penn, 1997, Author.
3. AORN: Recommended practices for use and selection of barrier materials for surgical gowns and drapes. In *Standards, recommended practices and guidelines,* Denver, 2000, Author, pp 267-270.
4. Association for the Advancement of Medical Instrumentation (AAMI): *Selection of surgical gowns and drapes in health care facilities,* AAMI Technical Information Report (TIR), No. 11-1994, Arlington, Va, 1994, Author.
5. Beck WC, Collette TS: False faith in the surgeon's gown and drape, *Am J Surg* 83:125-126, 1952.
6. Cruse PJE, Foord R: The epidemiology of wound infection: a 10-year prospective study of 62,939 wounds, *Surg Clin North Am* 60:27-40, 1980.
7. Fogg DM: Clinical issues, *AORN J* 69(1):272-274, 276, 1999.
8. Fortunato N: *Berry & Kohn's operating room technique,* ed 9, St Louis, 2000, Mosby.
9. Gruendemann BJ, Fernsebner B: *Comprehensive perioperative nursing,* vol 1, *Principles,* Boston, 1995, Jones & Bartlett.
10. Jackson DW, Pollock AV, Tindal DS: The value of a plastic adhesive drape in the prevention of wound infection: a controlled study, *Br J Surg* 58:340-342, 1971.
11. Lewis JA, Brown PL: Breaking the comfort barrier in impervious gowns, *Surgical Services Management* 4(2):29-38, 1998.
12. Lilly HA et al: Effects of adhesive drapes on contamination of operation wounds, *Lancet* 2:431-432, 1970.

13. Mangram AJ, Hospital Infection Control Practices Advisory Committee (HICPAC), Centers for Disease Control and Prevention: Guideline for prevention of surgical site infection, 1999, *Infect Control Hosp Epidemiol* 24(4):247-278, 1999. (Reprinted, in part, in Appendix B.)

14. Manz EA, Edgar, BL: Examining draping practices for cost-effectiveness, *Surgical Services Management* 4(8):41-47, 1998.

15. Mews PA: Establishing and maintaining a sterile field. In Phippen ML, Wells MP: *Patient care during operative and invasive procedures,* Philadelphia, 2000, WB Saunders, pp 61-93.

16. Patterson P: Draping: what's necessary, what's proven, *OR Manager* 6(7):1, 15-16, 1990.

17. Pournoor J: New scientific tools to expand the understanding of aseptic practices, *Surgical Services Management* 6(4):28, 31-32, 2000.

18. Roy MC: The operating theater: a special environmental area. In Wenzel RP, editor: *Prevention and control of nosocomial infections,* ed 3, Baltimore, 1997, Williams & Wilkins, pp 515-538.

19. Sommers JR: Flammability standards for surgical drapes and gowns, past, present, and future, *Surgical Services Management* 4(2):41-44, 1998.

20. Stull JO, Pournoor KJ: Using the ASTM test methods to select surgical gowns and drapes, *Surgical Services Management* 4(2):13-15, 19-22, 1998.

21. U.S. Food and Drug Administration (FDA): *Guidance on notification [510(k)] submissions for surgical gowns and surgical drapes,* Washington, DC, 1993, U.S. Government Printing Office.

22. Whyte W et al: The role of clothing and drapes in the operating room, *J Hosp Infect* 11(suppl C):2-17, 1988.

23. Wong ES: Surgical site infections. In Mayhall CG, editor: *Hospital epidemiology and infection control,* Baltimore, 1996, William & Wilkins, pp 154-175.

Suggested Reading

1. Koch F: Surgical gowns and drapes, selecting the best fit for your facility, *Surgical Services Management* 4(2):25-28, 1998.

2. Leonas KK, Jinkins RS: The relationship of selected fabric characteristics and the barrier effectiveness of surgical gown fabrics, *Am J Infect Control* 25(2):16-23, 1997.

3. McCullough EA: Methods for determining the barrier efficacy of surgical gowns, *Am J Infect Control* 21(12):368-374, 1993.

4. McCullough EA, Schoenberger LK: Liquid barrier properties of nine surgical gown fabrics, *INDA: The Journal of Nonwovens Research* 3(3rd quarter):14-20, 1991.

5. Smith JW, Nichols RL: Barrier efficiency of surgical gowns: are we really protected from our patients' pathogens? *Arch Surg* 126(6):756-763, 1991.

6. Telford GL, Quebbeman EJ: Assessing the risk of blood exposure in the operating room, *Am J Infect Control* 21(12):351-356, 1993.

N. Dressings and Drains

❖◆❖

Surgical team members often remove dressings before performing the surgical skin preparation and apply dressings to fresh wounds as soon as the incision is closed. Dry sterile dressings are most often used because the edges of a surgical wound are usually well approximated. However, dressings may also be applied to open wounds.

A surgical drain is used to evacuate fluid that may accumulate in a wound or body cavity after closure of the incision. If excess fluid accumulates and a drain is not in place, the fluid can exert pressure on the suture line. This creates swelling and increases the chance of dehiscence or infection.

Surgical personnel are responsible for using strict aseptic technique during drain placement and dressing application and and care to decrease the risk of surgical site infection (SSI).

PRIMARY WOUND HEALING

When skin is injured its normal barrier function is destroyed. A series of events and cascades initiate hemostasis. In a healthy, uncompromised host, acute wounds heal spontaneously without complications (15, p. 1). A closed wound or incision heals by primary intention and has accurately approximated edges. As an incision is made the vessel wall injury activates platelets and causes smooth muscle constriction. These events initiate clot formation and hemostasis. Healing continues during a proliferation phase that continues for about 21 days. Three major events occur during this phase: epithelialization, neovascularization, and collagen synthesis. This type of wound healing occurs in a sutured surgical incision with well-approximated edges.

1. During epithelialization, fixed basal cell mitosis and marginal basal cell migration act together to bridge the gap created by the incision. Epithelialization begins within 24 hours after the incision is made and is complete within 48 hours (13, p. 434).

2. During neovascularization, angiogenesis begins and reaches peak activity in 7 days. Endothelial cells of existing vessels proliferate to form new capillaries, which accounts for the bright pink color of the wound edges (13, p. 434).

3. During collagen synthesis, a function of fibroblasts, macrophages secrete angiogenesis factor (AGF) and fibroblast-stimulating factor combines with a growth factor released by dead platelets in the first moments after injury, resulting in

the influx of fibroblasts into the wound. Collagen fibers appear by the third day. The production of collagen, synthesized by fibroblasts, and ground substance peak by the fifth to seventh days. Newly formed collagen is weak but increases in strength after the fifth day (13, p. 434).

The maturation phase of healing begins about 21 days after incision and may last for a year or more. During this phase the collagen produced is thicker and more compact, and fibers begin to cross-link. Both of these processes increase the tensile strength of the wound. Significant remodeling occurs during the maturation phase, with scar tissue forming and resolving. Reabsorption of excess collagen remodels the scar, increases its pliability, and contracts the suture line (13, p. 434).

SECONDARY WOUND HEALING

The mechanism of secondary intention wound closure is granulation, reepithelialization, and contraction. Secondary wound healing is facilitated if the dermal layer is preserved. The wound is left open and allowed to heal from the inner toward the outer surface. Devitalized tissue must be repeatedly debrided and the wound packed with moist packing material. The risk of infection is proportional to the amount of necrotic tissue in the wound and the immune response of the patient (7, p. 562). An example of secondary wound healing is when the appendix has ruptured, the wound is contaminated, and the outer layers of the wound are left open.

Understanding the process of wound closure and healing is important to fully appreciate surgical personnel's infection prevention role in dressing application and incision care.

DRESSINGS
Removing Old Dressings

Patients often arrive in the operating room with dressings in place. These dressings must be removed before surgical skin preparation.

- Nonsterile examination gloves should be worn to loosen tape and remove the outer dressing. However, sterile gloves should be worn and sterile technique used to remove the remainder of the dressing. To prevent damage to the skin, the tape should be pulled back gently and tape remover used to moisten and separate the tape from the skin. Tape remover should be used to remove any tape debris from the skin (19).
- The dressing should be removed one layer at a time (5, p. 589).
- If the dressing adheres to the wound, a small amount of sterile normal saline can be poured on the dressing to loosen it and prevent disruption of healing tissue (4, p. 988).

- Used dressing and gloves should be discarded in a plastic bag (4, p. 988).
- The wound and surrounding tissue should be inspected for appearance, color, size, depth, drainage, and integrity (23, p. 24).
- Traumatic wounds may need copious irrigation to remove debris and microorganisms before surgical skin preparation (7, p. 507).

Dressing Application to Closed Wounds

Some manufacturers' instructions state that the prep solution should be left on the skin for additional bacteriostatic action. Others recommend removing solution at the end of the surgery, some with alcohol. General guidelines include the following:

- The skin may be cleansed of blood with a sterile saline-dampened sponge (7, p. 573).
- Mild cleansing agents such as hydrogen peroxide may be used for closed wounds.

NOTE: Surgical incisions are usually closed with sutures, clips, or special tapes. Presterilized zippers, with adhesive support strips attached to the sides of the incision, provide another method of closing clean incisions.

Dry dressings

Dry sterile dressings are applied to closed incisions. The purposes of the dressings are to:

- Absorb exudate and other drainage from the wound (10, p. 84)
- Protect the wound from exogenous contamination (10, p. 84)
- Protect the wound from injury or trauma and provide an optimal environment for wound healing (5, p. 585)
- Promote hemostasis by direct pressure and through absorption of drainage (5, p. 585)
- Reduce the discomfort associated with the wound, as well as conceal it aesthetically (5, p. 585)

All closed incisions should be covered with a dry sterile dressing for the first 24 to 48 hours and sterile technique should be used for wound care and dressing changes (22, p. 24BB; 18, p. 268).

- An x-ray sponge should not be used for a dressing because the radio-opaque strip could distort a postoperative x-ray film or cause an incorrect count at closure, or if the patient's incision must be reopened (7, p. 573).
- A layer of moist dressing may be placed over the wound. The dressing may contain petrolatum or a mixture of bismuth and petrolatum. The purpose of this layer of dressing is to protect the healing wound tissue. The porous mesh allows fluids to flow freely into the overlying absorbent dressing. The dressing

does not adhere to the wound and thus helps to reduce pain during dressing changes (14; 8, p. 61).

- An antibiotic ointment may be applied directly to the wound, followed by the gauze dressing. This ointment seals and protects the wound and reduces pain during dressing changes (7, p. 572).
- The sterile dressing should be applied with sterile gloves before the drape is removed (7, p. 573).
- The sterile dressing should be applied one layer at a time. Careful application of dressing sponges prevents introduction of microorganisms into the wound (4, p. 986).

A nonadherent contact layer such as Telfa can be placed closest to the surgical wound to prevent the gauze from sticking to the wound (6, p. 366). Wounds that have more drainage will require either more layers or a thicker absorbent dressing (5, p. 590; 6, p. 366; 13, p. 444).

- Single layer dressings can be used for a clean, uncomplicated surgical wound. Various polyurethane adhesive materials can also be used on a clean, uninfected wound (13, p. 444).
- Transparent film dressings can be used alone or over gauze dressings. This type of dressing serves as a barrier to bacteria and water, is permeable to oxygen, and promotes a moist environment for new granulation (8, p. 61). Other transparent dressings also allow oxygen and moisture to leave the covered wound while providing a barrier to bacteria and other contaminants (17).
- The dressing should be secured with tape so that it adheres to 5 to 8 cm of skin on all sides of the dressing (5, p. 590).
- The tape or adhesive covering should be applied gently without putting traction on the skin. This prevents skin blistering or damage (19).
- Before taping, the patient's allergies and skin condition must be assessed. If tape applied directly to the skin is contraindicated, an alternative such as Montgomery straps or elastic mesh can be used. If taping cannot be avoided, a protective barrier dressing can be placed first to provide an alternative contact for the tape (13, p. 444).
- After dressing the wound, sterile gloves should be removed and disposed of in the proper receptacle (4, p. 986).

Dressing Changes
Closed wounds

If a wound is not infected and has no drainage, the following is recommended:

- The dressing should be changed and the incision cleaned daily (23, p. 26)

- A nonadherent dressing should be changed every 24 hours (23, p. 26)
- The incision should be assessed for signs of infection (23, p. 26)
- The patient and caregivers should be instructed regarding incision care, symptoms of SSI, and the need to report such symptoms (18, p. 268)

Open wounds

Open wounds that will heal by secondary intention require the application of moist dressings in the wound bed, followed by a dry dressing. An absorbent pad used as the outer layer is secured by ties or tape (4, p. 990).

During the many dressing change procedures that will follow the initial application, a variety of wound care products can be used to keep the wound moist (24, pp. 68-69; 25, p. 51).

- Open wounds should be packed with antiseptics. However, agents like povidone-iodine, Dakin's solution, and hydrogen peroxide, thought to enhance wound healing, should never be used as cleansing or packing agents when treating open wounds such as pressure ulcers because the agents kill white blood cells (26, p. 33). Sterile normal saline solution should be used instead (19).
- Frequency of dressing change is determined by the wound status, type of dressing, amount of drainage, and protocols of the physician or agency (4, p. 982).
- It is imperative that good handwashing and sterile technique be used before and after every dressing change (4, p. 990).

DRAINS

A surgical drain is used to evacuate fluid that may accumulate in a wound or surgical site such as the brain, joints, or abdomen. If a large amount of drainage is anticipated from a wound, a drain is usually inserted. If a drain is not inserted, fluids can place pressure on the suture line, which creates swelling and can increase the chances of dehiscence or infection.

Specific procedures and protocols have been developed for proper insertion and maintenance of surgical drains. Following these procedures can decrease the potential risks and complications of SSI. The Centers for Disease Control and Prevention (CDC) states that drains placed through an operative incision increase SSI risk. Therefore drains should be placed distal to the incision site, through a separate incision. A closed-suction drain should be used (18, pp. 263, 268).

Purpose of Drains

The purpose of drains is to:
- Remove foreign or harmful materials (present or anticipated) that might lead to complications (13, p. 444)
- Decompress the structure of the G-I tract (13, p. 444)
- Act as a stent to promote healing and prevent scarring and stricture formation (13, p. 444)
- Decrease the amount of dead space, prevent hematoma and edema formation, minimize post-op pain, promote the healing process and tissue approximation, and decrease the risk of infection (2, p. 291; 7, p. 569)

Types of Drains

The type of drain used depends on the need for drainage, surgeon preference, and the area to be drained (13, p. 444).

Open and closed drains

A Penrose drain is an open-ended flat cylinder of varying size. It is made of soft latex and functions by passive, overflow, and capillary action, causing fluids to flow through the drain to the absorbent dressing. A Penrose drain may or may not have a gauze wick inserted in it, but only the ones without a gauze wick are rinsed in normal saline before insertion (7, pp. 569-570). Use of an open drain should be discouraged (18, p. 263).

Small tubes such as a T-tube, Malecot, or Pezzer catheters are also passive drainage devices and are inserted into organs to assist in gravity flow from the gallbladder or kidney. They are attached to a collection device that may be open or closed (7, p. 570).

Vacuum drains

Closed drains are attached to an external source of vacuum to create suction in the wound. These catheters are placed by use of a trocar that pierces the skin or by a small stab wound close to the incision. The catheter is attached to a plastic reservoir or collection chamber. The amount of suction in these systems depends on the method of creating the vacuum. Manually operated collection chambers have a preset vacuum level. Suction must be checked and the system reactivated by compression. Other collection systems may have a battery-powered adjustable suction device that sets a continuous vacuum level. This device may serve for autotransfusion that collects and filters blood and returns it to the patient (7, p. 570).

Drain Insertion and Fixation

- Drains, catheters, and tubes should be kept sterile, and sterile technique should be used during insertion. Drains, catheters,

drainage tubing, and adaptors should be single-use items (7, p. 571).
- The drain should be placed through a stab wound—a separate small incision close to the operative site. This placement decreases the chance of SSI, dehiscence, and incisional hernia. Research suggests that a drain placed through the operative site increases the risk of SSI (13, p. 445; 18, pp. 263, 268).
- The external portion of the drain is secured to the skin with a nonabsorbable suture (7, p. 569).
- The drain manufacturer's instructions must be followed to activate the device (7, p. 570).
- A drain can be left in place up to 10 days. However, bacterial colonization of initially sterile drain tracts increases with the number of days the drain is left in place. Therefore the drain should be removed as soon as possible once drainage has subsided or is very minimal (14, p. 445; 18, p. 263).
- A split dressing made of either gauze or nonadherent material should be placed around the drain. The remainder of the dressing is then applied to the incision (7, p. 571). NOTE: The split dressing fits directly around the drain and next to the skin.

Chest Tube Placement and Care

A chest tube is placed using strict aseptic technique to drain the pleural cavity and ensure complete reexpansion of the lung following procedures within the chest cavity. The tube or tubes are connected to a sterile, closed, water-seal drainage device. When the collection device is filled to the correct level with sterile water, outside air is sealed off instead of being drawn into the pleural space. Negative pressure within the system is maintained. Fluid drains by gravity from the chest into the drainage device. If gravity is not adequate to promote drainage, suction may be applied to the device (7, pp. 570-571).
- The tubing must be securely connected to the drainage device before transporting the patient from the operating room. The chest tube may be clamped before transporting as a safety measure. The surgeon should be consulted with regard to whether clamping is needed (7, p. 571).
- The chest drainage system should be checked for tidaling, bubbling, and fluid creep. Tidaling refers to fluctuations that occur with respiration and that reflect changes in intrapleural pressure and confirm chest tube patency. Tidaling decreases as an air leak resolves, and its absence indicates either occlusion or crimping of the tube or lung healing. Bubbling indicates the presence of an air leak and communication with the pleural

space. If the patient coughs and no bubbling occurs, reexpansion is present. Fluid creep results in the elevation of fluid level, loss of manometer function, or full lung expansion and pleural seal (12, p. 264).

- Measures to reduce potential buildup of fluid or air and promote flow include avoiding dependent loops of fluid-filled tubing (19; 21, p. 323) and kinks in the tubing, maintaining the patient tube clamp in the open position, and keeping the drainage unit in an upright position below the level of the patient (21, p. 321; 12, p. 266).
- Tube site care should include continuous assessment of the wound site. Agency policies may vary according to individual physician and nursing practice guidelines. Techniques for tube site care include using no protective covering; applying daily povidone-iodine ointment with sterile gauze dressing; and using petroleum occlusive dressing wrapped firmly around the tube, covered with a dressing. Petroleum gauze can cause skin maceration and increase the risk of infection. Principles of surgical wound care emphasize using aseptic technique when placing or changing the dressing around the chest tube. This should minimize the risk of bacterial colonization (12, p. 269).

Continuous Bladder Irrigation

Continuous bladder irrigation during surgery enables the surgeon to visualize the distended bladder walls. After surgery, continuous bladder irrigation is needed to wash out blood, bits of resected tissues, or stone fragments. A sterile closed irrigation system is used to prevent airborne contamination of the solution and the surgical site (7, p. 689). The closed method of irrigation during the postoperative period uses a triple-lumen indwelling urethral catheter. The first lumen is used to inflate the balloon, the second is used for the removal of urine, and the third is connected to a source of sterile solution for bladder irrigation. The type and amount of irrigant and the frequency of irrigation are prescribed by the surgeon. The lumen used for urinary drainage can either be clamped to allow the bladder to fill during irrigation and then opened to allow drainage, or it can be left open to allow outflow of urine throughout the procedure (4, pp. 1070-1071).

Autotransfusion Devices

An autotransfusion device is used to collect blood from wound drains. During collection the blood is filtered and reinfused into the patient. This device and method of blood administration is especially suited for use after surgery of the mediastinum and total knee arthroplasty (TKA). During TKA, tourniquet inflation prevents blood loss and allows all of the blood shed to be collected postoperatively (3, p. 272).

- Contamination of autotransfusion equipment or collected blood carries a potential risk of life-threatening infection. It is imperative that all caregivers who have direct contact with the equipment during setup or maintenance are familiar with the manufacturer's recommendations for safe handling. Aseptic technique and standard precautions must be used during the manipulation of infusion bags and handling of tubing connections and collection equipment (16, pp. 242-243).
- One study of autologous blood collection via an auto-transfusion device showed the blood to be of very high quality. The clinical safety and effectiveness of autotransfusion was based on hematologic parameters. Postoperative autotransfusion was shown to decrease postoperative transfusion requirements and the exposure to homologous transfusion (1, p. 22).
- Research supports the conclusion that unwashed shed blood effectively replaces lost blood and reduces the need for allogenic blood. Researchers also agree that the autotransfusion of shed blood should be limited to 2 units. Transfusion should be completed within 6 hours after commencement of collection (11, p. 11).

Documentation

- Documentation should include type and number of drains, location, how secured, drainage receptacle (if any), type of dressings, how dressings were secured, and characteristics and amount of drainage observed on transfer from the surgical area (13, p. 445).
- Drainage output should be recorded, and separate totals for each drain should be maintained (19; 20, p. 2).
- Drains should be assessed regularly for obstruction or changes in the character of the drainage (4, p. 992).

POSTOPERATIVE WOUND AND DRAIN CARE

- Assessment of drains and dressings should include checking for the amount, color, and consistency of drainage; any kinks or loose connections of tubing; and any signs of irritation or infection of the surrounding skin or insertion site (20, p. 1).
- Dressings around drains should be changed using strict sterile technique (18, p. 263).
- Gloves should be worn when emptying the drain reservoir. Contamination to the healthcare worker and the environmental

surfaces surrounding the patient are likely to occur with splashing (27, p. 346). The edge of the pour spout should be cleansed with an alcohol wipe before and after emptying, and the reservoir should be compressed and the cap reinserted tightly and aseptically into the reservoir to maintain sterility and vacuum pressure (19).

- The patient and family should be taught how to care for the wound and drain, including cleansing, monitoring for signs and symptoms of infection, changing the dressing, emptying the collection chamber, recording drainage amounts, and irrigating the drain if needed (20, pp. 1-2).

Potential Problems

- Problems can be caused by inadequate tube diameter, a kink or plug in the tubing, improper placement or displacement of tubing, loss of vacuum pressure (for closed drains), occlusion of the drain with clot or tissue, and retrograde contamination of the wound during emptying of the drainage reservoir (9, p. 244).
- Complications include hemorrhage, sepsis, loss of the drain inside the wound, and bowel herniation caused by an abdominal drain (6, p. 365).
- Because drains are foreign bodies, they can cause tissue damage to delicate adjacent structures (13, p. 445).

References

1. Berman AT: Postoperative autotransfusion after total knee arthroplasty, *Orthopedics* 19(1):15-22, 1996.
2. Briggs M: Principles of closed surgical wound care, *J Wound Care* 6(6):288-292, 1997.
3. Carstens VL, Earnshaw P: Postoperative orthopedic autotransfusion, *AORN J* 56(2):272-280, 1992.
4. Craven RF, Hirnle CJ: *Fundamentals of nursing: human health and function,* ed 3, Philadelphia, 2000, Lippincott.
5. Elkin MK, Perry AG, Potter PA: *Nursing interventions and clinical skills,* St Louis, 1996, Mosby.
6. Fairchild SS: *Perioperative nursing: principles and practice,* Boston, 1996, Little, Brown.
7. Fortunato N: *Berry & Kohn's operating room technique,* ed 9, St Louis, 2000, Mosby.
8. Fortunato N, McCullough SM: *Plastic and reconstructive surgery,* St Louis, 1998, Mosby.
9. Fox VJ: Facilitating care after the operative or invasive procedure. In Phippen M, Wells MP: *Patient care during operative and invasive procedures,* Philadelphia, 2000, WB Saunders, pp 229-247.
10. Galvani J: Not yet cut and dried, *Nurs Times* 93(16):84, 86, 1997.
11. Geier K: Perioperative blood management, *Orthopedic Nursing* 17(suppl):6-37, 1998.

12. Gross SB: Current challenges, concepts and controversies in chest tube management, *AACN Clin Issues Crit Care Nurs* 4(2):260-275, 1993.

13. Gruendemann BJ, Fernsebner B: *Comprehensive perioperative nursing,* vol 1, *Principles,* Boston, 1995, Jones & Bartlett.

14. Johnson & Johnson: *Adaptic non-adhering dressings,* Skillman, NJ, 1999, Author (product insert).

15. Kane DP, Krasner D: Wound healing and wound management. In Krasner D, Kane DP: *Chronic wound care: a source book for healthcare,* ed 2, Wayne, Pa, 1997, Health Management, pp 1-4.

16. Ley SJ: Intraoperative and postoperative blood salvage, *AACN Clin Issues* 7(2):238-248, 1996.

17. 3M Health Care: *Two new styles of absorbent adhesive dressings,* St. Paul, Minn, 1997, Author.

18. Mangram AJ, Hospital Infection Control Practices Advisory Committee (HICPAC), Centers for Disease Control and Prevention: Guideline for prevention of surgical site infection, 1999, *Infect Control Hosp Epidemiol* 20(4):247-278, 1999. (Reprinted, in part, in Appendix B.)

19. Mangum S: Sterile techniques. In *Encyclopedia of nursing skills,* Irvine, Ca, 2000, Concept Media (CD-ROM series).

20. Montgomery KL: SOP: care of patients with drains, *NIH Clinical Center Nursing Department,* 1996, www.cc.nih.gov/nursing/drains.html (accessed 2000).

21. Schmelz JO, et al: Effects of position of chest drainage tube on volume drained and pressure, *Am J Crit Care* 8(5):319-323, 1999.

22. Sterile vs. clean: a judgment call in home care, *RN* 60(9):24BB, 24DD, 1997.

23. Strimike CL, Wojcik JN, Stark BS: Incision care that really cuts it, *RN* 60(7):22-26, 1997.

24. Tallon RW: Wound care dressings, *Nurs Manage* 27(10):68-69, 1996.

25. Thompson J: A practical guide to wound care, *RN* 63(1):48-52, 2000.

26. Whittington K: Debunking wound care myths, *RN* pp 32-33, Aug 1995.

27. Zerbe M, McArdle A, Goldrick B: Exposure risk related to the management of three wound drainage systems, *Am J Infect Control* 24(5):346-352, 1996.

Suggested Reading

1. Briggs M, Wilson S, Fuller A: Infection control: the principles of aseptic technique in wound care, *Prof Nurse* 11(12):805, 806, 808, 810, 1996.

2. Bux M, Mahli JS: Assessing the use of dressings in practice, *J Wound Care* 5(7):305-308, 1996.

3. Carter L: Non-sterile dressings and infection risk, *J Wound Care* 1(1):14-16, 1992.

4. Cuzzell J: Choosing a wound dressing, *Geriatric Nursing: American Journal of Care for the Aging* 18(6):260-265, 1997.

5. Fay M: Drainage systems, their role in wound healing: *AORN J* 46(3):442-455, 1987.

6. Godden J, Hiley C: Managing the patient with a chest drain: a review, *Nurs Stand* 12:32, 35-39, 1998.

7. Hollinworth H: Nurses' assessment and management of pain at wound dressing changes, *J Wound Care* 4(2):77-83, 1995.

8. Low-tech zipper plays role in modern surgery, *Same Day Surg* pp 33-34, March 2000.

O. Care of Specimens

Providing the clinical laboratory with cultures and specimens demands conscientious effort on the part of surgical personnel. Specimens and cultures must be handled, prepared, labeled, and delivered to the appropriate department so that accurate results are obtained to aid in the diagnosis and treatment of the patient. Both direct and indirect contact with pathogens from patients' blood or sera can occur; therefore surgical personnel must protect themselves and others from potential contamination from these specimens.

Specimen handling and processing can put the healthcare worker (HCW) at risk because of the aerosolization of pathogen-contaminated specimens such as shigella, salmonella, hepatitis B and C, and tuberculosis. The exposure of skin or mucous membranes to body fluids containing pathogenic organisms also puts the HCW at risk. Specimen transport can place the HCW at risk for contamination via surfaces on transport vehicles, leaking specimen containers, and pneumatic tubes (7, p. 16).

HANDLING CULTURES AND SPECIMENS

- Cultures and specimens should be handed off the sterile field as soon as they are taken to prevent inadvertent discard during or at the end of the procedure (8, p. 188; 3, p. 362).
- Because cultures and specimens are considered potentially infectious—virtually all laboratory specimens are considered biohazardous material—all personnel should use gloves to handle them. Specimens should be put in leak-proof containers to ensure safe handling, processing, storage, transport, and shipping. Standard precautions should be followed during transportation to the laboratory (6, p. 280; 8, p. 183; 7, p. 16).
- A mask, protective eyewear (or a face shield), and gloves must be worn while handling specimens that are likely to generate droplets of blood or other body fluids (9, p. 131).
- Hands and other skin surfaces must be washed immediately and thoroughly if contaminated with blood or other body fluids (9, p. 131; 1, p. 335).
- After gloves are removed, hands should be washed thoroughly. Other personal protective equipment (PPE) should be worn when there is a risk of splash or spray (6, p. 280; 5, p. 474; 3, p. 364; 8, p. 183).
- Specimens of blood or other potentially infectious materials should be placed in a container that prevents leakage during

collection, handling, processing, storage, transport, and shipping. The container should be labeled or color-coded as biohazardous if the specimen is sent outside the facility. It should be closed before being stored, transported, or shipped (11, p. 64176).

- Contamination of the outside of culture and specimen containers with blood or other body fluids should be avoided. If contamination occurs, the exterior of the container should be disinfected with an agency-approved disinfectant before the specimen is removed from the surgical suite (3, p. 364; 5, p. 474; 8, p. 183).

- If a tube or container cannot be disinfected, it should be placed in a clear plastic bag for transportation to the lab. A note should be attached stating that the exterior surface of the inside container is contaminated. This practice alerts the person receiving the culture or specimen to use caution when handling the tube or container (8, p. 183; 5, p. 474). Another option is to place the contaminated container within a second container. This added step should prevent leakage. The outer (second) container should be labeled or color-coded as biohazardous (11, p. 64176).

- If there is a chance that a specimen could puncture the container, the container should be placed within a second container that is puncture resistant. Both containers should be labeled as biohazardous (11, p. 64176).

- Formalin, a water-based formaldehyde solution, is often used as a specimen preservative. Staff should be aware that formaldehyde is a potent allergen, mutagen, and carcinogen. The permissible exposure limit (PEL) is 1 ppm time-weighted average (TWA) (National Institute for Occupational Safety and Health [NIOSH]) to 3 ppm TWA (Occupational Safety and Health Administration [OSHA]) standard over 8 hours (5, p. 196).

Cultures

If possible, a culture is obtained before starting antimicrobial therapy. If the patient is already receiving antibiotic therapy, the antibiotic should be listed on the laboratory order. Aseptic technique should be used to prevent contamination from other tissues and fluids in the culture area and from the person collecting the culture (8, pp. 186-187).

The following is the procedure for collecting a culture:

- A sterile kit containing sterile cotton-tipped applicators and culture tube is opened. The package of long cotton-tipped applicators is delivered to the sterile field by the circulator. The scrub person opens the package and hands the cotton-tipped applicators to the surgeon, who obtains the specimen. The applicators are placed in the media inside the culture tube that is held by the circulator. The applicators are broken off and the lid is placed on the culture tube. When a culture is obtained, care is taken to obtain enough specimen for the laboratory to be able to perform all requested tests. Care is also taken to maintain the integrity of the specimen. Contact with a germicide or disinfectant may invalidate test results (8, pp. 186-187).

• If an anaerobic study is requested, every effort should be made to exclude oxygen either by evacuating air from the container or by closing it quickly if air cannot be evacuated. Exposure to room air may kill anaerobes in a few minutes. Special containers may be available that facilitate air evacuation. If the specimen contains purulent material, it should be collected in a disposable syringe through a disposable needle. This needle is removed and placed in the sharps container. After the specimen is collected, all of the air should be expelled from the syringe, away from the sterile field. The specimen should be marked with a biohazard label and immediately delivered to the laboratory (8, p. 187).

• If a Gram stain is ordered, the specimen is collected in an aerobic culture tube and is immediately sent for smear and fixation (8, p. 187).

• Spinal fluid removed during a spinal tap or the insertion of a catheter may be sent in sterile tubes. Separate tubes should be used for cell count or cell differentiation, glucose, and protein studies (8, p. 187).

• Acid-fast cultures are sent in an aerobic transport system. The specimen should be labeled and sent immediately after collection (8, p. 187).

• Studies needed on fungi may include the direct microscopic examination of a smear in addition to culturing. If microscopic examination is desired, the specimen can be sent in a Petri dish (8, p. 187).

Specimens

Tissue for single or multiple studies may be taken during surgery. These specimens may be for tests such as biopsy and frozen section, permanent studies, receptor site and cytology studies, or Papanicolaou (Pap) smear (8, p. 188). Specimens should not be shaken, crushed, or torn. They should arrive at the laboratory in a near-natural state, particularly tissues sent for frozen section (8, p. 188).

Frozen section and permanent study

• A specimen for frozen section should not be placed in normal saline or formalin because these solutions will cause moisture to form during the freezing process, which may interfere with the results of the examination (8, p. 188). The specimen should be placed on a moist towel or piece of nonabsorbent material. It should not be placed on a counted sponge. The circulator should always wear gloves when handling the specimen (8, p. 188).

- Tissue for permanent study may be placed in sterile normal saline or formalin solution according to laboratory protocol (8, p. 188).
- When pouring formalin or placing the specimen in the solution, splashing, contact with body surfaces, and breathing of vapors should be avoided by wearing the appropriate PPE and working in a properly ventilated area (8, pp. 183-184).
- Unless hospital policy dictates otherwise, all tissue or other objects removed from the patient are sent to the laboratory as specimens (8, p. 188).
- NOTE: Healthcare agencies may designate some tissue specimens as normal (e.g., foreskin from circumcision or a herniated disk) and set policy that these need not be sent for examination. Agency policy, the surgeon, or the operating room administration should be consulted before the tissue is discarded.
- Tissue for hormonal receptor study is taken from the primary tumor site. The specimen should be placed in normal saline solution, labeled, and sent to the laboratory (8, p. 188).
- Uterine and cervical cells sent for Pap smear are placed in fixative with the glass plate sides placed back to back so that they are exposed to the fixative. The specimen is placed in a special container, labeled, and sent to the laboratory (8, p. 189).
- Explants (e.g., plates and screws) are considered surgical specimens and are sent to the laboratory for identification, examination, and cataloging. They may be sent for gross examination only, thereby decreasing the cost to some degree. Explants must be thoroughly cleaned, sterilized, and judged to be safe before they can be released to the patient or surgeon. After an explant has been examined and cataloged in the laboratory, it may be given to the patient. If the patient does not wish to retain the device, it may be given to the surgeon for educational purposes. Any device with cracks, crevices, or any type of convoluted construction that makes it difficult to clean should be retained by the facility and disposed of in the same manner as other surgical specimens (4, p. 401; 8, p. 189).
- Explants that must be returned to the manufacturer and cannot be sterilized must be placed in a dry waterproof container, sealed and labeled both on the inner wrapper and outer packaging as containing biohazardous material (11, p. 64176).

- Foreign bodies (e.g., metal, glass, wood) are disposed of or preserved according to agency policy. A record is kept for legal purposes, and a description of the object is recorded. A foreign body such as a bullet may be given to the police, depending on legal implications. The bullet should not be allowed to touch metal, and care should be taken not to scratch it as this may interfere with ballistics testing. The foreign body must be placed in a dry impervious container before leaving the surgical area (5, p. 474; 8, p. 189).
- Amputated body parts are wrapped in plastic and labeled before being sent to the laboratory (5, p. 474).

DOCUMENTATION
Labeling of Cultures and Specimens
To ensure continuity of care, it is critical that specimens be labeled accurately. Proper documentation allows tracking of a specimen from its source to its disposition. Because laboratory results become part of the patient's permanent record, important information such as the patient's name, identification number, room number, physician's name, medical diagnosis, type of specimen, date and time of collection, and test requested should be documented (8, pp. 183, 185).

Establishing a Chain of Custody
A procedure to document a chain of custody ensures accountability for specimens. A log should be kept to track the specimen from the operative area to the laboratory or pathology department. A dual log system is recommended: one book is used to register specimens for culture and the other is used to register permanent and frozen section specimens and objects removed from the patient. Patient identification information should be recorded, including the patient's name, source of culture or type of tissue, date and time of specimen log-in, name and signature of person sending the specimen, name of person in laboratory to receive the specimen, and time of transfer of specimen to the laboratory (8, p. 185).

TRANSPORTING CULTURES AND SPECIMENS
HCWs should receive specific instructions regarding the handling and transportation of cultures and specimens. Any staff member sending a specimen to a laboratory must ensure that the transporter knows where and to whom the specimen is to be delivered (8, p. 189).

To prevent the potential spread of diseases, strict adherence to recommended safety practices when handling or processing laboratory specimens is required. Guidelines may be individually customized to meet the requirements of a specific laboratory. It is the responsibility of the employer, the laboratory director, and the HCWs to maintain a safe working environment at all times regardless of the anticipated risks (7, p. 24).

SPECIAL PRECAUTIONS FOR CREUTZFELDT-JAKOB DISEASE

Special handling is required for brain, cornea, cerebral spinal fluid, lymph node, and tonsil specimens that are suspected or confirmed to be infected with Creutzfeldt-Jakob disease (CJD).

- CJD is particularly virulent, and the prions are resistant to destruction by heat, chemicals, radiation, freezing, drying, and organic detergents (5, p. 214; 10, p. 951).
- PPE (gloves, eyewear, face mask, and impervious gown) should be worn to handle infected items (2, p. 13; 10, p. 956).
- Strict handwashing procedures should be followed (2, p. 13).
- Each specimen should be placed in an impervious plastic bag and labeled "suspected CJD." This bag should be placed in a clean secondary container also labeled "suspected CJD" (2, p. 13; 10, p. 956).
- Specimens should not be placed in formaldehyde. Pre-fixing will not render the specimen noninfectious (2, p. 13).
- Laboratory personnel should be notified before transporting the specimen to the laboratory (2, p. 13).
- The laboratory should use a formic acid-formalin procedure when processing specimens. Agency policy should be followed (10, p. 956).
- In the event of percutaneous exposure, the skin should be rinsed with 1 M (molar) sodium hydroxide for several minutes, then washed with soap and water. If the exposure was via mucous membrane, the area should be irrigated thoroughly with sterile saline or water for several minutes (10, p. 957).
- If eye exposure has occurred, the HCW should contact an ophthalmologist immediately. Sodium hydroxide is *not used* to decontaminate eyes (2, p. 14).
- For any exposure, the HCW should immediately contact the occupational health department for follow-up (2, p. 14; 10, p. 957).

References

1. AORN: Recommended practices for standard and transmission-based precautions in the perioperative practice setting. In *Standards, recommended practices and guidelines,* Denver, 2000, Author, pp 335-340.
2. Canola T, Becker L, Padilla S: Creutzfeldt-Jakob disease precautions, *Infection Control and Sterilization Technology* 4(7):12-14, 1998.

3. Fairchild SS: *Perioperative nursing: principles and practice,* Boston, 1996, Little, Brown.

4. Fogg D: Clinical issues, *AORN J* 71(2):401, 2000.

5. Fortunato N: *Berry & Kohn's operating room technique,* ed 9, St Louis, 2000, Mosby.

6. Gruendemann BJ, Fernsebner B: *Comprehensive perioperative nursing,* vol 1, *Principles,* Boston, 1995, Jones & Bartlett.

7. Hart PD: Occupational acquisition of infectious agents in the clinical laboratory, *Infection Control and Sterilization Technology* 4(12):14-24, 1999.

8. Hendricks S: Handling cultures and specimens. In Phippen M, Wells MA, editors: *Patient care during operative and invasive procedures,* Philadelphia, 2000, WB Saunders, pp 183-190.

9. Jennings J, Manian FA: *APIC handbook of infection control and epidemiology,* ed 2, Washington, DC, 1999, Association for Professionals in Infection Control and Epidemiology.

10. Steelman VM: Prion diseases: an evidence-based protocol for infection control, *AORN J* 69(5):946-967, 1999.

11. Occupational Safety and Health Administration: OSHA regulations, Dec 6, 1991: occupational exposure to bloodborne pathogens—final rule, *Federal Register* 56(235):64175-64182, 1991.

Suggested Reading

1. Rosenberg RN et al: Precautions in handling tissues, fluids and other contaminated materials from patients with documented or suspected Creutzfeldt-Jakob disease, *Ann of Neurol* 19(1):75-77, 1986.

2. Steelman VM: Activity of sterilization processes and disinfectants against prions (Creutzfeldt-Jakob disease agent). In Rutala WA, editor: *Disinfection, sterilization and antisepsis in health care,* Washington, DC, 1997, Association for Professionals in Infection Control and Epidemiology.

P. Waste Management

Officials of every healthcare facility and every surgical setting are concerned about waste management (WM). Increasing numbers of regulations, environmental issues, and healthcare worker (HCW) protection concerns are contributing to the heightened awareness of the need to focus on and be proactive in the management of wastes.

Issues in medical WM today include conflicting definitions of medical and infectious waste; increased surveillance of practices; mind-boggling local, state, and federal regulations; and dilemmas over perception versus reality regarding what is and what is not infectious waste.

WM is more than simple waste handling. It includes an overall assessment of wastes generated, analyses of how the waste stream itself can be minimized at points of generation, which wastes can be segregated properly, which wastes can be efficiently and safely recycled, and how disposal of wastes can be streamlined and made more cost effective.

A WM plan should be in place in every healthcare institution. The plan should be implemented by authorized personnel who can clearly focus on the total waste stream, both its segregation and disposal. A WM team consisting of those intimately involved with the most im-

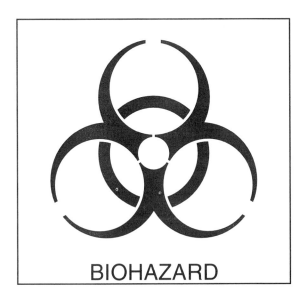

BIOHAZARD

portant aspects of the WM process should coordinate policies and procedures and be accountable for the outcomes of the plan and its goal. The following departments should be represented on the WM team:

- Environmental Services
- Infection Control/Epidemiology/Employee Health (including personnel with expertise on regulations)
- Risk Management/Safety
- Engineering
- Materials Management
- Nursing Services
- Quality Improvement
- Public Relations
- Administration

This chapter will discuss the background of WM issues, definitions of various types of waste, statements of several professional organizations and regulatory agencies, waste minimization and segregation, and technology options for treatment and disposal of waste.

BACKGROUND

The East Coast beach wash-ups of 1987-1988 triggered much of the furor of the past decade regarding waste. Wash-ups that were thought to be waste from healthcare facilities later were determined to be from commercial and military boats and to consist of drug user paraphernalia, discarded home care materials, and illegal intravenous drug supplies. In fact, the vast majority (99%) of waste on beaches has been determined to be debris such as plastic, glass, and paper, not medical waste (MW) (7, p. 35).

The AIDS epidemic has increased the focus on waste from healthcare facilities by prompting a change in thinking, emphasizing barrier protection for both patients and HCWs, and renewing the emphasis on blood, blood products, and bloodborne diseases. This epidemic has substantially increased public awareness of the potentially hazardous nature of exposure to blood, blood products, needles, and other sharps, but it has also spurred fear and irrationality, heightened media attention, and caused a rush to judgment on related voluntary and regulatory matters (7, p. 35).

Public perceptions prompted the U.S. Environmental Protection Agency (EPA) to establish the Medical Waste Tracking Act (MWTA) of 1988, establishing demonstration projects to regulate and track medical waste in four states and Puerto Rico. The MWTA project, which ended in June 1991, is only one example of overreaction to the issue of proper WM. The MWTA defined MW more broadly than necessary, resulting in disposal costs that were well beyond the original and realistic estimates. Even though short lived, the MWTA prompted state legislatures to enact a myriad of rules, some of which have been refined over the years and are based on sound scientific studies of waste. However, other rules enacted were primarily based on common perceptions and the public's fears about waste, landfills, and emissions. Some of this nonfactual information is still a part of the public consciousness, especially the information regarding the public health consequences of MW (7, pp. 35-36).

Because of intense and often misleading media coverage of this issue (e.g., the MWTA and the associated demonstration projects) and a lack of understanding of disease transmission, the states and the federal government have created strict regulations, which defined an increased amount of waste as infectious. To complicate matters further, some waste treatment options such as landfilling have been eliminated, and others such as incineration may be eliminated. The result is an extraordinary increase in cost with little environmental or public health benefit. The MW policies that have evolved from perceived risks over the past few years should be supplanted by rules based on scientific considerations (13, p. 581).

The MWTA demonstration projects produced no evidence of a public health need to create paper trails to track MW transported to off-site treatment or disposal facilities. Nevertheless, many states have established "cradle-to-grave" MW tracking requirements (3, p. 11).

The public perception of the potential hazards associated with MW has been one of fear that members of the public might become infected as a result of exposure to stray MW. Even though no scientific evidence of disease transmission from such exposure has been demonstrated, public perception of the dangers of exposure has driven regulatory responses (10, p. 727).

Over the years, there has been a growing concern over the volume of air pollutants released from numerous categories of emission sources. Title III of the Clean Air Act Amendments of 1990 (CAAA) instructed the EPA to protect public health by reducing emissions of hazardous air pollutants from the sources that release them. The CAAA singled out waste incineration for special attention. The EPA was directed to develop regulations for four categories of solid waste incinerators. Because some of this incineration included small amounts of hospital waste and/or medical/infectious waste, the EPA Final Rule of 1997 focused on incinerators whose primary purpose is the disposal of hospital waste and/or medical/infectious waste in an effort to avoid duplicative requirements. The U.S. EPA Final Rule ("Final Rule") regulating Hospital/Medical/Infectious Waste Incinerators (HMIWIs) became law in 1997 (7, pp. 6-7).

The EPA's goal in developing the Final Rule was the improvement of air quality and health through the reduction of air pollution from HMIWIs. One result of the regulation will likely be, out of necessity, a switch to alternative waste disposal methods for those incinerators that do not meet the emission standards. Because of the cost of retro-fitting existing systems with add-on pollution control systems, an estimated 50% to 80% of the existing incinerators will close. The Rule applies to incinerators used by hospitals and other healthcare facilities, as well as to incinerators used by commercial waste disposal companies that burn hospital and/or medical/infectious waste. The EPA estimates that there are approximately 2,400 of these facilities operating incinerators in the United States. Fewer than one half of U.S. hospitals operate their own incinerators, but in addition to this number are the 21,000 nursing homes and 4,200 commercial research laboratories operating in the United States, some of which may operate incinerators (7, pp. 6-8).

The 1997 Final Rule is only the beginning, a first phase, of a total regulatory analysis geared to the reduction of air pollution caused by all forms of incineration. Some wastes that are now excluded in this Rule (pathological, chemotherapeutic, low-level radioactive wastes) may not remain excluded in the future (7, pp. 2, 6-7).

The EPA estimates that the Final Rule will result in a reduction of at least 90% of mercury, particulate matter, hydrogen chloride, and dioxin/furan emissions in MW incinerators. To accomplish this, the Rule is expected to have a dramatic impact on MW disposal practices in the United States (3, p. 12). Personnel working in surgical settings should be familiar with the EPA Final Rule because it is the driving force behind many changes in WM and treatment today. The Rule is complex and comprehensive. It contains performance criteria, training and monitoring requirements, and very detailed guidelines for existing, new, and modified HMIWIs. State plans and regulations play a substantial role in the promulgation of this Rule. (See reference 14 for more details on the Final Rule.)

DEFINITIONS AND DISCUSSIONS

A healthcare facility must have a clear definition of regulated medical waste (RMW), also known as infectious waste, to create a WM plan. Since definitions for RMW are at variance, it behooves healthcare officials to create a definition for their facility, taking under consideration the local, state, and federal regulations with which the facility must comply. Many states have rules for MW that are very restrictive and define RMW too broadly, resulting in "over–red-bagging" that stems from the false belief that all patient-contact waste must be treated as infectious waste (7, p. 39).

Following are a number of definitions of RMW with accompanying discussions. These definitions are commonly part of an organization or agency position statement or regulation. The reader is urged to consult the references for the background information that led each of these groups and/or experts to formulate their respective definitions and positions.

- Despite the attention given to medical waste issues in the past decade or so, the terms *hospital waste, medical waste (MW), regulated medical waste (RMW),* and *infectious waste* are often thought to be synonymous. This is not true. Medical waste is a category of hospital waste; infectious waste, which is synonymous with regulated medical waste, is a category of medical waste.
  - *Hospital waste* refers to all waste, biologic or nonbiologic, that is discarded and not intended for further use in a hospital or other healthcare facility. Examples of hospital waste are paper, cardboard boxes, and food.
  - *Medical waste* is material generated as a result of the diagnosis or treatment of a patient, such as soiled dressings or intravenous tubing. Other examples of MW are disposable packaging of patient supplies and RMW.
  - *Infectious waste,* sometimes referred to as *red-bag waste* or *biohazardous waste,* is that portion of MW that might potentially transmit an infectious disease. Examples of infectious waste are contaminated sharps, microbiological stocks, and cultures of infectious agents.
  - *Regulated medical waste* is a term that has been used by Congress and the EPA in place of infectious waste because the possibility of transmission of disease by such waste is remote.
  Approximately 2% of the total solid (municipal) waste in the United States is hospital waste. About 0.3% of that solid waste (about 10% to 15% of hospital waste) can be classified as RMW or infectious waste (13, p. 579; 7, pp. 38-39).
- Besides hospitals, many types of healthcare facilities generate MW: physician, dental, and veterinary offices; neighborhood medical clinics; outpatient centers; long-term care institutions; funeral homes; and freestanding laboratories and blood banks. Each generates its own form of MW (7, p. 37).
- A uniform definition of what constitutes RMW has not been universally adopted. Factors that should be considered when deciding if something is RMW include the presence of pathogenic organisms in sufficient numbers to be capable of causing infection in living beings (many microorganisms are incapable

of causing infection) and the presence of a portal of entry into a susceptible host. A cut, needlestick, puncture wound, or skin lesion can provide this portal of entry (5, p. 197).

- The EPA defines *infectious waste* as waste capable of causing an infectious disease. This RMW must contain pathogens with enough virulence and quantity that exposure to them could result in an infectious disease in a susceptible host (14; 5, p. 197).

- The CDC defines *infectious waste* as waste that represents a sufficient potential risk of causing infection during handling and disposal and for which special precautions appear prudent. Four categories of infectious waste are:
  1. Microbiological cultures/stocks
  2. Pathological waste
  3. Human blood and blood products
  4. Used sharps

  Studies analyzing the microbial content of household waste versus that generated in a healthcare setting have consistently shown that municipal waste is more microbiologically contaminated than MW—in some cases 100 times more pathogenic. Thus there is no epidemiological evidence to suggest that most hospital waste is any more infectious than residential waste. Moreover, there is no epidemiological evidence that current hospital waste disposal practices have caused disease in the community. Therefore identifying wastes for which special precautions are necessary is largely a matter of judgment about the relative risk of disease transmission. Special precautions need to be taken with wastes in the four categories of infectious waste. In general, these wastes should be either incinerated or decontaminated before disposal in a sanitary landfill. Bulk blood, suctioned fluids, excretions, and secretions may be carefully poured down a drain connected to a sanitary sewer (check state regulations). Sanitary sewers may also be used to dispose of other potentially infectious wastes that can be ground and flushed into the sewer (6; 4; 7, pp. 37, 40; 9, p. 638). (NOTE: Liquid contaminated waste should not be poured into scrub sinks in the operating room [OR].)

- The OSHA Bloodborne Pathogen Final Rule designates certain types of MW as RMW:
  1. Liquid or semiliquid blood or other potentially infectious materials (OPIM); contaminated items that would release blood or OPIM in a liquid or semiliquid state if compressed; items that are caked with dried blood or OPIM and are capable of releasing these materials during handling

2. Contaminated sharps
3. Pathologicals
4. Microbiological wastes containing blood or OPIM (11)

- The Association of Professionals in Infection Control and Epidemiology (APIC) supports the definition of RMW put forth by the Agency for Toxic Substances and Disease Registry (ATSDR), an agency within the CDC, as the standard definition of RMW. According to the ATSDR:
  - From a public health standpoint, RMW should include the following categories: cultures and stocks, pathological waste, sharps, animal waste, selected isolation waste, and unused discarded sharps.
  - The health of the general public is not likely to be adversely affected by MW generated in the traditional healthcare setting (3, p. 11).
- The Society of Healthcare Epidemiology of America (SHEA) states that, based on epidemiological and microbiological data, only two types of MW would require special handling and treatment: sharps and microbiological waste (12; 7, p. 40).
- The Association of periOperative Registered Nurses (AORN) defines *RMW* in accordance with the 1991 OSHA bloodborne Pathogen Rule. The AORN document then lists four categories of RMW that should be included because of the risk to public health and the environment:
  1. Sharps, used and unused (includes needles, syringes with attached needles, trocars, pipettes, scalpel blades, blood vials, and broken or unbroken glassware that has been in contact with infectious agents)
  2. Cultures and stocks of infectious agents (includes wastes from the production of biologicals; discarded live and attenuated vaccines; and culture dishes and devices used to transfer, inoculate, and mix cultures of infectious agents)
  3. Animal waste (includes carcasses, body parts, blood, and bedding of animals known to have been in contact with infectious agents)
  4. Selected isolation waste (includes waste and discarded materials contaminated with blood, excretions, exudates, or secretions from humans or animals who are isolated to protect others from certain highly virulent diseases)

Two other categories of MW are included in the AORN document only because of the aesthetic concerns of the public, not because of public health risks: (1) pathological waste and

(2) human blood, blood products, and body fluids (1; 7, pp. 42-43).

- The Joint Commission on Accreditation of Healthcare Organizations (JCAHO) does not define *RMW* in its accreditation manual, but it does give directives for a waste management plan (7, p. 42).
- It is important to make a distinction between *contaminated* and *infectious* (pertaining to waste), even though some documents consider the terms synonymous. In an OR or other surgical setting where sterile technique is used, the word *contaminated* refers to items that are no longer sterile. An instrument set used during surgery is contaminated. If the set is opened for a surgical procedure and not used, it is still considered contaminated, regardless of whether it harbors infectious waste (7, p. 21).
- In regulatory parlance, the word *contaminated* refers to an object that has been in contact with an infectious agent, as in contaminated sharps. In the OSHA Bloodborne Pathogen Rule, *contaminated* is defined as "the presence or the reasonably anticipated presence of blood or other potentially infectious materials on an item or surface." It is important that staff recognize the two uses of the word *contaminated* and not consider, for example, items simply opened for sterile procedures as infectious or RMW. Many healthcare facilities use "red bags" excessively and thus incur extra costs, mainly because the meaning of the word *contaminated* is misunderstood (7, p. 21).

WASTE MINIMIZATION
Segregation and Disposal

- The definition that officials at each facility use for RMW will determine the exact nature of the policy that dictates red bag contents. Federal, state, and local regulations, as inherent parts of policies and procedures, must be carefully observed. A review of the professional literature, as well as an assessment of aesthetic considerations and community concerns, is necessary to ensure that good and appropriate information is used to determine what is and what is not RMW (7, p. 20).
- The disposal of RMW is at least 8 to 10 times more costly than the disposal of noninfectious waste; therefore it is important that only authentic RMW be placed in red bags or other approved or appropriate bags or containers. Many institutions have identified correct segregation processes as prime factors in immediate and visible cost reductions. Waste segregation undergirds most WM efforts (7, p. 20).

- Infectious waste (RMW) should be segregated from noninfectious waste in the general waste stream. Color-coded, labeled bags should be used to visually segregate infectious waste from noninfectious waste. Segregating waste at the point of generation reduces volume, cost, and the risk of unnecessary personnel exposure. Personal protective equipment (PPE) should be used when handling blood, body fluids, or other hazardous materials (2, p. 263).
- Fluid containers with blood, body fluids, and other hazardous wastes should be handled with extreme care. Fluid containers should be impermeable to moisture; resistant to puncture, rupture, or tears; and sealed for transport to prevent leakage (2, p. 263). NOTE: Solidification systems are available for liquid WM. Caution should be used in choosing these systems because some contain chemicals that are inappropriate for landfill or incineration. Also, some of the chemicals may cause airway reactions when used. For more information on liquid waste disposal, the reader is referred to the section on microencapsulation in this chapter.
- The following are general guidelines for setting up an appropriate waste segregation program:
  - Employees should be educated on the rationale for waste segregation.
  - Facility-specific goals and outcomes, such as the percentage reduction in RMW expected in the first year, should be established.
  - Facility-wide protocols should be established. (It may be helpful to document via videotape or photographs all protocols for 3 months. This documentation could then be used to educate employees in sessions that would also include safe handling and disposal of MW and the use of PPE.)
  - Receptacles for RMW and noninfectious waste should be easy to recognize and placed in convenient locations.
  - Receptacles and bags for RMW should be leak proof, puncture proof, and tear proof. Bags should be identified by color and/or the universal biohazard symbol.
  - Because the majority of facility waste is noninfectious (solid municipal waste), general waste containers should be the most plentiful and accessible containers (7, p. 20).

Source Reduction and Single-Use Versus Reusable Products

- One of the simplest methods for reducing the environmental impact of performing surgical procedures is to use fewer supplies.

The following guidelines may be helpful:

- Open only supplies that are routinely used when preparing the sterile field for a procedure. Supplies that *may* be needed should be readily available but should remain unopened until either they are requested or it is obvious that they will be used.
- Consider using custom sterile packs and sterilization containers, which can reduce the amount of packaging material generated during a procedure (8, p. 298).

- APIC agrees that one of the most effective methods of managing MW is to reduce the volume of waste generated and recommends that each healthcare provider evaluate its system for waste reduction opportunities (3, p. 12).
- Many single-use (disposable) products were developed out of a demonstrated patient care or infection control need. The following factors should be considered during product selection when choosing between single-use and reusable products:
  - Cost
  - Ease of delivery
  - Convenience
  - Quality
  - Comfort
  - Amount of waste generated
  - Environmental impact
  - Laundering costs
  - Labor costs
  - Inventory control

  For example, nonwoven, single-use drapes and gowns generate a significant amount of waste; however, the laundering and storage of reusable products can add to the environmental impact and affect inventory management. Thus there are pros and cons to the use of both reusable and single-use products, and the decision-making process is often difficult. A product selection committee can bring relevant, scientific information to the discussion (8, p. 298).
- The decision to purchase single-use or reusable products can be difficult for healthcare facilities that are trying to reduce both disposal costs and high labor costs related to the reprocessing of reusable products. When evaluating product performance, comfort, and cost, consideration should be given to the availability of resources and specific environmental issues in the geographic location of the healthcare facility (e.g., clean water supply availability and limitations on disposal of solid waste) (2, p. 262). NOTE: Choosing reusables versus disposables is discussed in the chapter "Gowning."

Recycling

- Recycling helps save natural resources. Many items and materials can be recycled in a healthcare facility. A number of communities and municipalities have mandatory recycling codes for certain items. Recycling efforts in a surgical setting should start small, perhaps with easy-to-segregate items such as office paper, cardboard, newspapers, aluminum cans, and solution bottles. Depending on the success of each effort, other items can be added to the list—plastics, glass, and fluorescent bulbs, for example (7, pp. 21-22).

- Many surgical supplies can be recycled. Recycling reduces air pollution, the amount of waste in landfills, and the amount of virgin resources that are consumed. Wrappers and many plastic items that are noninfectious, nonregulated trash can and should be recycled. Recycling in the surgical setting should be an integral part of the overall recycling program of a facility (5, p. 179).

- Healthcare facilities may encounter difficulties in recycling because of a perception that anything that comes from a healthcare facility, especially a hospital, is biohazardous or harmful. Recycling vendors may be cautious about accepting "hospital by-products" or items that have come in contact with patients. Also, healthcare facilities may not have sufficient quantities of recyclable items to make the effort worthwhile. Depending on the items, hospitals may have to pay for recyclable materials to be hauled away. Nevertheless, in spite of the need for education to dispel misperceptions, a hospital recycling program can be very successful and can promote a high level of satisfaction among surgical personnel. Donating clean, opened but unused items to charitable organizations and third-world healthcare foundations is a different yet worthwhile form of recycling (7, pp. 21-22).

WASTE TREATMENT OPTIONS

- According to AORN, the methods usually employed to decontaminate MW (for the four categories that pose some public health risk) are:
  - Heat treatment (incineration, autoclaving, microwaving, pyrolysis)
  - Chemical treatment (hypochlorite, chlorine dioxide)
  - Radiation treatment (gamma ray, electron beam)

  The efficacy and efficiency of each method depends on factors such as contact time, bioload, organic content and volume, and the physical state of the waste (e.g., liquid or solid). The presence of other waste products (e.g., radioisotopes, hazardous chemicals) also must be taken into account when determining the proper method of waste treatment (1, pp. 147-148).

• APIC encourages the design of new and efficient technologies for RMW treatment and disposal in which incineration may not be the preferred treatment method. New treatment technologies must effectively disinfect MW with minimal negative impact on the environment. Alternative treatment methods include dry heat, electrothermal deactivation, infrared, ultraviolet radiation, microwaving, chemical disinfection, and pyrolysis (3, p. 12).

• Each healthcare facility and surgical setting must carefully evaluate the various treatment options and determine the usefulness and value that fits the particular situation and setting. The evaluation must include federal, state, and local regulations and issues such as safety, effectiveness, efficiency, and cost. Certain factors must be considered before selecting alternative on-site and off-site processes:
  • Existing processes and equipment
  • The "fit" between wastes generated and capability of equipment being considered
  • Space, energy, and personnel requirements
  • Regulatory, quality management, and certification compliance
  • Maintenance, parts, and supplies needed; guarantees
  • Customer service, support, and training needed
  • Personnel and expertise available on-site as compared with off-site, with company and system being considered
  • Contingency plan in case of breakdown
  • Recommendations/advice of other facilities that are currently using/chose not to use a particular technology or process (7, p. 32)

• Management options for MW treatment and disposal include on-site treatment, off-site treatment and disposal, or a combination of both. On-site treatment is usually more convenient and controllable than off-site treatment; however, off-site treatment can allow more alternatives, cause less hassle to the institution, and address community concerns regarding waste disposal (7, p. 33). Mobile waste treatment systems are also available.

• Classic methods of MW disposal are:
  • *Landfill:* consignment to a sanitary landfill or other community waste disposal mechanism
  • *Sewer:* discharge into the sanitary sewer system (designed to treat biological wastes such as blood and body fluids)
  • *Autoclaving:* on-site steam sterilization or disinfection, rendering the waste noninfectious before disposal

- *Incineration:* combustion of waste materials
- *Transport:* transportation by a licensed hauler for off-site storage, treatment, or disposal (7, p. 33)
- The six categories of technologies for MW treatment and management are:
  1. *Mechanical:* Processes such as shredding and compacting are not, by themselves, sufficient to allow adequate treatment; subsequent treatment is needed to render the waste noninfectious. These methods allow for efficient treatment by first reducing size and volume of the waste.
  2. *Thermal:* Now the most commonly used modalities, these processes use heat to destroy microorganisms. The most common processes are incineration and autoclaving, but other technologies are available.
     - *Incineration:* The use of high-temperature combustion to destroy waste. Reduces weight and volume by as much as 95%. Preferred method for pathological waste.
     - *Autoclaving:* High-temperature steam under pressure that contacts waste and destroys pathogens. Gravity displacement is the preferred conventional autoclaving method. Heat distribution throughout the load may be a problem in some devices.
     - *Microwaving:* The use of microwave radiation that decontaminates by heat generated within the waste; usually involves shredding, moistening with steam, and then heating to reach disinfection temperatures.
     - *Thermal oxidation:* Uses high-temperature thermal dynamics to reduce waste volume and weight by up to 98%, guaranteeing complete sterilization. Waste is first prepared by a pretreatment system that reduces it to small particles and combines it to create a homogeneous mixture for the primary combustion chamber. In a secondary chamber, combustion vapors are mixed with additional oxygen and the temperature is raised to as high as 2200° F, ensuring complete oxidation of all particulate matter.
     - *Electrothermal deactivation:* Shredded waste is deactivated and heated by exposure to low-frequency radio waves; the material is reduced to an unrecognizable form.
     - *Pyrolysis:* A thermochemical conversion of waste that includes gasification, liquefaction, and thermal decomposition in the process, without using oxygen.
     - *Laser treatment:* Delivery of energy that rapidly vaporizes organic material.

- *Other:* Gas/vapor/plasma sterilization, dry heat, dry thermal inactivation, infrared treatment.

3. *Chemical:* In this process, disinfectants are used to destroy harmful microorganisms. The process is often accompanied by mechanical destruction or grinding for reduction to small particle size, and disfigurement. Waste can be shredded in the presence of a disinfectant solution under negative pressure. The most commonly used chemicals are chlorine, hypochlorites, chlorine derivatives, peracetic acid, and ozone. In some chemical processes the waste can be disposed of into the general waste stream after it has been disinfected and rendered unrecognizable. This process is most suited to wastes that are easily penetrable. Chemical treatment of suction canister contents is available. This method is also convenient for small quantities of waste.

4. *Irradiation:* These systems use electromagnetic or ionizing radiation to treat and sterilize MW. Radiation dosages can be calculated with great reliability, which makes the process highly predictable. The efficacy of gamma radiation is well documented. Irradiated waste looks identical to the pretreatment waste, although a secondary destructive process (e.g., grinding, shredding) can be added. This treated waste has no residual radiation.
   - *Ultraviolet:* Seldom used for MW.
   - *Cobalt 60:* Gamma rays are discharged by radioactive cobalt.
   - *Electron beam:* Irradiation through an accelerated, concentrated electron stream that kills microorganisms.
   - *Electrothermal radiation:* A process that shreds and disinfects with long-frequency radiation.

5. *Biologicals:* Although not widely used, some processes are available that add biological enzymes to the waste in order to destroy all organic constitutes. In the process, the waste is ground into a liquid slurry mixture and then treated with chemicals/enzymes.

6. *Other:* A few technologies are available:
   - *Microencapsulation:* A liquid treatment system at the point of generation; converts liquid waste into treated solid MW. A catalyst is added to decontaminate and gel the contents of sharps containers and suction receptacles that contain blood and fluids (both body and irrigation). A dissolvable pouch for preloading or after treatment dissolves and disperses powder uniformly. (This is not an approved process in all states.)

- *Conversion into waste blocks:* An on-site disposal system that transforms contaminated needles, blood-stained sharps, and soiled razors, for example, into harmless "bricks" of solid waste. The waste is decontaminated and the volume reduced by about 80% (7, pp. 33-35).

- Various technologies used to process MW are often combined for more effective results. Examples are chemical/mechanical, grinding/irradiation, and compacting/autoclaving processes. Newer systems may also be available as smaller units to facilitate waste treatment as close to the site of generation as possible, particularly in small surgical settings (7, p. 35).

As waste treatment options continue to increase, healthcare facility leaders will develop criteria to accurately assess needs and specifications for their particular types and amounts of waste. Cost effectiveness, convenience, and collaborative negotiations will be part of the contract considerations as WM planners continue to evaluate goals and outcomes (7, p. 35).

References

1. AORN Position Statement: Regulated medical waste definition and treatment: a collaborative document. In *Standards, recommended practices and guidelines,* Denver, 2000, Author, pp 145-148.
2. AORN: Recommended practices for environmental responsibility. In *Standards, recommended practices and guidelines,* Denver, 2000, Author, pp 261-265.
3. APIC Position Statement (revised): Infection control implications associated with medical waste, *APIC News* 18(6):11-12, 1998.
4. Centers for Disease Control and Prevention: Infectious waste, 1997, www.cdc.gov/ncidod/diseases/hip/waste.htm (accessed 2000).
5. Fortunato N: *Berry & Kohn's operating room technique,* ed 9, St Louis, 2000, Mosby.
6. Garner JS, Favero MS: *Infective waste: guideline for handwashing and hospital environmental control,* Atlanta, 1985, Centers for Disease Control and Prevention.
7. Gruendemann BJ: *Healthcare waste management, a template for action,* Cary, NC, 1999, INDA.
8. Gruendemann BJ, Fernsebner B: *Comprehensive perioperative nursing,* vol 1, *Principles,* Boston, 1995, Jones & Bartlett.
9. Keene JH: Medical waste: a minimal hazard, *Infect Control Hosp Epidemiol* 12(11):682-685, 1991.
10. Keene JH: Regulated medical waste. In Abrutyn E, Goldmann DA, Scheckler WE, editors: *Saunders infection control reference service,* Philadelphia, 1998, WB Saunders, pp 727-730.
11. Occupational Safety and Health Administration: Occupational exposure to bloodborne pathogens: final rule, *Federal Register* 56(235):64175-64182, December 6, 1991.
12. Rutala WA, Mayhall CG, SHEA (The Society for Healthcare Epidemiology of America) Position Paper: Medical waste, *Infect Control Hosp Epidemiol* 13(1):38-48, 1992.

13. Rutala WA, Weber DJ: Infectious waste: mismatch between science and policy, *N Engl J Med* 325(8):578-581, 1991.
14. U.S. Environmental Protection Agency (EPA): Standards of performance for new stationary sources and emission guidelines for existing sources: hospital/medical/infectious waste incinerators—Final Rule 40 CFR, Part 60, *Federal Register* pp 48347-48391, September 15, 1997. Online: www.epa.gov/ttn/uatw/129/hmiwi/rihmiwi.html

Suggested Reading

1. Agency for Toxic Substances & Disease Registry (ATSDR): *The public health implications of medical waste: a report to Congress,* Atlanta, 1990, ATSDR, Centers for Disease Control and Prevention, U.S. Department of Health and Human Services.
2. Doucet LG: The prognosis for medical waste incinerators, *Surgical Services Management* 5(2):39-48, 1999.
3. Garcia R: Effective cost-reduction strategies in the management of regulated medical waste, *Am J Infect Control* 27(2):165-175, 1999.
4. Glenn J: The state of garbage in America, *BioCycle* Part I, pp 32-43, April 1998; Part II, pp 48-52, May 1998.
5. Hedrick ER: Infectious waste management—will science prevail? *Infect Control Hosp Epidemiol* 9(11):488-490, 1988.
6. Jager E, Xander L, Ruden H: Hospital wastes: microbiological investigations of hospital wastes from various wards of a big and of smaller hospital in comparison to household refuse, *Zbl Hyg Umweltmed* 188:343-364, 1989.
7. Johnson & Johnson Medical: *In the bag: waste management in the OR,* Arlington, Tex, 1996, Author (videotape and study guide).
8. McGurk J: Preparing for future medical waste management challenges: lessons gleaned from implementing California's Medical Waste Management Act, *Infection Control Today* 2(10):26, 28, 32, 1998.
9. Pugliese G, Favero MS: Medical news: TB transmission from medical waste, *Infect Control Hosp Epidemiol* 19(5):370-371, 1998.
10. Rutala WA, Odette RL, Samsa GP: Management of infectious waste by U.S. hospitals, *JAMA* 262(12):1635-1640, 1989.
11. Shaner H: *Becoming a mercury free facility: a priority to be achieved by the year 2000,* Chicago, 1997, American Society for Healthcare Environmental Services, American Hospital Association.
12. Shaner H, McRae G: *Managing wastes in merger conditions: optimizing systems,* Chicago, 1995, American Society for Healthcare Environmental Services, American Hospital Association.
13. Spitzley J: We all win with single barrier packaging, *Surgical Services Management* 4(5):36-40, 1998.

5

Special Considerations

A. Standard Precautions

Because of its importance, the Centers for Disease Control and Prevention (CDC) document, "Guideline for Isolation Precautions in Hospitals," is reprinted, in part, in Appendix A. Commonly known as *Standard Precautions (SP)*, the guidelines in this document, as well as the guidelines for Airborne, Droplet, and Contact Precautions (labeled as *Transmission-Based Precautions*), have applicability for the care of patients in surgical settings.

Transmission-Based Precautions, in addition to SP, are to be used in situations in which patients are either known or suspected to be infected with highly transmissible pathogens known to contribute to nosocomial infection (3, pp. 60-65).

STANDARD PRECAUTIONS

Topics covered in the SP document include the following that apply to surgical settings:

- Gowns and protective apparel
- Masks, respiratory protection, eye protection, and face shields
- Handwashing and gloving
- Linen and laundry
- Transport of infected patients
- Patient care equipment and articles
- Routine and terminal cleaning (3, pp. 60-65)

SP synthesize the major features of Universal Precautions (UP)—Blood and Body Fluid Precautions, designed to reduce the risk of transmission of bloodborne pathogens, and Body Substance Isolation (BSI), designed to reduce the transmission of pathogens from moist body substances—and apply them to *all patients* receiving care in hospitals, regardless of their diagnosis or presumed infection status (3, p. 64).

SP apply to blood; all other body fluids, secretions, and excretions (except sweat), regardless of whether they contain visible blood; nonintact skin; and mucous membranes. SP are designed to reduce the risk of transmission of microorganisms from both recognized and unrecognized sources of infection in hospitals (3, p. 64).

SP were devised because of the confusion that arose with the use and interpretation of previous approaches such as UP, BSI, and the CDC isolation guidelines. SP are a synthesis of these various systems, intended to provide guidelines with logistically reasonable recommendations for preventing the many infections that occur in hospitals through diverse modes of transmission. In addition, SP address the problems of emerging multidrug-resistant microorganisms and offer appropriate precautions for containment (3, p. 59).

TRANSMISSION-BASED PRECAUTIONS

SP apply to all patients. Transmission-Based Precautions, the second tier of guidelines, are designed only for the care of specified patients, those documented or suspected to be infected or colonized with highly transmissible or epidemiologically significant pathogens for which *additional precautions beyond SP* are needed to interrupt transmission in hospitals. When used singularly or in combination, the Transmission-Based Precautions are to be used *in addition to* SP. Implementation of SP is the primary strategy for successful nosocomial infection control (3, p. 55).

Airborne Precautions

Airborne Precautions are used with patients who have tuberculosis (TB), measles, or varicella (chicken pox)—diseases that are spread by airborne droplet nuclei 5 μ or smaller. Recommendations for Airborne Precautions that are of special interest to surgical personnel include the following:

- Placing a surgical mask on a patient during transport
- Wearing respiratory protection when entering the room of a patient with pulmonary TB
- Keeping the door to the room of a patient closed
- Having appropriate discharge or filtration of air in negative-pressure patient rooms (3, pp. 69-70)

NOTE: Operating rooms (ORs) are positive-pressure rooms. If a TB patient must undergo a surgical procedure, the OR may have to remain vacant for a time after surgery to allow for appropriate ventilation air changes. More information on this topic is included in the chapter "Tuberculosis."

Droplet Precautions

Droplet Precautions are used with patients undergoing bronchoscopy who are known or suspected to have respiratory illnesses transmitted by large particle droplets, larger than 5 μ. These precautions are also used with patients who have influenza, pneumonia, diphtheria, pertussis, mumps, rubella, certain types of meningitis, or streptococcal pharyngitis. Recommendations for Droplet Precautions include wearing a mask when working within 3 feet of the patient and masking the patient during transport to minimize dispersal of droplets (3, pp. 69-70).

Contact Precautions

Contact Precautions are used with patients who have the following: gastrointestinal or enteric infections such as hepatitis A, shigellosis, and those caused by *Escherichia coli* and *Clostridium difficile;* respiratory syncytial and parainfluenza viruses; skin infections such as herpes simplex, impetigo, and scabies; wound infections such as major abscesses, cellulitis, and decubiti; pediculosis; viral hemorrhagic infections; and colonization with multidrug-resistant bacteria (3, p. 66). Recommendations for Contact Precautions include the following:

- Wearing gloves when touching the patient
- Washing hands after removing gloves
- Gowning if clothing will have direct contact with the patient
- Dedicating equipment if possible
- Cleaning and disinfecting common equipment before use on another patient (3, pp. 69-70)

NOTE: The reader is urged to refer to the SP document for aspects of care in addition to the examples of Transmission-Based Precautions provided in this chapter.

WHY STANDARD PRECAUTIONS?

SP identify practices that can be employed to protect patients and healthcare workers from exposure to bloodborne and body fluid pathogens, which are primary potential sources for transmission of disease (1, p. 335).

In surgical settings, staff members have historically relied on UP to protect themselves and others from bloodborne infections. Little attention has been routinely given to protecting healthcare providers or other patients from non–human immunodeficiency virus or non–hepatitis B infectious diseases. Staff in surgical services should be knowledgeable in application criteria and in practicing both SP and the additional Transmission-Based Precautions (2).

References

1. AORN: Recommended practices for Standard and Transmission-Based Precautions in the perioperative practice setting. In *Standards, recommended practices and guidelines,* Denver, 2000, Author, pp 335-340.
2. AORN Online Clinical Practice FAQ Database, 1999: www.aorn.org/_results/clinical.asp (accessed 2000).
3. Garner JS, Hospital Infection Control Practices Advisory Committee (HICPAC), Centers for Disease Control and Prevention: Guideline for isolation precautions in hospitals, *Infect Control Hosp Epidemiol* 17(1):53-80, 1996. (Reprinted, in part, in Appendix A.)

B. Bloodborne Pathogens and Safety Issues

This chapter focuses on bloodborne pathogens and diseases, and the measures necessary to prevent transmission of these pathogens to either surgical personnel or patients.

The chapter begins with a brief review of two well-known bloodborne diseases, acquired immunodeficiency syndrome (AIDS) and hepatitis B virus (HBV), and a third bloodborne disease, hepatitis C virus (HCV), which has emerged as a major source of morbidity, mortality, and chronic liver disease. A table comparing and contrasting the forms of viral hepatitis follows.

The emphasis in the chapter is on practices in surgical settings that reduce or eliminate injury risk to personnel and patients from bloodborne pathogens. Safety is the foremost concern addressed.

Standard Precautions (SP), discussed in the chapter "Standard Precautions," and Universal Precautions (UP), discussed in this chapter, still form the basis for the care of patients with known or sus-

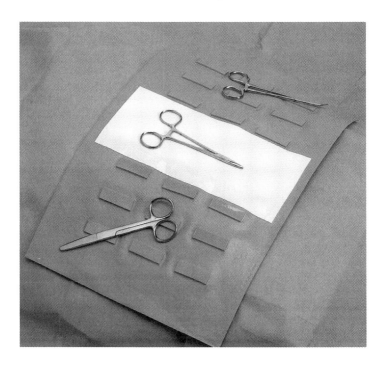

pected infections caused by bloodborne pathogens. UP are an integral part of the Occupational Safety and Health Administration (OSHA) regulation, "Occupational Exposure to Bloodborne Pathogens" (11) (also known as the OSHA Bloodborne Pathogen Rule). The discussion in this chapter includes supplementary measures that can be taken to enhance the care of patients with known or suspected infections caused by bloodborne pathogens and to reduce the risk of transmission of any pathogens.

BLOODBORNE DISEASES
Acquired Immunodeficiency Syndrome

The human immunodeficiency viruses, known collectively as human immunodeficiency virus (HIV), are ribonucleic acid (RNA) retroviruses. HIV will survive in blood and any body fluid that contains white blood cells, including semen; cervical and vaginal secretions; saliva; tears; cerebrospinal, synovial, pleural, pericardial, peritoneal, and amniotic fluids; and breast milk (2, p. 192). The primary routes of transmission are by direct contact with blood and blood products and through sexual intercourse. HIV may be transferred to the fetus by the blood of an infected mother or to the neonate via breast milk. *HIV is not transmitted by casual contact with an infected person.* In fact, the virus is relatively fragile and easily destroyed when it is outside of the body (2, p. 192).

As the acute stage of infection and the syndrome progress, and as the concentration of virus gradually increases, the patient becomes symptomatic for clinical manifestation of AIDS. AIDS is not a well-defined disease but rather a state of immune system dysfunction. Clinical diagnosis of AIDS requires a positive test for HIV antibodies and the presence of one of the specified opportunistic infections (2, p. 192).

Patients with known HIV infection or AIDS, or those who test positive for HIV antibodies but are asymptomatic, may come to a surgical setting for diagnostic or palliative procedures. In some cases HIV-infected patients may not be aware of their HIV status because either they have not been tested or they have not yet tested positive for HIV antibodies. Therefore it is important to regard *all* patients as potentially infectious (2, p. 193).

Most cases of occupational HIV have been contracted through the inadvertent injection of blood by deep hollow-bore needlesticks, not through superficial scratches. Although there is concern about the risk of HIV through mucous membrane exposure, this risk remains much lower than that posed by hollow-bore needles (8, p. 247). (See the chapter "Employee Health" for the Centers for Disease Control and Prevention [CDC] guidelines for post-exposure prophylaxis.)

Hepatitis B Virus

Formerly known as serum hepatitis, HBV is transmitted percutaneously or permucosally by blood, serum, and other body fluids. HBV is a major nosocomial problem for both patients and healthcare workers (HCWs). The average incubation period is 6 weeks, and mild to severe symptoms start to appear, on average, 60 days after exposure. Approximately 10% of infected patients become carriers, which are a main source of cross-infection. Chronic hepatitis, cirrhosis, or liver carcinoma may develop if HBV is left untreated (2, p. 191).

The HBV surface antigen is easily transmitted by direct contact with blood and body fluids by a needlestick or scalpel cut; by a break in the skin such as a minor cut or hangnail; or by a splash into the mucosa of the eye, nose, or mouth. HBV can also be transmitted via fomites (nonliving materials such as bed linen that may transmit microorganisms), sexual intercourse, and an infected mother to a neonate during birth (2, p. 191).

- HBV immunization is recommended for high-risk healthcare professionals and should be given before exposure. After exposure, such as following an accidental needlestick, both the vaccine and hepatitis B immune globulin may be given (see the chapter "Employee Health") (2, p. 191).
- All surgical and perioperative personnel should receive the hepatitis B vaccine because HBV presents a high risk of occupational disease to these professionals. The vaccine is both safe and cost effective (8, pp. 247-248).

Comparing Human Immunodeficiency Virus with Hepatitis B Virus

It was apparent at the beginning of the HIV epidemic that HBV and HIV have similar modes of transmission. This led many to erroneously believe that HIV and HBV are equally transmissible; however, this is not true (8, p. 247).

- The risk of transmission of HBV from a known hepatitis B surface antigen–positive person from a hollow-bore needlestick is between 27% and 43%, according to OSHA. The risk of occupational HIV infection from a hollow-bore needlestick from a known HIV-positive person is approximately 0.31%, or 1 in 310 needlesticks (8, p. 247; 11).
- In the United States the incidence of HBV in HCWs each year is between 10,000 and 18,000 reported cases, which results in 200 to 300 deaths and hundreds of cases of chronic liver disease, according to OSHA (8, p. 247; 11).

- Although the risk of being infected with HIV and acquiring AIDS is relatively low compared with that of HBV, it is not zero. Even for those who are only occasionally exposed to HIV through an accidental needlestick, scalpel wound, or splash to a mucous membrane, the risk is significant, no matter what the statistics say (8, p. 247).

Hepatitis C Virus

This silent killer is the most common chronic bloodborne infection in the United States. There is no vaccine for HCV (4, p. 1; 14, p. 229).

Many Americans (3.9 million) have chronic HCV, but most do not know it because the disease often has no detectable symptoms. Patients with HCV are at risk for developing chronic liver diseases for 2 or more decades following initial infection. Most HCV-infected persons are ages 20 to 39 years (4, pp. 1, 5).

Of persons with acute HCV infection, 60% to 70% are asymptomatic. Of those with symptoms, malaise may be the only symptom at first, followed possibly by loss of appetite and abdominal pain. However, some persons may experience jaundice. The overall lack of overt symptoms represents a risk to HCWs who do not follow SP when caring for all patients (5, p. 12).

The most extraordinary hallmark of HCV infection is its propensity to develop chronicity, with approximately 85% of the individuals demonstrating evidence of infection 6 months or more after acute infection (14, p. 229).

HCV-associated end-stage liver disease is the most frequent indication for liver transplantation among adults. Forty percent of chronic liver disease is HCV related, resulting in an estimated 8,000 to 10,000 deaths each year (4, p. 1; 14, p. 229).

HCV is transmitted primarily through large or repeated direct percutaneous exposures to blood. Blood transfusion, which accounted for a substantial proportion of HCV infections acquired before 10 years ago, rarely accounts for recently acquired infections. Injection-drug use currently accounts for 60% of HCV transmission in the United States. Injection-drug use is currently the single most important risk factor for HCV in the United States. It has been demonstrated that 50% to 94% of injection-drug users are infected with HCV, which is four times greater than the rates for either HIV or HBV (14, pp. 230-231).

Both incidence and prevalence studies have documented an association between levels of antibodies to HCV and increasing years of dialysis. An estimated 10% of people who have received hemodialysis treatments have HCV infection (4, pp. 1-2, 6, 9).

Nosocomial transmission of HCV has been unequivocally confirmed and underscores the need for strict infection control practices; SP should always be followed (14, p. 233).

Currently postexposure immunoglobulin prophylaxis following exposure to an HCV-infected individual is not recommended. Moreover, there are no data regarding the use of antiviral therapy (e.g., alpha-interferon) after exposure but before seroconversion (14, p. 233). (See the chapter "Employee Health.")

It is likely that the number of deaths attributable to HCV-related chronic liver disease will increase substantially during the next 2 decades. The potential economic and clinical burden resulting from HCV infection is staggering (14, p. 229).

Table 5-1 compares and contrasts forms of viral hepatitis. Both bloodborne (hepatitis B, C, and D) and nonbloodborne (hepatitis A and E [for informational purposes only]) forms are included in this table.

OSHA BLOODBORNE PATHOGEN RULE

OSHA's primary responsibility is to ensure that employers in all states and U.S. territories, including hospitals and other healthcare facilities, provide a safe and healthy work environment for employees. Some states have petitioned OSHA and have implemented state OSHA programs. Their laws are at least as strict as the federal OSHA regulations (8, p. 249).

The OSHA Bloodborne Pathogen Rule, published in 1991, is based on the CDC's concept of UP. The purpose of the Rule is to prevent bloodborne pathogen transmission in the workplace (11). Employers who are not in compliance with these regulations are subject to heavy fines and penalties. The objective of the OSHA Bloodborne Pathogen Rule is sound, and some of the requirements represent commonsense practices that have been in place in healthcare facilities for many years. Surgical and perioperative personnel have always been concerned with protecting themselves from exposure to infectious agents; therefore they share OSHA's goal (8, p. 249).

OSHA DIRECTIVE

The 1999 OSHA Bloodborne Directive updates an earlier directive issued in 1992 and reflects the availability of improved devices, better treatment following exposure, plus OSHA policy interpretations. The revised directive emphasizes the importance of an annual review of the employer's bloodborne pathogens program and requires that employers provide hands-on training in the use of safe needle devices. The directive also emphasizes the use of safer medical devices to help reduce needlesticks and other sharps injuries. OSHA inspec-

TABLE 5-1	Viral Hepatitis: An Overview				
	Hepatitis A (HAV)	**Hepatitis B (HBV)**	**Hepatitis C (HCV)**	**Hepatitis D (HDV)**	**Hepatitis E (HEV)**
Other names	Infectious hepatitis	Serum hepatitis	Post-transfusion non-A non-B hepatitis	Hepatitis delta virus	Enterically transmitted non-A non-B hepatitis
Source of virus	Feces; contaminated drinking water	Blood or blood-derived body fluids	Blood or blood-derived body fluids	Blood or blood-derived body fluids	Feces; contaminated drinking water
Route of transmission	Fecal-oral	Bloodborne; percutaneous, mucosal, sexual contact, perinatal	Bloodborne; percutaneous, mucosal, sexual contact, perinatal	Bloodborne; percutaneous, mucosal; occurs as either a co-infection with HBV or as a superinfection	Fecal-oral (similar to HAV)
Incubation period	30 days average	60-90 days average	6-9 weeks average	2-8 weeks average	26-42 days average

Modified from Phillips D: *Hepatitis and you as a healthcare worker*, part I (syllabus), Carrollton, Tex, 2000, Health & Sciences Television Network, PRIMEDIA Healthcare.

Continued

TABLE 5-1	Viral Hepatitis: An Overview—cont'd				
	Hepatitis A (HAV)	**Hepatitis B (HBV)**	**Hepatitis C (HCV)**	**Hepatitis D (HDV)**	**Hepatitis E (HEV)**
Signs and symptoms	*Abrupt onset* Influenza-like symptoms; myalgia, headache, fever, fatigue, malaise, anorexia, nausea, abdominal discomfort, dark urine, jaundice	*Insidious onset* Anorexia, vague abdominal discomfort, nausea and vomiting, sometimes arthralgias and rash, jaundice, dark urine and clay-colored stool	*Insidious onset* Malaise, anorexia, vague abdominal discomfort, nausea and vomiting, jaundice (less frequent than with HBV)	*Abrupt onset* Symptomology similar to HBV, but may be more severe; must have HBV to acquire this co-infection	Similar to HAV
Chronic complications likely?	No	Yes	Yes	Yes	No
Treatment	Symptomatic and supportive	Alpha-interferon therapy beneficial in approximately 40% of patients; should only be used to treat serious disease	Alpha-interferon and ribavirin therapy effective in some chronic disease patients; this therapy may be questionable, however	Symptomatic and supportive	Supportive

Healthcare worker prevention	Standard Precautions	Standard Precautions and sharps safety	Standard Precautions and sharps safety	Standard Precautions and sharps safety	Standard Precautions
Public health and patient education issues	Hygiene and sanitation; handwashing; preexposure/postexposure immune globulin therapy	Safe sex practices; avoidance of shared needles, razors, toothbrushes, nail clippers; preexposure/post-exposure immune globulin therapy; immunization	Same as for HBV but immune globulin therapy not recommended; no vaccine available (but hepatitis B immunization may be recommended)	Same as for HBV, but no vaccine available	Hygiene and sanitation; handwashing; safe drinking water; no vaccine available; does not occur often in the United States

Modified from Phillips D: *Hepatitis and you as a healthcare worker*, part I (syllabus), Carrollton, Tex, 2000, Health & Sciences Television Network, PRIMEDIA Healthcare.

tors have the authority to cite healthcare employers for failing to evaluate and implement the use of devices that can reduce these injuries. OSHA does not advocate one particular medical device over another but instead emphasizes safe work practices, the use of personal protective equipment, and administrative controls (12; 13). Surgical personnel should become familiar with this directive and its implications for surgical settings. An example of an applicable work practice would be the use of neutral zones (discussed later in this chapter) at the sterile field for handling sharps and sharp instruments.

UNIVERSAL PRECAUTIONS

As stated earlier, UP form the basis for care of patients with known or suspected infections caused by bloodborne pathogens; therefore their application is limited to body fluids that transmit pathogens. Following the publication of the SP document (see Appendix A), UP were considered, conceptually at least, to fit into the broader category of SP (i.e., to be a subset of "Guidelines for Isolation Precautions in Hospitals"). However, the fact is that both UP and SP have their place in today's infection control climate; both serve a purpose with their somewhat different emphases, and both are necessary. It must be remembered, though, that the SP document is a CDC guideline only—heavy in credibility and a respected authority, but not enforceable as law—as opposed to the OSHA Bloodborne Pathogen Rule, which is an enforceable regulation.

- With UP a bold step was taken that eliminated a previous category of precautions and recommended that precautions be taken for *all patients,* regardless of their bloodborne pathogen (infectious) status. With UP all human blood, and certain body fluids, are treated as if known to be infectious for HIV, HBV, and other bloodborne pathogens (8, p. 245).
- Body fluids to which UP apply are blood; amniotic, cerebrospinal, pericardial, peritoneal, pleural, spinal, and synovial fluids; semen; vaginal secretions; and saliva during dental procedures. Body fluids to which UP *do not apply* (unless they contain visible blood) are feces, nasal secretions, saliva (except as previously noted), sputum, sweat, tears, urine, and vomitus (8, p. 245; 11).
- UP advocate the use of specific barriers whenever it is likely that exposure to blood or one of the other body fluids to which UP apply will occur. Examples of these barriers include gloves, gowns, masks, and protective eyewear (8, p. 245; 11).
- In a surgical setting, circulating nurses should wear protective eyewear when there is a risk of exposure to splattering blood

and body fluids. Nonsterile gloves should also be readily available to prevent contact with blood or body fluids (8, p. 245).

- Gloves should be worn when touching blood and other body fluids, mucous membranes, nonintact skin, and items or surfaces soiled with blood or body fluids. Gloves should be changed after contact with each patient, and hands should be washed immediately after gloves are removed. Single-use gloves should not be washed or decontaminated for reuse. A gown or apron should be worn whenever performing invasive procedures that are likely to result in the splashing of blood, other body fluids, or potentially infectious materials. Protective eyewear and a mask or face shield must be worn for procedures that commonly result in the generation of droplets, splashing of blood or other body fluids, or chipping of bones (8, p. 246; 11; 12).

- It is not unusual in the operating room (OR) environment for personnel to be exposed to blood even when they are not near the patient. Products commonly used in the OR that are potential sources of blood exposure are devices that pump blood under pressure; suction canisters; irrigation devices; and blood-contaminated sponges, drapes, and instruments (9, p. 990).

- Sharps safety to prevent injuries from needles, scalpels, and other sharp instruments or devices during procedures, cleaning, disposal, and handling after procedures is a major component of UP and the OSHA Bloodborne Pathogen Rule (7, p. 245; 11).

- UP are not particularly difficult to implement in surgical and perioperative areas. The concept of treating all patients as though they are infectious has been the impetus for eliminating the practice of "dirty case" management (8, p. 246).

- With the exception of the use of protective eyewear (which is now becoming commonplace), surgical personnel have long been using the barrier techniques advocated by UP when the splashing of blood and other body fluids is likely. Although historically surgical attire has been worn to protect patients, not surgical personnel, UP are designed to protect HCWs. Now protective items are looked at in a broader sense, and their protective value to both patients and surgical personnel (dual protection) is stressed (8, p. 246).

- A recent survey found that the surgical team has a mixed record in protecting its members from bloodborne pathogens.

OR personnel have made good progress in adopting "safe needle" alternatives for intravenous access systems and syringes—a hot issue with lawmakers and regulators—but less progress in using scalpels with safety features or hands-free transfer (3, p. 9).

SAFETY PRACTICES
Exposure Study

A surveillance study of occupational blood exposures in the ORs of six hospitals was conducted to identify risk patterns and prevention strategies (9). Following are some of the findings of this study.

- Factors that were identified as setting the OR apart from other healthcare settings include prolonged contact of surgical personnel with open surgical sites, frequent manipulation of sharp instruments, and the presence of relatively large quantities of blood (9, p. 979).
- The types of surgeries with highest exposure risk were cardiovascular, general, and orthopedic (9, p. 984).
- Personnel at highest risk were resident and attending surgeons and scrub persons. Although scrub persons had a significantly greater frequency of percutaneous injuries than circulating nurses, the frequency of blood exposures were similar for these two groups (9, p. 984).
- Of the 481 exposure events that were reported in this study, 386 (80%) were percutaneous injuries and 95 (20%) were mucocutaneous blood exposures (9, p. 984).
- Suture needles and scalpel blades were the leading causes of percutaneous injuries, with suture needles alone accounting for more than 50% of the sticks. Most of these sticks were from needles used to sew muscle or fascia, a task for which blunt needles were designed. A majority of the scalpel injuries occurred while passing or disassembling the scalpel, or disposing of the blade (9, p. 992).
- More than 75% of the OR injuries in this study were caused by five types of devices: suture needles (most frequent), scalpel blades, syringes and needles, retractors/skin or bone hooks, and electrosurgical units. Although suture needle injuries were most common, scalpel blade injuries were more to likely to cause moderate to severe injuries (9, pp. 987, 989).
- Hollow-bore needles presented a higher risk than solid needles for bloodborne pathogen transmission because of the larger blood inoculum associated with this type of injury. Anesthesia personnel are at highest risk for this type of injury in surgical

settings. However, when nursing personnel initiate IV therapy, they are also at high risk for exposure (9, p. 990).

- Blood contact via the mucocutaneous routes of eyes, mouth, nose, and skin presents a serious hazard to surgical personnel. Blood contact with the mucosa of the eyes was the most common mucocutaneous exposure in this study. This information suggests that the surgical personnel wore barrier protection for the mouth and nose more consistently than they wore eye protection, or that the eye protection worn may not have been adequate (9, p. 991).

- Although it is well documented that conjunctiva serve as a transmission route for HIV, HBV, and HCV, and it is not uncommon for blood to spray or splash significant distances from the surgical site, protective eyewear often is worn only by those working in closest proximity to the surgical site. All personnel, regardless of their proximity to the surgical site, should wear protective eyewear as routinely as surgical masks. The warning "Eye protection when splashing or splattering is expected" means goggles, glasses with side shields, or a chin-length face shield should be worn. In the referenced study, circulating nurses had nearly the same number of eye exposures as scrub persons (9, p. 994).

- To protect the hands from percutaneous injuries, alternatives such as stapling devices, adhesive strips, and tissue adhesives should be considered for skin closure when feasible. The selective use of puncture-resistant gloves or finger guards during high-risk procedures should be evaluated, and retractors rather than hands should be used during incision or suturing (9, pp. 992, 994).

- Increased use of barrier precautions and the improved liquid resistance of barrier materials are important factors in reducing mucocutaneous blood contact (9, p. 994).

- A high proportion of blood contact events was associated with the inadequate liquid resistance of surgical gowns worn, the failure to double glove, and the failure to use protective eyewear (9, p. 981).

- Infection control experts recommend the practice of double gloving to help prevent exposures; however, some surgeons have found the practice to be cumbersome and double gloves to interfere with manual dexterity (9, p. 994).

- Exposure surveillance, as well as a demand for safer products and procedures, should be an important prevention strategy (9, p. 995).

General Safety Practice Guidelines

General safety practice guidelines for surgical settings include the following (8, p. 248; 7, p. 228):

- Sharps should not be manipulated by hand. An instrument should be used to attach a blade to a knife handle.
- Suture needles should be armed directly from suture packets and needles passed in a needleholder.
- Sharp instruments and needles should be passed on a tray or magnetic pad using a hands-free technique rather than passing from hand to hand.
- Used injection needles should not be recapped except by using a recapping safety device or a one-handed "scoop" technique that keeps hands and fingers away from the sharp point of the needle.
- Needles should not be removed from a disposable syringe after use. Instead, needles and syringes should be disposed of as a unit.
- Needles and sutures should be manipulated with forceps rather than gloved fingers, and instruments should be held by the handle rather than by the tips. Procedures should always be modified whenever exposures are likely.
- All blades and needles should be placed in a puncture-resistant container (8, p. 248; 7, p. 228).

Use of Neutral Zones

Neutral zones are used for the placement of sharps during a surgical procedure so that no person-to-person transfer of sharps occurs (8, p. 248). The "no-pass" (or "no-touch") technique ensures that two or more people—the surgeon, the assistant, and the scrub person—do not touch the same sharp instrument at the same time. A neutral zone is established between the operative field and the Mayo stand. An emesis basin or a magnetic pad can be used for this purpose. Instruments are placed in the neutral zone by the scrub person and then picked up by the surgeon or the assistant, and vice versa (1).

The purpose of a recent study conducted in a 1200-bed facility in Sweden was to investigate whether changes in working methods (e.g., reducing the use of sharp instruments, introducing a neutral zone, using the no-touch technique) during orthopedic procedures reduced the risk of intraoperative exposure to blood for the scrub person, surgeon, first assistant, and patient. To avoid hand-to-hand contact, three strategies were implemented: (1) the use of a tray specifically designed for the study, (2) the designation of a specific area on the back table, and (3) the use of an emesis basin (when few sharp instruments were used or when a mobile neutral zone was required). Circumstances in which the no-touch technique were used were: (1) picking up and holding suture needles while suturing, (2) manipulating suture needles in needle carriers, (3) tying sutures while holding needles, (4) holding and retracting tissue, and (5) pulling sharp drainage trocars through tissue. The study results indicated that the introduction of a neutral zone and the use of the no-touch technique reduced the number of intraoperative incidents during orthopedic surgical procedures. However, the authors state that changing *only* work methods will *not* reduce the total number of incidents to OR personnel. *Specific preventive strategies* for handling suture needles, scalpel blades, and sharp instruments, and for cutting AO wires, are needed (6).

Several processes have been recommended for reducing sharps injuries in the OR and other surgical settings, most notably at the sterile field. Because most operative procedures involve the use of sharps (e.g., scalpel blades, suture and hypodermic needles [solid and hollow-bore], sharp skin retractors, sharp-tipped electrosurgical pencils), it is incumbent upon the scrubbed OR team to avoid improper and unsafe handling of these devices, thereby preventing injuries. Among the processes recommended are the implementation of neutral zones or other work practices that aim to reduce sharps injuries. Following is a sample work practice, to which modifications can be made:

- Sharps are placed by the scrub person or surgeon in an intermediate "neutral" basin or on a designated drape, instrument mat, magnetic pad, or part of a drape that is used only for sharps transfers.
- The hand-to-hand passing of *any* sharps is prohibited. Instead, a zone is designated for sharps to be placed by the scrub person and then picked up by the surgeon or assistant. Used sharps are placed in this zone and then picked up by the scrub person to return to the Mayo stand or back table. In this way the direct passing of sharp instruments is avoided.
- The surgeon or assistant returns used suture needles to the neutral zone, still mounted on a needle holder. Closed needle holder jaws may be used to return used suture needles.
- Before transfer or placement of a sharp, audible announcements (e.g., "needle back" or "knife in basin") are given. Only one sharp at a time should be in the neutral zone.
- All sharps are passed to the surgeon and received by the scrub person only by way of the neutral zone.
- Communication is the most important part of this work practice. Communication includes the audible announcements mentioned and also the discussions that take place before and

after instituting neutral zone practices. These discussions should involve surgical personnel and should cover the roles and responsibilities of scrubbed team members, objectives, expectations, anticipated improvements, projected outcomes, and evaluations.

SAFETY ALERT

A National Institute for Occupational Safety and Health (NIOSH) alert, *Preventing Needlestick Injuries in Health Care Settings,* was issued in late 1999. This alert came at almost the same time that OSHA issued a revised compliance directive for its Bloodborne Pathogens Standard (see the section on the OSHA directive in this chapter). Both the NIOSH alert and the OSHA directive are directly applicable to infection prevention practices in surgical settings (15, p. 12).

The NIOSH alert states the following regarding the prevention of needlestick injuries:

1. Employers should establish a comprehensive program to reduce needlestick injuries by eliminating needles where feasible and implementing the use of devices with safety features
2. Employers should ensure that workers are properly trained in the safe use and disposal of needles
3. HCWs should use the devices with safety features provided by their employers (10)

The alert discusses information on bloodborne diseases, risk of infection after a needlestick injury, how needlestick injuries occur, federal and state regulations, case reports, preventive engineering controls, and recommendations. The report noted that 600,000 to 800,000 workers are injured by needlesticks each year (10).

NIOSH states that, although exposure to HBV poses a high risk for infection, administration of preexposure vaccination or postexposure prophylaxis to workers can dramatically reduce this risk; such is not the case with HCV and HIV. Preventing needlestick injuries is the best approach to preventing these diseases in HCWs and is an important part of any bloodborne pathogen prevention program in the workplace (10).

As outlined in the alert, the desirable characteristics of safety devices include the following:

- The device is needleless.
- The safety feature is integral to the device.
- Preferably the device works passively (i.e., requires no activation by the user). If user activation is necessary, the safety feature can be engaged using a single-handed technique and allows the worker's hands to remain behind the exposed sharp.

- The user can easily tell whether the safety feature is activated.
- The safety feature cannot be deactivated and remains protective through disposal.
- The device performs reliably.
- The device is easy to use, practical, safe, and effective for patient care (10).

The measures outlined in the alert should be part of a comprehensive program to prevent the transmission of bloodborne pathogens. Several states have enacted needlestick legislation, and this trend is likely to continue. NOTE: The reader is encouraged to refer to the sections on needlesticks, percutaneous injuries and mucocutaneous exposures, post-exposure follow-up for needlestick and percutaneous incidents, and use of safety devices in the chapter "Employee Health."

References

1. AORN Online Clinical Practice FAQ Database, 1999: www.aorn.org/_results/clinical.asp (accessed 2000).
2. Atkinson LJ, Fortunato NH: *Berry & Kohn's operating room technique,* ed 8, St Louis, 1996, Mosby.
3. Blood safety survey shows room for improvement, *OR Manager* 15(11):9-11, 1999.
4. Centers for Disease Control and Prevention: Recommendations for prevention and control of hepatitis C virus (HCV) infection and the HCV-related chronic disease, *MMWR* 47(No. RR-19):1-39, 1998.
5. Emmett P: Hepatitis C: the silent epidemic, *HealthWeek* pp 12-13, April 26, 1999.
6. Folin A, Nyberg B, Nordstrom G: Reducing blood exposures during orthopedic surgical procedures, *AORN J* 71(3):573-582.
7. Fortunato N: *Berry & Kohn's operating room technique,* ed 9, St Louis, 2000, Mosby.
8. Gruendemann BJ, Fernsebner B: *Comprehensive perioperative nursing,* vol 1, *Principles,* Boston, 1995, Jones & Bartlett.
9. Jagger J, Bentley M, Tereskerz P: A study of patterns and prevention of blood exposures in OR personnel, *AORN J* 67(5):979-996, 1998.
10. National Institute for Occupational Safety and Health: *NIOSH Alert: preventing needlestick injuries in health care settings,* Cincinnati, Ohio, 1999, Author. Online: www.cdc.gov/niosh
11. Occupational Safety and Health Administration: Occupational exposure to bloodborne pathogens: final rule, *Federal Register* 56(235):64175-64182, December 6, 1991.
12. Occupational Safety and Health Administration: *OSHA Directives 2-2.44D: Enforcement procedures for the occupational exposure to bloodborne pathogens,* Washington, DC, November 11, 1999, U.S. Department of Labor, OSHA. Online: www.osha-slc.gov/OshDoc/Directive_data/CPL_2-2_44D.html
13. OSHA bloodborne revision, *Infection Control Today* 4(1):12, 2000.
14. Rosen HR: Primer on hepatitis C for hospital epidemiologists, *Infect Control Hosp Epidemiol* 21(3):229-234, 2000.
15. RN News Watch: Government turns up the heat on employer needlestick efforts, *RN* 63(1):12, 2000.

Suggested Reading

1. Cardo DM, Bell DM: Bloodborne pathogen transmission in health care workers: risks and prevention strategies, *Infect Dis Clin North Am* 11:331-346, 1997.

2. Centers for Disease Control and Prevention: Exposure to blood: what health-care workers need to know, 1999.

3. Culver J: Preventing transmission of blood-borne pathogens: a compelling argument for effective device-selection strategies, *Am J Infect Control* 25(5):431-433, 1997.

4. Davis M: *Advanced precautions for today's OR: the operating room professional's handbook for the prevention of sharps injuries and bloodborne exposures,* Atlanta, 1999, Sweinbinder.

5. Finney J: When a needle stick occurs, *Surgical Services Management* 6(3):41-43, 2000.

6. Jagger J, Perry J: Shield staff from occupational exposure, *Nurs Manage* 30(6):53-55, 1999.

7. Marx JF: Understanding the varieties of viral hepatitis, *Nursing 98* 28(7):43-49, 1998.

8. Pugliese G, Salahuddin M, editors: *Sharps injury prevention program: a step-by-step guide,* Chicago, 1999, American Hospital Association.

9. Tokars JI et al: Percutaneous injuries during surgical procedures, *JAMA* 267:2899-2904, 1992.

10. Tokars JI et al: Skin and mucous membrane contacts with blood during surgical procedures: risk and prevention, *Infect Control Hosp Epidemiol* 16:703-711, 1995.

11. Wilburn S: Preventing needlesticks in your facility, *Am J Nurs* 100(2):96, 2000.

C. Antibiotic-Resistant Organisms

It is not uncommon these days for people either colonized or infected with antibiotic-resistant organisms (AROs) to become surgical patients. Underlying the care of ARO patients are basic infection prevention and control procedures (Standard Precautions [SP]) that are used with all patients. However, sometimes, as discussed in the chapter "Standard Precautions" and also in the SP document itself, additional steps (Contact Precautions) are taken in the care of these patients.

This chapter includes a brief overview of antibiotic resistance and key points in the care of two representative types of patients—those with methicillin-resistant *Staphylococcus aureus* (MRSA) and those with vancomycin-resistant enterococcus (VRE)—during their stay in a surgical, perioperative setting. These two types of patients were chosen because MRSA and VRE are the most prominent of the AROs and because the care of these patients is commonly questioned and discussed among surgical personnel.

RESISTANT ORGANISMS

- Multidrug resistance has increased as a result of the overuse of prescription antibiotics, the increasing prevalence of debilitated (immunocompromised) patients requiring frequent and/or prolonged antibiotic treatment, the availability of over-the-counter antibiotics in developing countries, and the lack of compliance with handwashing and barrier precautions. Infections from multidrug-resistant microorganisms pose a risk of significant morbidity and mortality to patients (10, p. 76).
- AROs can be transmitted to patients via the hands of personnel who have come in contact with, or via direct contact with, other patients or contaminated surfaces or devices (10, p. 76).
- The progression of antibiotic resistance has been unrelenting among hospitalized patients. In the United States alone, there has been a twentyfold increase in the frequency of VRE as nosocomial pathogens. Antibiotic resistance knows no boundaries and is observed worldwide and across the spectrum of care delivery (6, p. 504). An increasing proportion of surgical site infections are caused by antimicrobial-resistant pathogens such as MRSA and by *Candida albicans* (11, p. 253).
- Inappropriate use of antibiotics is the root cause of the emergence of most ARO strains. Prudent use of antibiotics and antimicrobials is fundamental to the control and prevention of AROs (6, p. 504).

- AROs are diminishing our ability to control the spread of infectious diseases. The rate at which resistant organisms develop is not solely a function of the use of antimicrobials in humans; it is also highly influenced by the use of these agents in veterinary medicine, animal husbandry, agriculture, and aquaculture (16, p. 303).
- Antibiotic resistance is a global public health crisis with the potential for adversely affecting health and leading, perhaps, to a "post-antibiotic era." Global perspectives and actions are urgently needed (6, p. 504).
- While the intense selective pressure of antimicrobial use and abuse has been an important factor in the rapid emergence of resistance, the inconsistent application of basic infection control techniques by hospital personnel largely accounts for the dissemination of resistant strains in hospitals. Caregivers neglect handwashing before or after the majority of contacts with their patients, despite extensive efforts to modify caregiver behavior. Gloves are not used when indicated and hands are not washed after glove removal. In some cases, caregivers go from patient to patient without changing their gloves, apparently confusing self-protection with patient protection. Both of these concepts are emphasized by SP, along with Contact Precautions and Universal Precautions (UP) (7, pp. 235-236).
- It has been said that antibiotic-resistant bacteria tend to be less virulent than their susceptible parents; this is not necessarily true because even less virulent bacteria can be dangerous pathogens for some hospitalized patients. An example of a resistant pathogen that appears to be just as virulent as the susceptible parent is MRSA. Antimicrobial resistance per se may not render pathogenic bacteria easier to clear from infected sites (15, p. 279).
- There is evidence that resistant pathogens are transmitted from patient to patient in much the same way as susceptible bacteria (e.g., through contact and sometimes by airborne droplets) (15, p. 279).
- There is no evidence that AROs are less susceptible to soap/detergent products or antiseptic agents when compared with antibiotic-sensitive organisms. Currently there is no evidence for the resistance of AROs to antiseptic agents at recommended concentrations. Antiseptic agents act in a nonspecific manner and at multiple target sites in/on microorganisms (6, p. 506).
- MRSA and VRE are no more resistant to inactivation by germicides than are sensitive isolates (6, p. 507).
- During the 1970s and 1980s, many antibiotic-resistant gram-negative bacilli emerged as nosocomial pathogens. More re-

cently, resistant gram-positive cocci, including MRSA and VRE, have emerged as major nosocomial pathogens. A study evaluated the germicidal activity of two disinfectants (a phenolic and a quaternary ammonium product) on the basis of whether hospital strains of antibiotic-resistant bacteria exhibited altered susceptibility to disinfectants. The researchers concluded that the development of antibiotic resistance does not appear to be correlated with increased resistance to disinfectants. Current standard routine disinfection and housekeeping protocols do not need to be altered. Also, routine monitoring of antibiotic-resistant bacteria for susceptibility to disinfectants is unnecessary (14).

METHICILLIN-RESISTANT *STAPHYLOCOCCUS AUREUS*

- MRSA emerged in the late 1970s and became endemic in hospitals. MRSA has also emerged as a problem in long-term care facilities, nursing homes, and outpatient clinics. Common risk factors for in-patients include severe underlying disease, prolonged hospitalization, previous antibiotic therapy, location in an intensive care unit (ICU) or burn unit, proximity to an infected patient, and intravascular catheterization (5, p. 56).
- MRSA is frequently introduced into a setting by a colonized or infected patient or healthcare provider. It is then transmitted from a colonized or infected patient to another patient by way of the healthcare provider (5, p. 56).
- The main mode of transmission of MRSA is via hands, especially the hands of healthcare workers, which may become contaminated by contact with colonized or infected patients; colonized or infected body sites of the personnel themselves; or devices, items, or environmental surfaces contaminated with body fluids containing MRSA (1).
- Using SP such as appropriate handwashing, gloving, masking, gowning, device handling, and handling of laundry should control the spread of MRSA in most instances. If MRSA is judged by the infection control program of a hospital to be of special clinical or epidemiological significance (e.g., if an open wound is present) then Contact Precautions should also be considered (see Appendix A) (1).
- *S. aureus* isolates with decreased or low-level resistance to vancomycin have also been reported (3; 4).
- Recommendations for the care of MRSA patients requiring surgical procedures include the following:
  - Clear communications between nursing units and surgical suite personnel.

- Adherence to routine infection control practices (SP) by all healthcare team members, with adherence to Contact Precautions as necessary.
- Proper handwashing practices using antimicrobial soaps followed by all healthcare team members.
- "Contact Precautions" sign placed outside the operating room (OR) and on the transport gurney or bed.
- Removal of unneeded OR and anesthesia equipment and supplies from room before arrival of patient.
- Table set up outside of room with clean garb such as a gown or gloves; shoe covers if large amounts of fluids are to be used (e.g., irrigation).
- Gowns and gloves worn by transporters when transporting patients.
- Special rooms or areas designated in preoperative holding area, or patients taken directly to OR.
- Linen from gurney removed in room after patient transfer; gurney then cleaned immediately.
- Traffic controlled by circulating nurse.
- Healthcare team members, especially nonscrubbed personnel such as the anesthesia provider and circulating nurse, follow barrier precautions, using gowns, gloves, and masks as required by Contact Precautions.
- Gown, gloves, mask, and shoe covers removed when leaving OR; hands washed before touching any surface; clean attire donned before reentering OR.
- Following surgical procedure, patient transferred to designated isolation room or area in postanesthesia care unit (PACU); PACU personnel wear gown and gloves. Dedicated patient equipment used in PACU, or patient recovers in OR or is transferred directly back to clinical unit or ICU to recover.
- At completion of procedure, and before leaving department, all healthcare team members change scrubs (unless wearing surgical or cover gowns, in which case these gowns are removed and discarded).
- Contaminated instruments and items taken directly to "dirty" utility room or decontamination section of central processing.
- All surfaces and OR equipment, including anesthesia equipment, blood pressure cuffs, pulse oximeters, and monitors, are cleaned with a facility-approved disinfectant.
- OR is terminally cleaned.
- OR may be used immediately after cleaning (12, pp. 21-23).
- No additional procedures are required for cleaning, disinfecting, and sterilizing critical and semicritical items in the presence of

MRSA or VRE. And when detergent-disinfectants are used for environmental cleaning, no additional or different products are required (6, p. 508).

VANCOMYCIN-RESISTANT ENTEROCOCCUS

- Enterococci are the second most common cause of nosocomial infections in the United States. They primarily cause urinary tract, surgical wound, soft tissue, and bloodstream infections. In 1989 the incidence of VRE infection was 0.3% of patients in large inner-city university hospitals. By 1998 the incidence had increased to 20% to 25% of these patients. This growth is significant for OR personnel because surgical patients particularly are at risk for acquiring nosocomial infections (13, p. 14).

- Reports of VRE infections began in the 1980s in Europe and are now a significant problem in the United States (17, p. 306).

- VRE infections are difficult to treat. Most clinical enterococcal isolates are *Enterococcus faecalis;* however, *Enterococcus faecium,* the second most common species, tends to exhibit even more antibiotic resistance. Infections that can be caused by enterococci include urinary tract, bacteremia, wound, abdominal-pelvic, and endocarditis. Enterococci are part of the normal gastrointestinal (G-I) and genital tract flora (8).

- Certain populations of patients are at increased risk for VRE infection or colonization: the critically ill; those with severe underlying disease or immunosuppression such as ICU, oncology, or transplant patients; those who have had an intra-abdominal or cardiothoracic surgical procedure or who have an indwelling urinary or central venous catheter; and those who have had prolonged hospital stays or received multi-antimicrobial and/or vancomycin therapy (2, p. 106). NOTE: In some institutions, transplant patients compose the vast majority of patients with VRE.

- Because enterococci are part of the normal flora of the G-I and female genital tracts, most VRE infections have been attributed to the patient's endogenous flora. However, VRE can be spread directly via patient-to-patient contact or indirectly via transient carriage on the hands of personnel or on contaminated environmental surfaces and patient care equipment (2, p. 106).

- VRE has also been of concern because of its potential for transmitting resistance to other organisms such as *S. aureus* and *Staphylococcus epidermidis* (2, p. 106).

- Widespread environmental contamination is likely in the room of someone infected with VRE. There is sufficient evidence that inanimate surfaces play a role in transmission. VRE has been found to survive for considerable periods on intravenous pumps,

blood pressure cuffs, electrocardiogram machines, computer tables, doorknobs, and floors. VRE has also survived on telephone
headsets for an hour and on countertops for a week. Recontamination of the patient environment is rapid, even after routine disinfection. The most effective disinfectants are quaternary ammonium compounds, phenolics, and alcohol. Healthcare provider
compliance with currently recommended handwashing and barrier precautions should be improved (17).

- Unlike most pathogens, VRE can extensively contaminate environmental surfaces such as doorknobs, curtains, charts, bedside
commodes, and faucet handles (9, p. 68).

- Clean, nonsterile gloves should be used when caring for a VRE
patient. If substantial contact with the patient or objects in the
room is expected, a gown should also be worn. Gloves should be
changed after contact with VRE-contaminated sources such as a
draining wound or stool. Hands should be meticulously washed
with an antiseptic soap or waterless antiseptic agent after glove
and gown removal. Single-use equipment such as thermometers
and blood pressure cuffs, or dedicated equipment such as stethoscopes, should be used whenever possible with patients who have
VRE (9, p. 68).

- Recommendations for the care of VRE patients who require procedures in a surgical setting are very similar to the recommendations for MRSA patients that were listed in the previous section
of this chapter. Contact Precautions are recommended, and the
use of good handwashing practices can minimize the risk of
transmitting VRE. Equipment (e.g., blood pressure cuffs and
monitoring equipment) should either be considered as one-time
use or should be terminally cleaned after the patient leaves the
surgical suite (13, p. 15).

- As stated previously, no additional procedures are required for
cleaning, disinfecting, and sterilizing critical and semicritical
items in the presence of MRSA or VRE. And when detergent-
disinfectants are used for environmental cleaning, no additional
or different products are required (6, p. 508).

References

1. Centers for Disease Control and Prevention (CDC): Methicillin-resistant *Staphylococcus aureus,* facts for healthcare workers, 1999, www.cdc.gov/ncidod/hip/
aresist/mrsa.htm (accessed 2000).
2. Centers for Disease Control and Prevention (CDC) Hospital Infection Control
Practices Advisory Board (HICPAC): Recommendations for preventing the
spread of vancomycin resistance, *Infect Control Hosp Epidemiol* 16(2):105-113,
1995.

3. Centers for Disease Control and Prevention (CDC): *Staphylococcus aureus* with decreased susceptibility to vancomycin, June 1997, www.cdc.gov/ncidod/hip/vrsa.htm (accessed 2000).

4. Centers for Disease Control and Prevention (CDC): "Staph" isolate with low-level resistance to vancomycin reported in the U.S., August 1997, www.cdc.gov/ncidod/hip/vrsa.htm (accessed 2000).

5. Cohen FL, Tartasky D: Microbial resistance to drug therapy: a review, *Am J Infect Control* 25(1):51-64, 1997.

6. Global consensus conference: Final recommendations, *Am J Infect Control* 27(6):503-513, 1999.

7. Goldmann DA et al: Strategies to prevent and control the emergence and spread of antimicrobial-resistant microorganisms in hospitals, *JAMA* 275(3):234-240, 1996.

8. Henning I, Brown AE: Vancomycin-resistant enterococci, *Infections in Urology* 8(6):185-187, 1995.

9. Jacobson AF: Controlling VRE, *Am J Nurs* 99(6):68, 1999.

10. Jennings J, Manian FA, editors: *APIC handbook of infection control and epidemiology,* ed 2, Washington, DC, 1999, Association for Professionals in Infection Control and Epidemiology.

11. Mangram AJ, Hospital Infection Control Practices Advisory Committee (HICPAC), Centers for Disease Control and Prevention: Guideline for prevention of surgical site infection, 1999, *Infect Control Hosp Epidemiol* 24(4):247-278, 1999. (Reprinted, in part, in Appendix B.)

12. Mikos-Schild S: MRSA—what every health care provider should know, *Today's Surg Nurse* 20(2):20-24, 1998.

13. Mikos-Schild S: VRE—what every health care provider needs to know, *Today's Surg Nurse* 20(3):13-16, 1998.

14. Rutala WA et al: Susceptibility of antibiotic-susceptible and antibiotic-resistant hospital bacteria to disinfectants, *Infect Control Hosp Epidemiol* 18(6):417-421, 1997.

15. Shales DM et al: Society for Healthcare Epidemiology of America and Infectious Diseases Society of America Joint Committee on the Prevention of Antimicrobial Resistance: guidelines for the prevention of antimicrobial resistance in hospitals, *Infect Control Hosp Epidemiol* 18(4):275-291, 1997.

16. Tenover FC, Hughes JM: The challenge of emerging infectious diseases: development and spread of multiply-resistant bacterial pathogens, JAMA 275(4):300-304, 1996.

17. Weber DJ, Rutala WA: Role of environmental contamination in the transmission of vancomycin-resistant enterococci, *Infect Control Hosp Epidemiol* 18(5):306-309, 1997.

Suggested Reading

1. A guide to TB, VRE, and MRSA, *RN* 61(7):24, 1998.

2. Bartkus JM: Confronting antibiotic resistance, an increasing threat to public health, *Surgical Services Management* 4(9):42-45, 1998.

3. Centers for Disease Control and Prevention (CDC): Interim guidelines for prevention and control of staphylococcal infection associated with reduced susceptibility to vancomycin, *MMWR* 27:626-635, 1997.

4. Levy SB: Confronting multi-drug resistance: a role for each of us, *JAMA* 269 (14):1840-1842, 1993.

5. Nosocomial infection rates rise 36%, *OR Manager* 14(6):19-20, 1998.
6. Sarver-Steffensen JA: When MRSA reaches into long-term care, *RN* 62(3):39-41, 1999.
7. Sheff B: VRE and MRSA—putting bad bugs out of business, *Nursing 98* 28(3):40-44, 1998.
8. Troillet N et al: Carriage of methicillin-resistant *Staphylococcus aureus* at hospital admission, *Infect Control Hosp Epidemiol* 19(3):181-185, 1998.
9. Tucci V, Haran MA, Isenberg HD: Epidemiology and control of vancomycin-resistant enterococci in an adult and children's hospital, *Am J Infect Control* 25(5):371-376, 1997.

D. Tuberculosis

The etiologic agent of tuberculosis (TB) is *Mycobacterium tuberculosis.* TB occurs worldwide, and the incidence is especially high in developing countries (6, p. 81).

Worldwide, 8 million new cases of and 3 million deaths from TB occur annually. In the United States, a steady decline in the number of new cases of TB was seen from 1950 through 1984. From 1985 through 1992, a steady 20% increase occurred. Causative factors included the HIV epidemic, large outbreaks of multidrug-resistant tuberculosis (MDR-TB), and an increase in active transmission because of inadequate healthcare resources. However, since 1993 the number of overall new cases of TB in the United States has been declining. In 1997 the rate of new cases was the lowest since U.S. national TB surveillance began in 1953 (7, p. 1). NOTE: Although the overall rate of new cases of TB has declined, there are some isolated U.S. cities where TB is on the increase in certain foreign-born populations (e.g., immigrants from countries where TB is a major public health concern).

Regardless of the declining rate of new TB cases in the United States, TB patients are still seen in surgical settings, prompting the use of infection control strategies that reduce risk of transmission to other patients and to staff. The guidelines outlined in the 1994 Centers for Disease Control and Prevention (CDC) document "Guidelines for Preventing the Transmission of *Mycobacterium tuberculosis* in Health-Care Facilities" (2) are still in effect and are discussed in this chapter. A proposed Occupational Safety and Health Administration (OSHA) standard for TB control was published in 1997; however, it is not yet finalized. Until this standard is finalized, OSHA will continue to inspect facilities for TB control using its authority under the General Duty Clause of the Occupational Safety and Health Act.

MODES OF TRANSMISSION

There have been dramatic outbreaks of both MDR-TB and drug susceptible strains of TB in hospitals, with transmission to both patients and healthcare workers (7, p. 3).

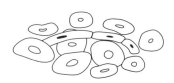

The mode of TB transmission is airborne droplet nuclei (1 to 5 μm in size) that are produced when a person with pulmonary or laryngeal TB coughs, sneezes, speaks or otherwise forcibly exhales air from his or her lungs (7, pp. 1-2).

Although nosocomial transmission occurs primarily via the airborne route, there are occasional reports of transmission via other routes such as primary cutaneous inoculation from needlesticks and lacerations, contaminated bronchoscopes, and organ transplantation (7, p. 2). Extrapulmonary TB has also been transmitted via surgical drainage and by aerosolization during wound irrigation of an abscess using a "water-pik" spray device (5).

PRECAUTIONS

In addition to Standard Precautions (SP), *Airborne Precautions* are instituted for patients known or suspected to be infected with microorganisms transmitted by airborne droplet nuclei that are smaller than 5 μm. This includes TB. Special air handling and ventilation are required, as well as patient placement in a room with either monitored negative air pressure (6 to 12 air changes per hour) and appropriate discharge of air outdoors or monitored high-efficiency filtration of room air before the air is circulated to other parts of the hospital. Respiratory protection (e.g., an N-95 mask) is required of those entering the room of a patient with known or suspected infectious pulmonary TB. Patient transport is limited; however, if transport is necessary, the patient wears a surgical mask to minimize the dispersal of droplet nuclei (4, pp. 68-69).

NOTE: The hierarchy of controls in the overall care of TB patients is (1) administrative (early identification of patients, beginning anti-TB therapy); (2) engineering (isolation in negative-pressure rooms); and (3) use of personal protective equipment (PPE), including masks.

TERMINOLOGY

The following definitions may assist the reader to understand references to respiratory protection in this chapter:

N-95 respiratory masks: Have the ability to filter 95% of particles down to the 0.3 μm size. NIOSH-approved N-95 masks are the minimum requirement for care of patients with TB.

Particulate respirator masks: Have high filtration levels; include the N-95 mask.

High-efficiency particulate air (HEPA) filters: Commonly used and required in hospitals; used in ventilation systems and with portable units; are capable of filtering 99.7% of particles.

Powered air purifying respirators (PAP... higher protection than N-95 masks b... not necessary for TB control; have a l... age. PAPR masks are used only with l...

Dust-mist-fume masks: Some of the fir... pirator masks used in hospitals at the... TB controls; are used today in industr... such as agriculture. NIOSH-approved ...... are the stan- dard masks used today for TB control.

SURGICAL SETTINGS

NOTE: When a TB patient requires a surgical procedure, it is best to admit the patient directly to the operating room (OR), eliminating a stop in the holding area where special TB room and ventilation requirements may not exist.

- Elective operative procedures on TB patients should be delayed until the patient is no longer infectious (2, p. 54269). However, high-risk procedures, such as bronchoscopy, drainage of TB abscess, or cutting of tissues, may need to be performed on a TB patient (7, p. 14).
- The TB patient should wear a surgical mask if transported outside of the isolation area/room (to the OR, for example) (7, p. 13).
- If an operative procedure must be performed, it should be done in an OR with an anteroom. If the OR does not have an anteroom, doors should be closed and minimal traffic maintained to lessen the opening and closing of doors (2, p. 54269).
- Procedures should be performed at times when other patients are not present and when a minimum number of personnel are present (e.g., end of day) (2, p. 54269).
- During postoperative recovery, the patient should be monitored in a private room or area that meets recommended standards for TB isolation rooms, including negative pressure (2, pp. 54269-54270). NOTE: Patients may also recover in the OR or in their room if there are no negative-pressure rooms in the postanesthesia care unit (PACU).

Personnel Respiratory Protection

- Respiratory protective masks must be worn by personnel when operative procedures are performed (and when patients are recovering after surgery). These masks (NOTE: a standard surgical mask worn over an N-95 respiratory mask or a commercially available combination particulate respirator/surgical mask) not

ect the sterile field and surgical site from the respiratory
ons of the healthcare worker (HCW) but also protect the
W from the infectious droplet nuclei generated both by the
patient and from fluid splashes (2, pp. 54261, 54270).

- Disposable N-95 respiratory masks are used strictly for TB control, and they may be reused by the same HCW as long as the respirator remains structurally intact and is not damaged or soiled
  (7, p. 13). NOTE: The mask should be replaced when breathing becomes difficult, which indicates that the filter has become
  obstructed.
- Infection control personnel should develop standard operating
  procedures for storing, reusing, and disposing of respirators that
  are designated to be disposable (2, p. 54293). NOTE: Good judgment should guide decisions regarding storage of these used respirators, especially storage in lockers after repeated use. Each surgical setting should establish policies that give guidance on the
  inspection of respirators before and after each use, including
  lengths of time before discard. However, the recommendation is
  to discard used disposable masks (surgical and N-95) after each
  use/procedure.
- For a bronchoscopy performed on a patient with MDR-TB, respirators with a higher than normal level of protection, such as a
  HEPA respirator or powered air-purifying respirator (PAPR),
  may be used (7, p. 14).

  See the chapter "Employee Health" for information on employee
TB-exposure reporting.

Fit Testing

- Fit testing is part of the respiratory protection program required
  by OSHA for all respiratory protective devices used in the workplace (2, p. 54292).
- The CDC recommends fit testing prior to issuance of a respirator
  and fit checking each time the respirator is donned. Fit checking
  of the face piece should detect any leaks. Manufacturers' recommendations should be followed (7, p. 14).
- Fit testing is a procedure used to evaluate how well a respirator
  fits a person by assessing leakage around the face seal. Fit testing
  can be either qualitative (i.e., relying on the subjective response of
  the wearer) or quantitative (i.e., using a measurement of actual
  leakage). (The qualitative method is commonly carried out by
  spraying a saccharin solution into an opening of the hood. If saccharin is tasted, the mask is not properly fitted and the test fails.)
  NIOSH explains that fit testing is needed to ensure at least the expected level of protection (i.e., that the concentration of airborne

contaminants inside the respirator is ≤10% of ambient levels). Fit testing does identify those wearers who have poor fit (8, p. 145).

- The requirement for fit testing of the N-95 respirators continues to be a controversial topic. OSHA's proposed TB standard requires initial fit testing; however, if the standard is enacted, employers will be allowed to determine the need for annual fit testing through an annual person-to-person evaluation consisting of a questionnaire and personal observation (8, p. 145).

Patient Masks

- For transport to the OR, a standard surgical mask is placed on the patient. The transporter wears a TB-filtering (N-95) mask (3, p. 216).
- Standard surgical masks are designed to prevent the respiratory secretions of the person wearing the mask from entering the air. To reduce the expulsion of droplet nuclei into the air, patients suspected of having TB should wear surgical masks when not in TB isolation rooms. These patients do not need to wear particulate respirators (N-95 masks), which are designed to filter the air before it is inhaled by the person wearing the respirator. Patients with suspected or confirmed TB should never wear a respirator that has an exhalation valve because this type of respirator does not prevent the expulsion of droplet nuclei into the air (2, p. 54262).

Anesthesia Equipment

NOTE: The information in the first two bulleted items is specific to TB patients. The information in the next two bulleted items applies to the care of all patients, including those with TB.

- Disposable anesthesia equipment should be used when possible. Reusable equipment must be sterilized or high-level disinfected immediately after use (3, p. 216).
- Placing a bacterial filter on the patient's endotracheal tube or at the expiratory side of the anesthesia breathing circuit when operating on a patient who has confirmed or suspected TB may help reduce the risk for contaminating anesthesia equipment or discharging tubercle bacilli into the ambient air (2, p. 54269).
- Although sterilization is preferred for semicritical items including anesthesia breathing circuits, high-level disinfection (HLD) that destroys vegetative microorganisms, most fungal spores, tubercle bacilli, and small nonlipid viruses may be used. Meticulous physical cleaning of such items before sterilization or HLD is essential (2, p. 54294).

- Reusable anesthesia equipment that comes in contact with mucous membranes, blood, or body fluids (e.g., laryngeal mask airways, masks, breathing circuits, airways, and laryngoscope blades) is considered semicritical and should be cleaned and then processed by HLD, pasteurization, or sterilization between each patient use. (Pasteurization is a process that uses time and hot water [160° to 170° F for 30 minutes] to establish a technique that offers HLD.) If pasteurization is the chosen disinfection method, manufacturers' instructions should be followed (1, pp. 195, 197).

Decontamination of Room, Equipment, and Environmental Surfaces

- Equipment used on TB patients is usually not involved in transmission of the tubercle bacillus, although transmission by contaminated bronchoscopes has been demonstrated. Selection of chemical disinfectants depends on the intended use, the level of disinfection required, and the structure and material of the item to be disinfected (2, pp. 54293-54294).
- Walls, floors, and other environmental surfaces are rarely associated with transmission of infections to patients or HCWs. Because TB infections generally require inhalation by the host, extraordinary attempts to disinfect or sterilize environmental surfaces are not indicated. A hospital-grade EPA-approved germicide/disinfectant that is not tuberculocidal can be used. The same daily cleaning procedures used in other rooms in the facility should be used to clean TB isolation rooms (2, p. 54294).

    NOTE: The question of how long an OR should remain vacant, if at all, following a procedure on a TB patient often arises. The answer is dependent on the specifications of each particular OR, including its ventilation system. Reference 2, pp. 54279-54284 (also available online), particularly Table S3-1, "Air Changes Per Hour (1-50) and Respective Time in Minutes Required for Removal Efficiencies of 90%, 99%, and 99.9% of Airborne Contaminants," p. 54279, can be very helpful. Additional information can be found in the American Institute of Architects Academy of Architecture for Health (AIAAAH) publication *Guidelines for Design and Construction of Hospital and Healthcare Facilities,* cited in the suggested reading list at the end of this chapter.

Exhaust Systems and Filtration Units

- The use of enclosures such as tents, booths, or hoods may be necessary alternatives when a PACU is not available or other required TB engineering controls cannot be met. A HEPA filter should be used on the discharge vent of any enclosure device. There are other types of local exhaust systems, such as smoke evacuation devices, that can be used during surgical procedures or during bronchoscopy (7, p. 11).

- HEPA filters can be used in exhaust ducts or in fixed or portable HEPA room air cleaners in TB isolation rooms or areas. These filtration units can be mounted on the wall or ceiling of the isolation room. Some HEPA filtration units use ultraviolet germicidal irradiation for disinfection of the air after HEPA filtration (7, p. 11). NOTE: Portable filtration units may not be appropriate for the OR because as they are used, the airflow in the OR is disrupted.

References

1. AORN: Recommended practices for cleaning and processing anesthesia equipment. In *Standards, recommended practices and guidelines,* Denver, 2000, Author, pp 195-198.
2. Centers for Disease Control and Prevention (CDC): Guidelines for preventing transmission of *Mycobacterium tuberculosis* in health-care facilities, 1994, *Federal Register* 59(208):54202-54303, 1994. Online: www.cdc.gov/nchstp/tb/pubs/mmwr/rr4313.pdf
3. Fortunato N: *Berry & Kohn's operating room technique,* ed 9, St Louis, 2000, Mosby.
4. Garner JS, Hospital Infection Control Practices Advisory Committee (HICPAC): Guideline for isolation precautions in hospitals, *Infect Control Hosp Epidemiol* 17(1):53-80, 1996. (Reprinted, in part, in Appendix A.)
5. Hutton MD et al: Nosocomial transmission of tuberculosis associated with a draining abscess, *J Infect Dis* 161(2):286-295, 1990.
6. Jennings J, Manian FA, editors: *APIC handbook of infection control and epidemiology,* ed 2, Washington, DC, 1999, Association for Professionals in Infection Control and Epidemiology.
7. Pugliese G: Preventing transmission of tuberculosis in healthcare facilities, *Asepsis* 20(4):1-22, 1999, www.asepsis.com (accessed 2000).
8. Pugliese G, Favero MS, editors: Is fit testing necessary? (medical news), *Infect Control Hosp Epidemiol* 20(2):145, 1999.

Suggested Reading

1. Agerton T et al: Transmission of a highly drug-resistant strain (strain W1) of *Mycobacterium tuberculosis, JAMA* 278:1073-1077, 1997.
2. American Institute of Architects Academy of Architecture for Health, U.S. Department of Health and Human Services: *Guidelines for design and construction of hospital and healthcare facilities, 1996-1997,* Washington, DC, 1996, American Institute of Architects Press.
3. Castro KG: Global tuberculosis challenges, *Emerg Infect Dis* 4(3):408-409, 1998.
4. Centers for Disease Control and Prevention (CDC): Laboratory performance evaluation of N-95 filtering face-piece respirators, *MMWR* 47:1045-1049, 1996.
5. Centers for Disease Control and Prevention (CDC): Prevention and treatment of tuberculosis among patients infected with human immunodeficiency virus: principles of therapy and revised recommendations, *MMWR* 47(RR-20):1-51, 1998.

6. Cohen FL, Tartasky D: Microbial resistance to drug therapy: a review, *Am J Infect Control* 25(1):51-69, 1997.

7. Hedrick E: Where's the science? *Am J Infect Control* 28(1):66-67, 2000.

8. King MA, Tomasic DM: Treating TB today, *RN* 62(6):26-30, 1999.

9. Michele TM et al: Transmission of *Mycobacterium tuberculosis* by a fiberoptic bronchoscope, *JAMA* 278:1073-1077, 1997.

10. Pugliese G, Tapper M: TB control in hospitals, *Infect Control Hosp Epidemiol* 17:819-827, 1996.

E. Creutzfeldt-Jakob Disease

Although rare, Creutzfeldt-Jakob disease (CJD) is a progressive, fatal disease characterized by dementia, myoclonus (muscle spasms), and multifocal neurologic symptoms. The condition may lie dormant for more than 30 years before the onset of symptoms. The disease then progresses rapidly, leading to coma and death usually within 2 years of onset. A new variant of CJD (nvCJD) has resulted from ingestion of beef contaminated with bovine spongiform encephalopathy (BSE) in the United Kingdom (3, p. 214).

The incidence of CJD is one in 1 million persons, and the disease is always fatal. Little is known about the natural transmission of CJD, but iatrogenic cases have occurred as a result of brain tissue transplants, injection of contaminated human pituitary–derived growth hormone, and contaminated surgical instruments (e.g., neurosurgical instruments, cortical electrodes, dura mater grafts, and corneal transplants (2, p. 873).

Because the CJD agent is proteinaceous and infectious, it is considered to be a *prion*. Prions cause a number of diseases in animals and humans including BSE, commonly referred to as "mad cow disease" in the United Kingdom. Prions accumulate in the brain, where they trigger symptoms. Although little is known about the human prion diseases, CJD is the most studied (7, p. 61).

Prion diseases are infectious, but not contagious. They are not transmitted by direct contact, droplet, or airborne routes. Rather, they are transmitted by direct inoculation past the natural defense skin barriers via transplanted tissue, contaminated drugs derived from highly infectious material, and surgical instruments (7, p. 73). Ocular infection following corneal transplantation and intracerebral infection from contaminated stereotactic electrodes have been documented. Cerebrospinal fluid, organs (especially corneas and brain tissue), and other body substances are considered hazardous materials; blood, feces, skin, and saliva are considered to be less hazardous (1, p. 194).

SURGICAL GUIDELINES

- Careful planning must be done to minimize the risks of CJD transmission. Disposable drapes and linens should be used during surgical procedures. Surgical team members should double glove and wear a face shield. No power tools should be used. A neutral zone for sharp instruments should be established to eliminate hand-to-hand passing of instruments. At the end of the procedure, all contaminated supplies should be carefully collected and spills wiped up (7, p. 74).

- Special isolation precautions (Contact Precautions) are needed in the operating room (OR) and decontamination areas to prevent transmission of CJD. Methods of choice recommended by Steelman for decontaminating the environment or equipment include chemical disinfection with either full-strength bleach (sodium hypochlorite) or 1N sodium hydroxide for a 1-hour contact time. However, full-strength bleach is very caustic, damaging both fabric and metal and irritating the airway of healthcare workers; therefore the use of sodium hydroxide, a hazardous substance that is less caustic than bleach, is more highly recommended. The use of protective apparel is a necessity (7, pp. 61, 73). NOTE: *Readers are cautioned to not confuse sodium hypochlorite with sodium hydroxide.*

- Destroying the infectious prions of CJD is a serious concern. Sodium hydroxide has been found to be the most effective agent for decreasing or eliminating the infectivity of the CJD prion. Other agents are either ineffective or only partially effective. Steam sterilization in either a gravity-displacement sterilizer for 60 minutes at 270° F (132° C) or a prevacuum sterilizer for 18 minutes at 274° F (134° C) after a 60-minute exposure to sodium hydroxide has been shown to be effective (2, p. 873).

- Steam sterilization for 1 hour at 270° F (132° C) has been recommended by Rutala as the preferred treatment of contaminated material. Immersion in 1N sodium hydroxide for 1 hour at room temperature is an alternative procedure for critical and semicritical items when autoclaving is not possible. Because noncritical patient care items and surfaces (e.g., autopsy tables, floors) have not been involved in disease transmission, they may be disinfected with either bleach (either undiluted or up to 1:10 dilution) or 1N sodium hydroxide at room temperature for 15 minutes or less. A formalin-formic acid procedure is required for inactivating virus infectivity in tissue samples from patients with CJD. The need for such recommendations is due to the existence of an extremely resistant subpopulation of CJD-like viruses (prions) and the protection afforded the tissue-associated virus (5, pp. 918-919).

- Because low-temperature sterilization does not eliminate infectivity or prions, instruments requiring sterilization with ethylene oxide, hydrogen peroxide, peracetic acid, or glutaraldehyde should not be used (7, p. 73).

- CJD is particularly virulent. The prions are resistant to destruction via heat, chemicals, radiation, freezing, drying, and organic detergents. Instruments should be steam sterilized for 1 hour in a gravity-displacement sterilizer, or for 18 minutes in a prevacuum sterilizer (both are longer than normal cycles) before routine cleaning. Sterilization of tissue that has been fixed with formalin is impossible (3, p. 214).

- Surgical instruments should be cleaned and placed in a container, then sterilized. The outside of the container should be kept clean. Manufacturers' instructions must be followed with regard to the sterilization cycle and type of container used. After sterilization, the instruments should be washed in a washer/decontaminator using the "heavily soiled" cycle and then packaged and sterilized in a routine fashion. Sodium hydroxide should be applied to contaminated equipment and floors and should be left standing for 1 hour. (NOTE: The reader is alerted that there are two recommendations in this chapter for duration for decontamination of surfaces: 15 minutes and 1 hour.) Liquid waste should be solidified. Because prions remain infectious in the environment for years, all disposable items should be carefully contained and incinerated (7, p. 74).

A detailed infection protocol for identifying high-risk patients, decontamination of the OR, treatment of staff exposure, and protection of healthcare personnel is discussed in a highly recommended article (see reference 6). The CDC may be proposing new guidelines for the treatment/disinfection of items contaminated with the CJD prion. A draft CDC statement is being reviewed (4).

References

1. Atkinson LJ, Fortunato NH: *Berry & Kohn's operating room technique,* ed 8, St Louis, 1996, Mosby.
2. Fogg DM: Clinical issues, *AORN J* 67(4):870-874, 1998.
3. Fortunato N: *Berry & Kohn's operating room technique,* ed 9, St Louis, 2000, Mosby.
4. Rutala WA: Changing practices in disinfection and sterilization (notes from lecture), APIC Annual Conference, Baltimore, June 1999, and personal communication with Dr. LM Sehulster, CDC, February 2000.
5. Rutala WA: Selection and use of disinfectants in health care. In Mayhall CG, editor: *Hospital epidemiology and infection control,* Baltimore, 1996, Williams & Wilkins, pp 913-936.
6. Steelman VM: Prion diseases—an evidence-based protocol for infection control, *AORN J* 69(5):946-967, 1999.
7. Steelman VM, Elliott C: Preventing transmission of Creutzfeldt-Jakob disease, *Infection Control Today* 3(1):61, 72-74, 1999.

Suggested Reading

1. Centers for Disease Control and Prevention (CDC): Bovine spongiform encephalopathy (BSE) in the United Kingdom and Creutzfeldt-Jakob disease (CJD) in the United States, 1996, www.cdc.gov/ncidod/diseases/cjd/qa96bse.htm (accessed 2000).

2. Pattison J: The emergence of bovine spongiform encephalopathy and related diseases, *Emerg Infect Dis* 4(3):390-394, 1998.

3. Rutala WA: APIC guideline for selection and use of disinfectants, *Am J Infect Control* 24(4):313-342, 1996.

4. Steelman VM: Activity of sterilization processes and disinfectants against prions (Creutzfeldt-Jakob disease agent). In Rutala WA, editor: *Disinfection, sterilization and antisepsis in health care,* Washington, DC, Association for Professionals in Infection Control and Epidemiology; Champlain, NY, Polyscience, 1998.

Appendix A
Summary of Standard Precautions and Transmission-Based Precautions

————◆ ◆ ◆————

STANDARD PRECAUTIONS

Standard Precautions synthesize the major features of UP (Blood and Body Fluid Precautions) . . . (designed to reduce the risk of transmission of bloodborne pathogens) and BSI . . . (designed to reduce the risk of transmission of pathogens from moist body substances) and applies them to all patients receiving care in hospitals, regardless of their diagnosis or presumed infection status. Standard Precautions apply to (1) blood; (2) all body fluids, secretions, and excretions *except sweat,* regardless of whether or not they contain visible blood; (3) nonintact skin; and (4) mucous membranes. Standard Precautions are designed to reduce the risk of transmission of microorganisms from both recognized and unrecognized sources of infection in hospitals.

TRANSMISSION-BASED PRECAUTIONS

Transmission-Based Precautions are designed for patients documented or suspected to be infected with highly transmissible or epidemiologically important pathogens for which additional precautions beyond Standard Precautions are needed to interrupt transmission in hospitals. There are three types of Transmission-Based Precautions: Airborne Precautions, Droplet Precautions, and Contact Precautions. They may be combined for diseases that have multiple routes of transmission. When used either singularly or in combination, they are to be used in addition to Standard Precautions.

   Airborne Precautions are designed to reduce the risk of airborne transmission of infectious agents. Airborne transmission occurs by dissemination of either airborne droplet nuclei (small-particle residue [5 µm or smaller in size] of evaporated droplets that may remain suspended in the air for long periods

From the Public Health Service, U.S. Department of Health and Human Services, Centers for Disease Control and Prevention, Atlanta.
Reprinted from Garner JS, Hospital Infection Control Practices Advisory Committee: Guideline for isolation precautions in hospitals, *Infect Control Hosp Epidemiol* 17:53-80, 1996, and *Am J Infect Control* 24:24-52, 1996. Also available online: www.cdc.gov/ncidod/hip/isolat/isolat.htm

of time) or dust particles containing the infectious agent. Microorganisms carried in this manner can be dispersed widely by air currents and may become inhaled by or deposited on a susceptible host within the same room or over a longer distance from the source patient, depending on environmental factors; therefore, special air handling and ventilation are required to prevent airborne transmission. Airborne Precautions apply to patients known or suspected to be infected with epidemiologically important pathogens that can be transmitted by the airborne route.

Droplet Precautions are designed to reduce the risk of droplet transmission of infectious agents. Droplet transmission involves contact of the conjunctivae or the mucous membranes of the nose or mouth of a susceptible person with large-particle droplets (larger than 5 µm in size) containing microorganisms generated from a person who has a clinical disease or who is a carrier of the microorganism. Droplets are generated from the source person primarily during coughing, sneezing, or talking and during the performance of certain procedures such as suctioning and bronchoscopy. Transmission via large-particle droplets requires close contact between source and recipient persons, because droplets do not remain suspended in the air and generally travel only short distances, usually 3 ft or less, through the air. Because droplets do not remain suspended in the air, special air handling and ventilation are not required to prevent droplet transmission. Droplet Precautions apply to any patient known or suspected to be infected with epidemiologically important pathogens that can be transmitted by infectious droplets.

Contact Precautions are designed to reduce the risk of transmission of epidemiologically important microorganisms by direct or indirect contact. Direct-contact transmission involves skin-to-skin contact and physical transfer of microorganisms to a susceptible host from an infected or colonized person, such as occurs when personnel turn patients, bathe patients, or perform other patient-care activities that require physical contact. Direct-contact transmission also can occur between two patients (e.g., by hand contact), with one serving as the source of infectious microorganisms and the other as a susceptible host. Indirect-contact transmission involves contact of a susceptible host with a contaminated intermediate object, usually inanimate, in the patient's environment. Contact Precautions apply to specified patients known or suspected to be infected or colonized (presence of microorganism in or on patient but without clinical signs and symptoms of infection) with epidemiologically important microorganisms than can be transmitted by direct or indirect contact.

A synopsis of the types of precautions and the patients requiring the precautions is listed in Table A-1.

TABLE A-1	Synopsis of Types of Precautions and Patients Requiring the Precautions

Standard Precautions
Use Standard Precautions for the care of all patients

Airborne Precautions
In addition to Standard Precautions, use Airborne Precautions for patients known or suspected to have serious illnesses transmitted by airborne droplet nuclei. Examples of such illnesses include:
- Measles
- Varicella (including disseminated zoster)*
- Tuberculosis†

Droplet Precautions
In addition to Standard Precautions, use Droplet Precautions for patients known or suspected to have serious illnesses transmitted by large particle droplets. Examples of such illnesses include:
- Invasive *Haemophilus influenzae* type b disease, including meningitis, pneumonia, epiglottitis, and sepsis
- Invasive *Neisseria meningitidis* disease, including meningitis, pneumonia, and sepsis
- Other serious bacterial respiratory infections spread by droplet transmission, including:
  - Diphtheria (pharyngeal)
  - Mycoplasma pneumonia
  - Pertussis
  - Pneumonic plague
  - Streptococcal (group A) pharyngitis, pneumonia, or scarlet fever in infants and young children
- Serious viral infections spread by droplet transmission, including:
  - Adenovirus*
  - Influenza
  - Mumps
  - Parvovirus B19
  - Rubella

*Certain infections require more than one type of precaution.
†See CDC "Guidelines for Preventing the Transmission of *Mycobacterium tuberculosis* in Health-Care Facilities."   *Continued*

TABLE A-1	Synopsis of Types of Precautions and Patients Requiring the Precautions—cont'd

Contact Precautions

In addition to Standard Precautions, use Contact Precautions for patients known or suspected to have serious illnesses easily transmitted by direct patient contact or by contact with items in the patient's environment. Examples of such illnesses include:

- Gastrointestinal, respiratory, skin, or wound infections or colonization with multidrug-resistant bacteria judged by the infection control program, based on current state, regional, or national recommendations, to be of special clinical and epidemiologic significance
- Enteric infections with a low infectious dose or prolonged environmental survival, including:
  - *Clostridium difficile*
  - For diapered or incontinent patients: enterohemorrhagic *Escherichia coli* O157:H7, *Shigella,* hepatitis A, or rotavirus
- Respiratory syncytial virus, parainfluenza virus, or enteroviral infections in infants and young children
- Skin infections that are highly contagious or that may occur on dry skin, including:
  - Diphtheria (cutaneous)
  - Herpes simplex virus (neonatal or mucocutaneous)
  - Impetigo
  - Major (noncontained) abscesses, cellulitis, or decubiti
  - Pediculosis
  - Scabies
  - Staphylococcal furunculosis in infants and young children
  - Zoster (disseminated or in the immunocompromised host)*
- Viral/hemorrhagic conjunctivitis
- Viral hemorrhagic infections (Ebola, Lassa, or Marburg)

EMPIRIC USE OF AIRBORNE, DROPLET, OR CONTACT PRECAUTIONS

In many instances, the risk of nosocomial transmission of infection may be highest before a definitive diagnosis can be made and before precautions based on that diagnosis can be implemented. The routine use of Standard Precautions for all patients should reduce greatly this risk for conditions other than those requiring Airborne, Droplet, or Contact Precautions. While it is not possible to prospectively identify all patients needing these enhanced precautions, certain clinical syndromes and conditions carry a sufficiently high risk to warrant the empiric addition of enhanced precautions while a more definitive diagnosis is pursued. A listing of such conditions and the recommended precautions beyond Standard Precautions is presented in Table A-2.

The organisms listed under the column "Potential Pathogens" are not intended to represent the complete or even most likely diagnoses,

TABLE A-2 | **Clinical Syndromes or Conditions Warranting Additional Empiric Precautions to Prevent Transmission of Epidemiologically Important Pathogens Pending Confirmation of Diagnosis***

Clinical Syndrome or Condition†	Potential Pathogens‡	Empiric Precautions
Diarrhea		
Acute diarrhea with a likely infectious cause in an incontinent or diapered patient	Enteric pathogens§	Contact
Diarrhea in an adult with a history of recent antibiotic use	*Clostridium difficile*	Contact
Meningitis	*Neisseria meningitidis*	Droplet
Rash or exanthems, generalized, etiology unknown		
Petechial/ecchymotic with fever	*Neisseria meningitidis*	Droplet
Vesicular	Varicella	Airborne and Contact
Maculopapular with coryza and fever	Rubeola (measles)	Airborne
Respiratory infections		
Cough/fever/upper lobe pulmonary infiltrate in an HIV-negative patient or a patient at low risk for HIV infection	*Mycobacterium tuberculosis*	Airborne

*Infection control professionals are encouraged to modify or adapt this table according to local conditions. To ensure that appropriate empiric precautions are implemented always, hospitals must have systems in place to evaluate patients routinely according to these criteria as part of their preadmission and admission care.

†Patients with the syndromes or conditions listed below may present with atypical signs or symptoms (e.g., pertussis in neonates and adults may not have paroxysmal or severe cough). The clinician's index of suspicion should be guided by the prevalence of specific conditions in the community, as well as clinical judgment.

‡The organisms listed under the column "Potential Pathogens" are not intended to represent the complete, or even most likely, diagnoses, but rather possible etiologic agents that require additional precautions beyond Standard Precautions until they can be ruled out.

§These pathogens include enterohemorrhagic *Escherichia coli* O157:H7, *Shigella*, hepatitis A, and rotavirus. *Continued*

	Clinical Syndromes or Conditions Warranting Additional Empiric Precautions to Prevent Transmission of Epidemiologically Important Pathogens Pending Confirmation of Diagnosis—cont'd
TABLE A-2	

Clinical Syndrome or Conditions†	Potential Pathogens‡	Empiric Precautions
Respiratory infections— cont'd		
Cough/fever/pulmonary infiltrate in any lung location in a HIV-infected patient or a patient at high risk for HIV infection	*Mycobacterium tuberculosis*	Airborne
Paroxysmal or severe persistent cough during periods of pertussis activity	*Bordetella pertussis*	Droplet
Respiratory infections, particularly bronchiolitis and croup, in infants and young children	Respiratory syncytial or parainfluenza virus	Contact
Risk of multidrug- resistant microorganisms		
History of infection or colonization with multidrug-resistant organisms‖	Resistant bacteria‖	Contact
Skin, wound, or urinary tract infection in a patient with a recent hospital or nursing home stay in a facility where multidrug- resistant organisms are prevalent‖	Resistant bacteria‖	Contact
Skin or wound infection Abscess or draining wound that cannot be covered	*Staphylococcus aureus,* group A streptococcus	Contact

‖Resistant bacteria judged by the infection control program, based on current state, regional, or national recommendations, to be of special clinical or epidemiological significance.

but rather possible etiologic agents that require additional precautions beyond Standard Precautions until they can be ruled out. Infection control professionals are encouraged to modify or adapt this table according to local conditions. To ensure that appropriate empiric precautions are implemented always, hospitals must have systems in place to evaluate patients routinely, according to these criteria as part of their preadmission and admission care.

Appendix B
CDC Recommendations for Prevention
of Surgical Site Infection

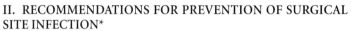

II. RECOMMENDATIONS FOR PREVENTION OF SURGICAL SITE INFECTION*

A. RATIONALE

The Guideline for Prevention of Surgical Site Infection, 1999, provides recommendations concerning reduction of surgical site infection risk. Each recommendation is categorized on the basis of existing scientific data, theoretical rationale, and applicability. However, the previous CDC system for categorizing recommendations has been modified slightly.

Category I recommendations, including IA and IB, are those recommendations that are viewed as effective by HICPAC and experts in the fields of surgery, infectious diseases, and infection control. Both Category IA and IB recommendations are applicable for, and should be adopted by, all healthcare facilities; IA and IB recommendations differ only in the strength of the supporting scientific evidence.

Category II recommendations are supported by less scientific data than Category I recommendations; such recommendations may be appropriate for addressing specific nosocomial problems or specific patient populations.

No recommendation is offered for some practices, either because there is a lack of consensus regarding their efficacy or because the available scientific evidence is insufficient to support their adoption. For such unresolved issues, practitioners should use judgement to determine a policy regarding these practices within their organization. Recommendations that are based on federal regulation are denoted with a dagger†.

B. RANKINGS

Category IA. Strongly recommended for implementation and supported by well-designed experimental, clinical, or epidemiological studies.

———
Reprinted from Mangram AJ, Hospital Infection Control Practices Advisory Committee (HICPAC), Centers for Disease Control and Prevention: Guideline for prevention of surgical site infection, 1999, *Infect Control Hosp Epidemiol* 24(4):247-278, 1999. Also available online: www.cdc.gov/ncidod/hip/SSI/SSI_guideline.htm
*Part I is not included in this reprint.

Category IB. Strongly recommended for implementation and supported by some experimental, clinical, or epidemiological studies and strong theoretical rationale.

Category II. Suggested for implementation and supported by suggestive clinical or epidemiological studies or theoretical rationale.

No recommendation; unresolved issue. Practices for which insufficient evidence or no consensus regarding efficacy exists.

Practices required by federal regulation are denoted with a dagger (†).

C. RECOMMENDATIONS

1. Preoperative

a. Preparation of the patient

1. Whenever possible, identify and treat all infections remote to the surgical site before elective operation and postpone elective operations on patients with remote site infections until the infection has resolved. *Category IA*

2. Do not remove hair preoperatively unless the hair at or around the incision site will interfere with the operation. *Category IA*

3. If hair is removed, remove immediately before the operation, preferably with electric clippers. *Category IA*

4. Adequately control serum blood glucose levels in all diabetic patients and particularly avoid hyperglycemia perioperatively. *Category IB*

5. Encourage tobacco cessation. At minimum, instruct patients to abstain for at least 30 days before elective operation from smoking cigarettes, cigars, pipes, or any other form of tobacco consumption (e.g., chewing/dipping). *Category IB*

6. Do not withhold necessary blood products from surgical patients as a means to prevent SSI. *Category IB*

7. Require patients to shower or bathe with an antiseptic agent on at least the night before the operative day. *Category IB*

8. Thoroughly wash and clean at and around the incision site to remove gross contamination before performing antiseptic skin preparation. *Category IB*

9. Use an appropriate antiseptic agent for skin preparation. *Category IB*

10. Apply preoperative antiseptic skin preparation in concentric circles moving toward the periphery. The prepared area must be large enough to extend the incision or create new incisions or drain sites, if necessary. *Category II*

11. Keep preoperative hospital stay as short as possible while allowing for adequate preoperative preparation of the patient. *Category II*

---

†Federal regulation: OSHA.

12. No recommendation to taper or discontinue systemic steroid use (when medically permissible) before elective operation. *Unresolved issue*

13. No recommendation to enhance nutritional support for surgical patients solely as a means to prevent SSI. *Unresolved issue*

14. No recommendation to preoperatively apply mupirocin to nares to prevent SSI. *Unresolved issue*

15. No recommendation to provide measures that enhance wound space oxygenation to prevent SSI. *Unresolved issue*

b. Hand/forearm antisepsis for surgical team members

1. Keep nails short and do not wear artificial nails. *Category IB*

2. Perform a preoperative surgical scrub for at least 2 to 5 minutes using an appropriate antiseptic. Scrub the hands and forearms up to the elbows. *Category IB*

3. After performing the surgical scrub, keep hands up and away from the body (elbows in flexed position) so that water runs from the tips of the fingers toward the elbows. Dry hands with a sterile towel and don a sterile gown and gloves. *Category IB*

4. Clean underneath each fingernail prior to performing the first surgical scrub of the day. *Category II*

5. Do not wear hand or arm jewelry. *Category II*

6. No recommendation on wearing nail polish. *Unresolved issue*

c. Management of infected or colonized surgical personnel

1. Educate and encourage surgical personnel who have signs and symptoms of a transmissible infectious illness to report conditions promptly to their supervisory and occupational health service personnel. *Category IB*

2. Develop well-defined policies concerning patient-care responsibilities when personnel have potentially transmissible infectious conditions. These policies should govern (a) personnel responsibility in using the health service and reporting illness, (b) work restrictions, and (c) clearance to resume work after an illness that required work restriction. The policies also should identify persons who have the authority to remove personnel from duty. *Category IB*

3. Obtain appropriate cultures from, and exclude from duty surgical personnel who have draining skin lesions until infection has been ruled out or personnel have received adequate therapy and infection has resolved. *Category IB*

4. Do not routinely exclude surgical personnel who are colonized with organisms such as *S. aureus* (nose, hands, or other body site) or group A *Streptococcus,* unless such personnel have been linked epidemiologically to dissemination of the organism in the healthcare setting. *Category IB*

d. **Antimicrobial prophylaxis**

1. Administer a prophylactic antimicrobial agent only when indicated, and select it based on its efficacy against the most common pathogens causing SSI for a specific operation and published recommendations. *Category IA*

2. Administer by the intravenous route the initial dose of prophylactic antimicrobial agent, timed such that a bactericidal concentration of the drug is established in serum and tissues when the incision is made. Maintain therapeutic levels of the agent in serum and tissues throughout the operation and until, at most, a few hours alter the incision is closed in the operating room. *Category IA*

3. Before elective colorectal operations in addition to d2 above, mechanically prepare the colon by use of enemas and cathartic agents. Administer nonabsorbable oral antimicrobial agents in divided doses on the day before the operation. *Category IA*

4. For high-risk cesarean section, administer the prophylactic antimicrobial agent immediately after the umbilical cord is clamped. *Category IA*

5. Do not routinely use vancomycin for antimicrobial prophylaxis. *Category IB*

2. **Intraoperative**

a. **Ventilation**

1. Maintain positive-pressure ventilation in the operating room with respect to the corridors and adjacent areas. *Category IB*

2. Maintain a minimum of 15 air changes per hour, of which at least 3 should be fresh air. *Category IB*

3. Filter all air, recirculated and fresh, through the appropriate filters per the American Institute of Architects' recommendations. *Category IB*

4. Introduce all air at the ceiling, and exhaust near the floor. *Category IB*

5. Do not use UV radiation in the operating room to prevent SSI. *Category IB*

6. Keep operating room doors closed except as needed for passage of equipment, personnel, and the patient. *Category IB*

7. Consider performing orthopedic implant operations in operating rooms supplied with ultraclean air. *Category II*

8. Limit the number of personnel entering the operating room to necessary personnel. *Category II*

b. **Cleaning and disinfection of environmental surfaces**

1. When visible soiling or contamination with blood or other body fluids of surfaces or equipment occurs during an operation, use

an EPA-approved hospital disinfectant to clean the affected areas before the next operation. *Category IB†*

2. Do not perform special cleaning or closing of operating rooms after contaminated or dirty operations. *Category IB*

3. Do not use tacky mats at the entrance to the operating room suite or individual operating rooms for infection control. *Category IB*

4. Wet vacuum the operating room floor after the last operation of the day or night with an EPA-approved hospital disinfectant. *Category II*

5. No recommendation on disinfecting environmental surfaces or equipment used in operating rooms between operations in the absence of visible soiling. *Unresolved issue*

c. Microbiologic sampling

1. Do not perform routine environmental sampling of the operating room. Perform microbiologic sampling of operating room environmental surfaces or air only as part of an epidemiologic investigation. *Category IB*

d. Sterilization of surgical instruments

1. Sterilize all surgical instruments according to published guidelines. *Category IB*

2. Perform flash sterilization only for patient care items that will be used immediately (e.g., to reprocess an inadvertently dropped instrument). Do not use flash sterilization for reasons of convenience, as an alternative to purchasing additional instrument sets, or to save time. *Category IB*

e. Surgical attire and drapes

1. Wear a surgical mask that fully covers the mouth and nose when entering the operating room if an operation is about to begin or already under way, or if sterile instruments are exposed. Wear the mask throughout the operation. *Category IB†*

2. Wear a cap or hood to fully cover hair on the head and face when entering the operating room. *Category IB†*

3. Do not wear shoe covers for the prevention of SSI. *Category IB†*

4. Wear sterile gloves if a scrubbed surgical team member. Put on gloves after donning a sterile gown. *Category IB†*

5. Use surgical gowns and drapes that are effective barriers when wet (i.e., materials that resist liquid penetration). *Category IB*

6. Change scrub suits that are visibly soiled, contaminated, and/or penetrated by blood or other potentially infectious materials. *Category IB†*

7. No recommendations on how or where to launder scrub suits, on restricting use of scrub suits to the operating suite, or for covering scrub suits when out of the operating suite. *Unresolved issue*

f. Asepsis and surgical technique

1. Adhere to principles of asepsis when placing intravascular devices (e.g., central venous catheters), spinal or epidural anesthesia catheters, or when dispensing and administering intravenous drugs. *Category IA*

2. Assemble sterile equipment and solutions immediately prior to use. *Category II*

3. Handle tissue gently, maintain effective hemostasis, minimize devitalized tissue and foreign bodies (i.e., sutures, charred tissues, necrotic debris), and eradicate dead space at the surgical site. *Category IB*

4. Use delayed primary skin closure or leave an incision open to heal by second intention if the surgeon considers the surgical site to be heavily contaminated (e.g., Class III and Class IV). *Category IB*

5. If drainage is necessary, use a closed suction drain. Place a drain through a separate incision distant from the operative incision. Remove the drain as soon as possible. *Category IB*

3. Postoperative incision care

a. Protect with a sterile dressing for 24 to 48 hours postoperatively an incision that has been closed primarily. *Category IB*

b. Wash hands before and after dressing changes and any contact with the surgical site. *Category IB*

c. When an incision dressing must be changed, use sterile technique. *Category II*

d. Educate the patient and family regarding proper incision care, symptoms of SSI, and the need to report such symptoms. *Category II*

e. No recommendation to cover an incision closed primarily beyond 48 hours, nor on the appropriate time to shower or bathe with an uncovered incision. *Unresolved issue*

4. Surveillance

a. Use CDC definitions of SSI without modification for identifying SSI among surgical inpatients and outpatients. *Category IB*

b. For inpatient case-finding (including readmissions), use direct prospective observation, indirect prospective detection, or a combination of both direct and indirect methods for the duration of the patients hospitalization. *Category IB*

c. When postdischarge surveillance is performed for detecting SSI following certain operations (e.g., coronary artery bypass graft), use a method that accommodates available resources and data needs. *Category II*

d. For outpatient case-finding, use a method that accommodates available resources and data needs. *Category IB*

e. Assign the surgical wound classification upon completion of an operation. A surgical team member should make the assignment. *Category II*

f. For each patient undergoing an operation chosen for surveillance, record those variables shown to be associated with increased SSI risk (e.g., surgical wound class, ASA class, and duration of operation). *Category IB*

g. Periodically calculate operation-specific SSI rates stratified by variables shown to be associated with increased SSI risk (e.g., NNIS risk index). *Category IB*

h. Report appropriately stratified, operation-specific SSI rates to surgical team members. The optimum frequency and format for such rate computations will be determined by stratified case-load sizes (denominators) and the objectives of local, continuous quality improvement initiatives. *Category IB*

i. No recommendation to make available to the infection control committee coded surgeon-specific data. *Unresolved issue*

Illustration Credits

Section Three

A, From Fortunato N: *Berry & Kohn's operating room technique,* ed 9, St Louis, 2000, Mosby; **B,** From Fortunato N: *Berry & Kohn's operating room technique,* ed 9, St Louis, 2000, Mosby; **D,** From Phippen M, Wells M: *Patient care during operative and invasive procedures,* Philadelphia, 2000, WB Saunders; **E,** From Fortunato N: *Berry & Kohn's operating room technique,* ed 9, St Louis, 2000, Mosby; **F,** From Fortunato N: *Berry & Kohn's operating room technique,* ed 9, St Louis, 2000, Mosby.

Section Four

A, From Fortunato N: *Berry & Kohn's operating room technique,* ed 9, St Louis, 2000, Mosby; **C,** From Cotton PB, Williams CB: *Practical gastrointestinal endoscopy,* ed 4, Boston, 1996, Blackwell Science; **E,** From Fortunato N: *Berry & Kohn's operating room technique,* ed 9, St Louis, 2000, Mosby; **K,** From Fortunato N: *Berry & Kohn's operating room technique,* ed 9, St Louis, 2000, Mosby; **M,** From Fortunato N: *Berry & Kohn's operating room technique,* ed 9, St Louis, 2000, Mosby.

Section Five

B, Photo courtesy DeRoyal, Powell, Tenn.

Index